Prebiotics and Probiotics - From Food to Health

Edited by Elena Franco Robles

Published in London, United Kingdom

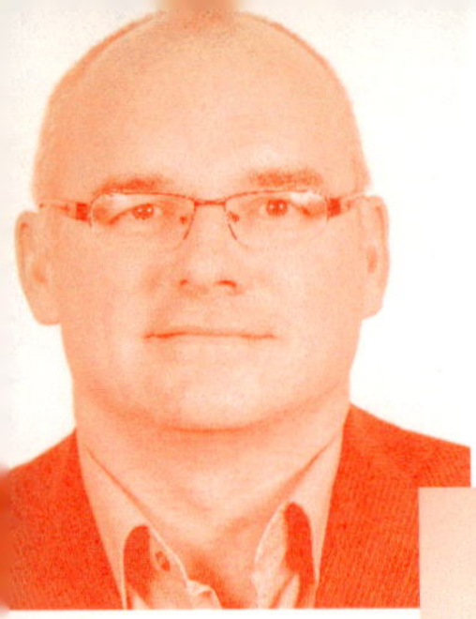
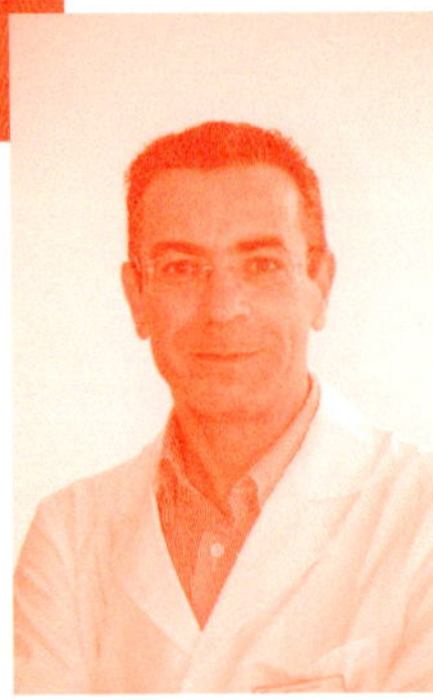
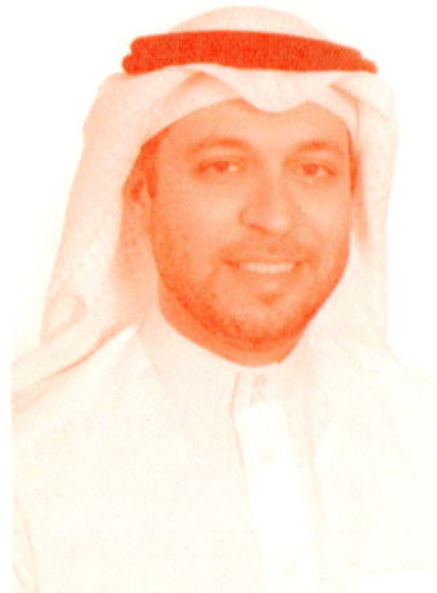
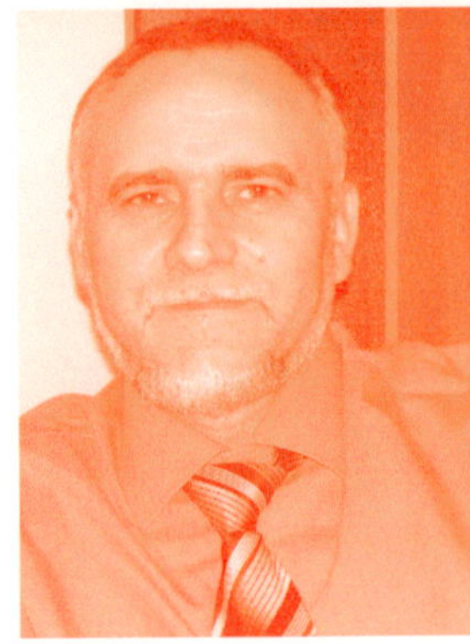
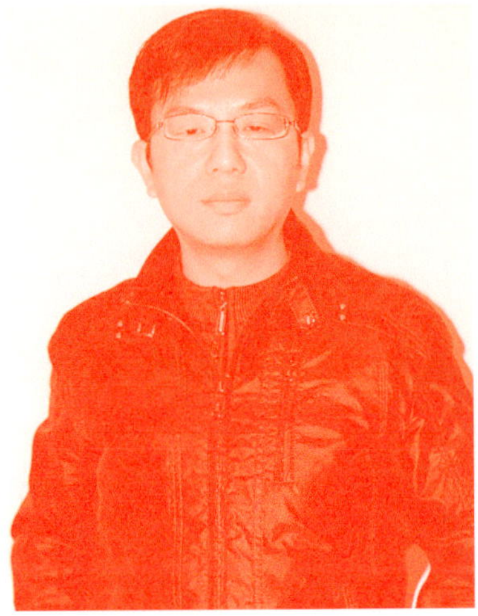
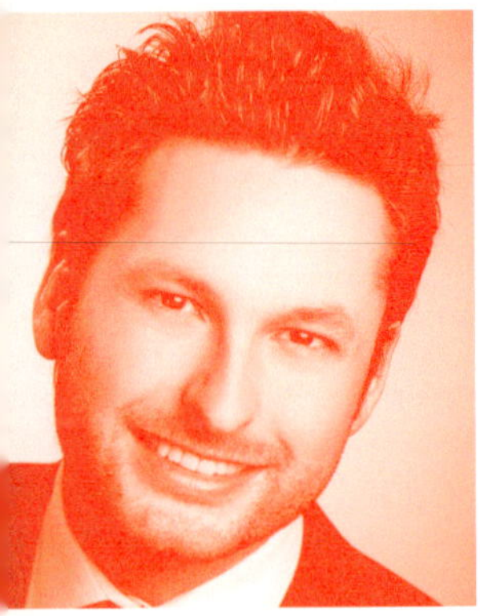
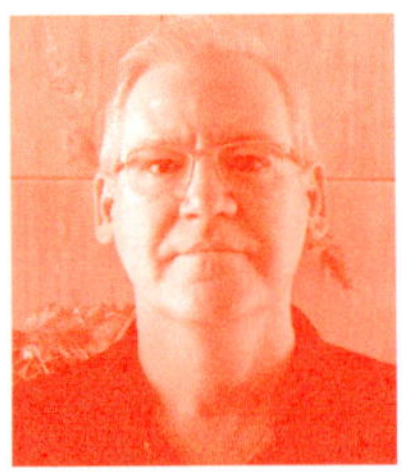

IntechOpen

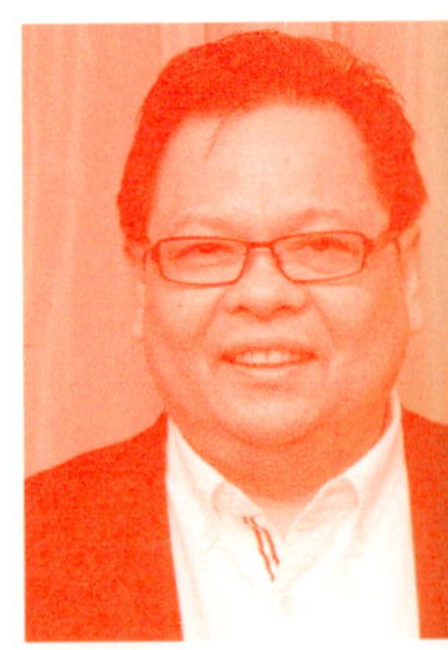
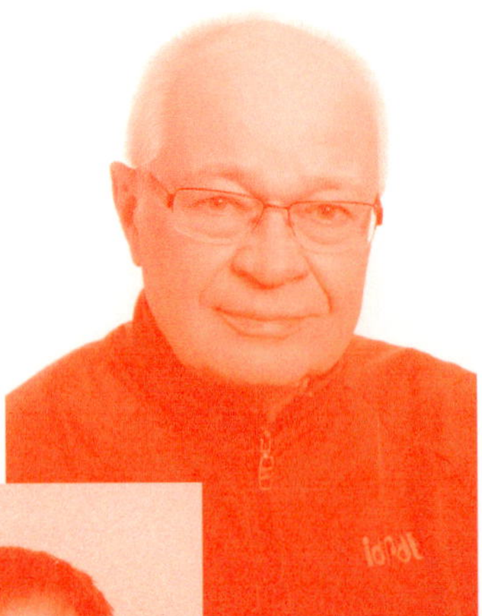
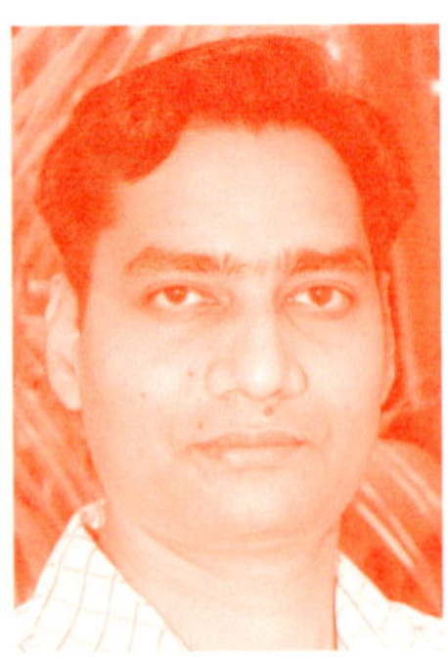
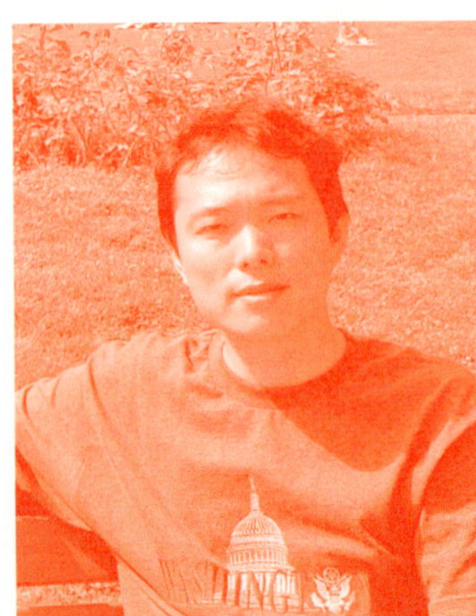
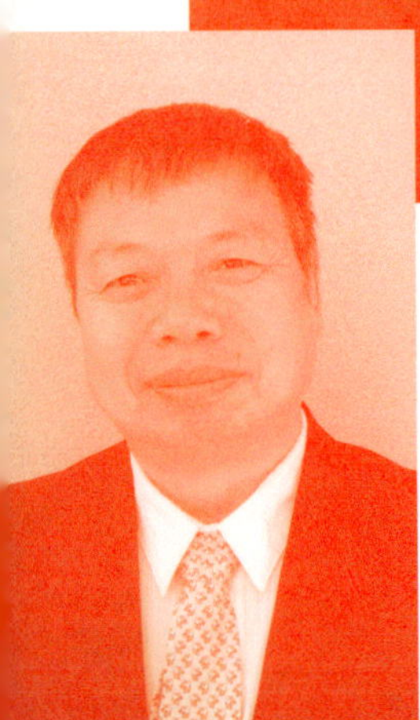
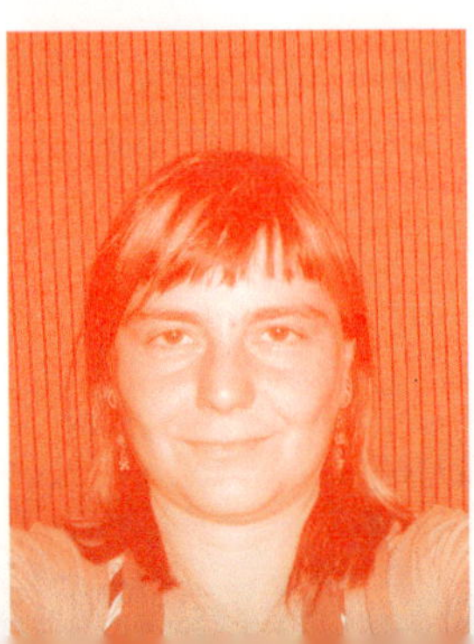

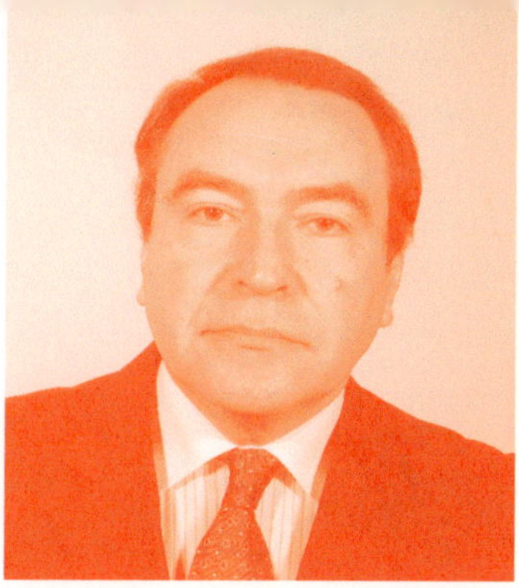
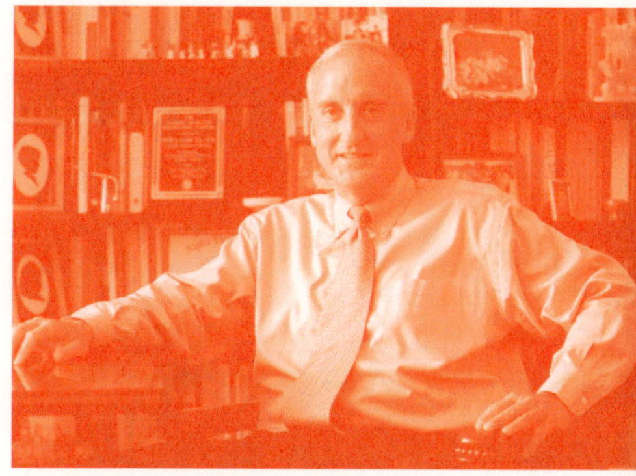
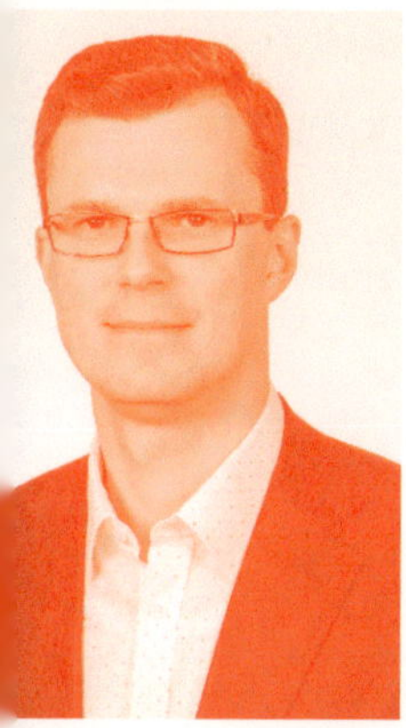
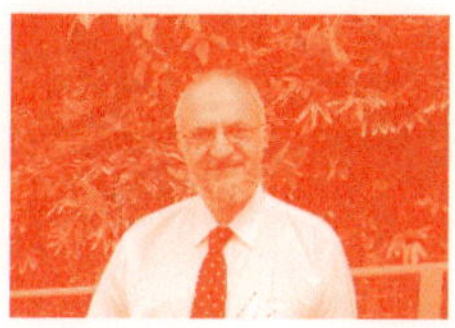
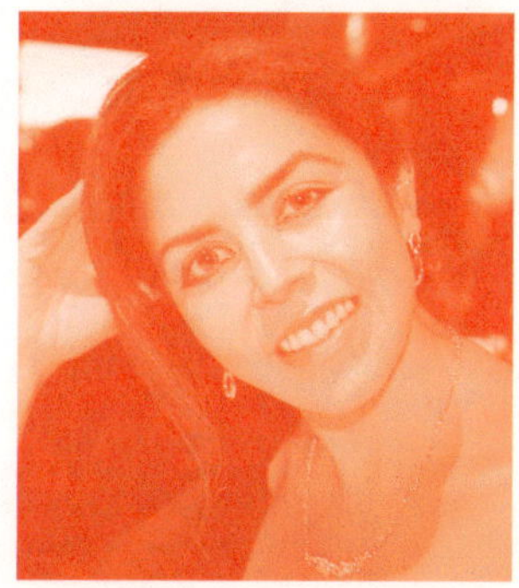

Supporting open minds since 2005

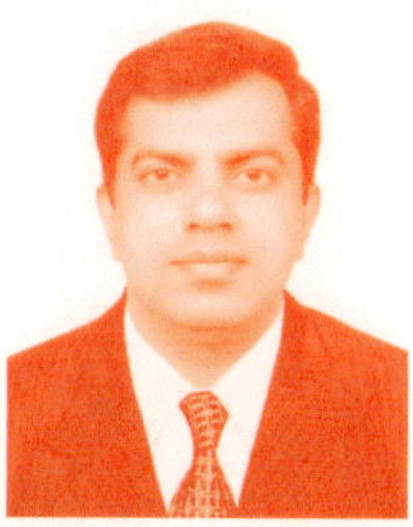
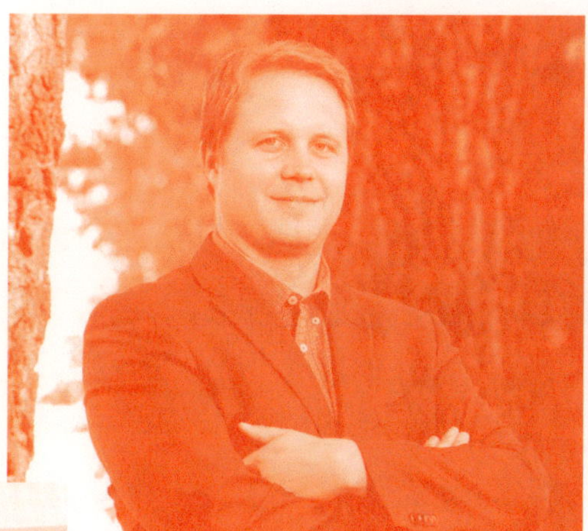
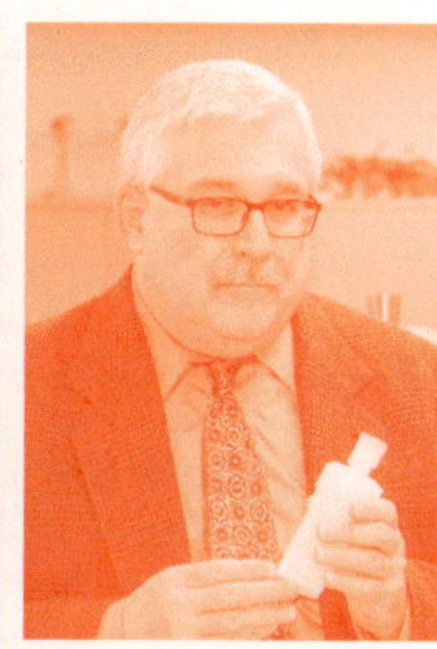
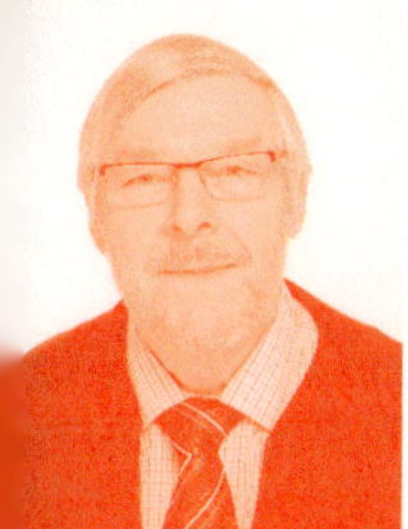
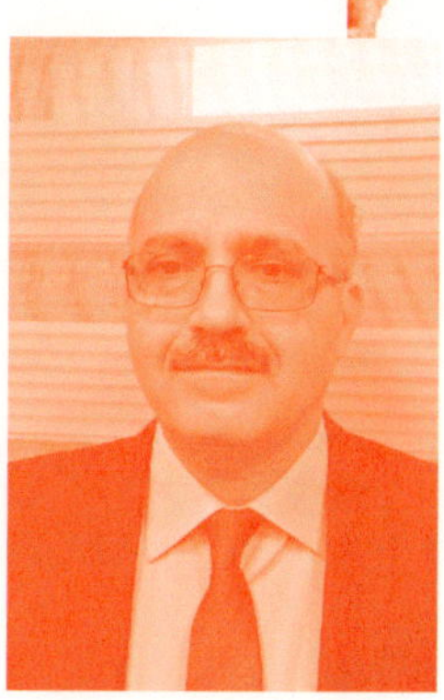
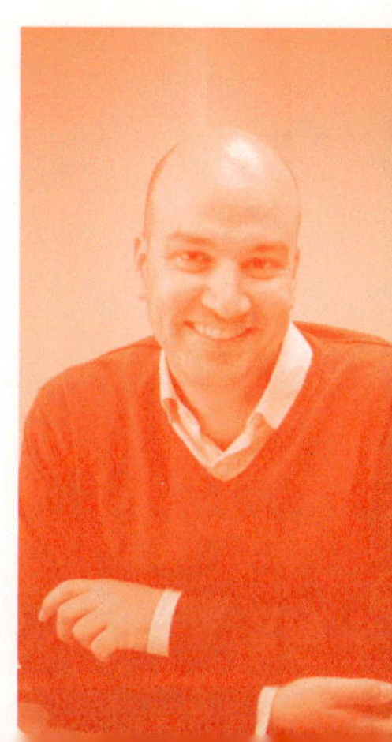
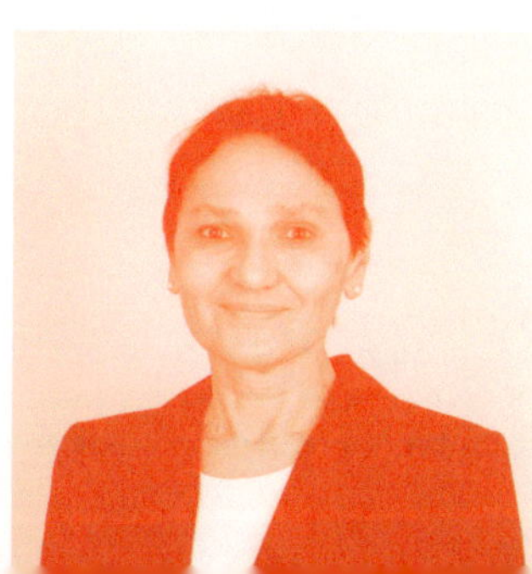

Prebiotics and Probiotics - From Food to Health
http://dx.doi.org/10.5772/intechopen.94725
Edited by Elena Franco Robles

Contributors
Vinícius De Rezende Rodovalho, Eric Guédon, Yves Le-Loir, Vasco Ariston de Carvalho Azevedo, Gwenaël Jan, Diego Lucas Neres Rodrigues, Hüseyin Sancar Bozkurt, Havva Bozkurt, Kaushal Sood, Nilofar Yasmin, Khushboo Kaur, Bolaji Lilian Ilesanmi-Oyelere, Marlena Cathorina Kruger, Muhammed Jimoh Ibrahim, Fateme Mahya Shoaei, Flávia Porto Pelá, Janet Cheruiyot Kosgey, Mercy W. Mwaniki, Fengmin Zhang, Ramesh Kothari, Amishi Bhatt, Charmy Kothari, Dhyey Kothari, Diego Romario-Silva, Edja Maria Melo de Brito Costa, Letícia Targino Campos, Rodrigo Barros Esteves Lins, Lincoln Pires Silva Borges, Sindy Magri Roque, Rafaela Parolina de Carvalho, Janaína Orlandi Sardi, Andréa Cristina Barbosa da Silva, Otávio Akira Souza Sakaguchi, Saeed Sepehrnia, Faisal Siddique, Kashif Akram, Etab Saleh Alghamdi, Qandeel Arshad, Ayesha Siddique, Anielle C.A. Almeida Silva, Ilza Fernanda Barboza Duarte, Valdemir da Costa Silva, Naianny Lívia Oliveira Nascimento Mergulhão, Laisa Carolina Gomes De Bulhões, Irinaldo Diniz Basílio Júnior

First published in London, United Kingdom, 2022 by IntechOpen
IntechOpen is the global imprint of INTECHOPEN LIMITED, registered in England and Wales, registration number: 11086078, 5 Princes Gate Court, London, SW7 2QJ, United Kingdom
Printed in Croatia

British Library Cataloguing-in-Publication Data
A catalogue record for this book is available from the British Library

Additional hard and PDF copies can be obtained from orders@intechopen.com

Prebiotics and Probiotics - From Food to Health
Edited by Elena Franco Robles
p. cm.
Print ISBN 978-1-83969-575-9
Online ISBN 978-1-83969-576-6
eBook (PDF) ISBN 978-1-83969-577-3

For EU product safety concerns:
IN TECH d.o.o., Prolaz Marije Krucifikse Kozulić 3, 51000 Rijeka, Croatia, info@intechopen.com or visit our website at intechopen.com.

Meet the editor

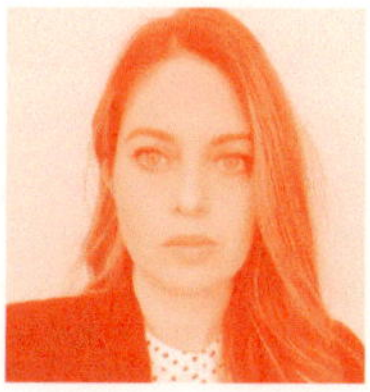

Dr. Elena Franco-Robles has an MMSc and DMSc from the Department of Medical Sciences, University of Guanajuato, Mexico. She also has a BS in Pharmaceutical Chemistry from the Faculty of Chemistry at the same university. She completed a post-doctorate in Biochemistry and Biotechnology at the Center for Research and Advanced Studies of the National Polytechnic Institute (CINVESTAV-IPN). In recent years, she has published more than fifteen scientific articles in international indexed and peer-reviewed journals on in vitro and in vivo studies, mainly in laboratory animals, which have been widely cited. She has been an evaluator of scientific articles and manuscripts for various international scientific publishers. The line of research that she develops is multidisciplinary in the areas of animal health, mucosal immunology, clinical diagnosis, and functional ingredients. She has collaborated with various educational institutions and research centers, as well as with the industrial sector. Dr. Franco has taught various courses and seminars and has participated in various national and international scientific conferences. Likewise, she has advised various students for the development and completion of bachelor's degrees, Master of Science degrees, and Doctor of Science theses in the health discipline.

Contents

Preface

This book discusses the most recent advances in probiotics and prebiotics, which are functional ingredients used as food additives to preserve human and animal health.

The volume contains thirteen chapters that explain the mechanisms of probiotics, prebiotics, and symbiotics from their interaction with the intestinal microbiota as antimicrobials and immunomodulators and their effect on human and animal health.

Importantly, the book covers proposals for new probiotic strains and new materials for the preservation of probiotics during their passage through the gastrointestinal tract.

This book is designed for students, researchers, teachers, and scientists in the fields of health and food.

I want to thank all the authors for their contribution to this book. I also thank IntechOpen and Author Service Manager Ms. Karmen Đaleta for their support.

Dr. Elena Franco-Robles
Associate Profesor,
Departamento de Veterinaria y Zootecnia,
División de Ciencias de la Vida,
Campus Irapuato-Salamanca,
Universidad de Guanajuato,
Irapuato, Guanajuato, Mexico

Chapter 1

Mucosal Immunology

Saeed Sepehrnia

Abstract

Approximately 80% of the pathogens that lead to deadly infections in humans choose mucosal tissue as the first site of infection. The mucosal surfaces of the body include the gastrointestinal tract, airways, oral cavity, and urogenital mucosa, which provide a large area conducive to the invasion and accumulation of many microorganisms and are of great importance in this regard. The large extent of mucus, as well as the accumulation of bacteria and countless foreign antigens in these areas, are the most important reasons for the importance of mucosal tissues. In addition to the myriad of symbiotic bacteria, large amounts of oral antigens (both pathogenic and non-pathogenic) enter a person's body daily and human mucosal tissues are exposed to these antigens. The function of the mucosal immune system is to distinguish pathogenic antigens from non-pathogenic ones. In this way, against a large number of oral antigens or co-tolerant microorganisms, and pathogenic antigens, a favorable (and even non-inflammatory, possible) immune response is produced. Mucosal tissue, as the largest lymphatic organ in the body, is home to 75% of the lymphocyte population and produces the highest amount of immunoglobulin. The amount of secreted IgA (slgA) produced daily by mucosal surfaces is much higher than the IgG produced in the bloodstream. A 70 kg person produces more than 3 grams of IgA per day, which is about 70–60% of the total antibodies produced in the body. The first embryonic organ in which immune system cells are located in the intestine. Some researchers consider this organ (and specifically mucosal lymph nodes) to be the source of the human immune system.

Keywords: mucosal immunology, mucosa associated lymphoid tissues, organized mucosal associated lymphoid tissue, diffuse mucosal associated lymphoid tissue, innate lymphoid cells, M cell, poly immunoglobulin receptor, mucosal vaccination

1. Introduction

Mucosal surfaces interact directly with the outside of the body and interact with countless antigens. The need to establish an immune system in this tissue to fight pathogens is obvious, but the development of an immune response against native antigens or bacterial bacteria is an undesirable response. Therefore, the immune system in the mucosal tissues must be tolerant of many antigens, while maintaining the ability to respond to a small number of pathogenic antigens. Any tissue that can secrete mucus on the surface of the epithelial layer and can participate in the immune response is considered part of the mucosal lymphatic tissue (MALT). MALT is present in the gastrointestinal tract, airways, urogenital tract, conjunctiva, and endocrine glands (salivary and sweat glands), but has been studied mainly in the gastrointestinal tract, respiratory tract, and urogenital tract. Both innate and adaptive immune systems (humoral and cellular) are seen in these tissues. One of the defense mechanisms in the mucosa is the physical and mechanical defense that acts as a non-specific barrier against infections, including the mucosal epithelial layer, intestinal peristaltic activity, and the mechanism of mucosal-mucosal clearance in the airways. The first line of defense in the mucosa is physical defense and innate immunity. Innate immune cells, such as tissue-resident macrophages and migrating neutrophils, are the first cells to act upon the onset of pathogen exposure. After innate immunity, adaptive immunity and its cells are activated by dendritic cells in the marginal lymph nodes (or in organized mucosal-associated lymphoid tissue) and called to the sites of infection. B cells in mucosal tissues produce and secrete antibodies, especially IgA. T lymphocytes also play a role in secreting pro-inflammatory cytokines or inducing cytotoxic activity. Moreover, mucosal tissues contain populations of $T\alpha\beta$ and $T\gamma\delta$ [1, 2].

1.1 Lymphatic tissues in the gastrointestinal tract

The human gastrointestinal tract consists of a tubular structure covered by a mucosal epithelial layer. Beneath the epithelial cells is the lamina propria, or lining of the mucosa, which contains the mucosal connective tissue (MALT), blood vessels, and lymph vessels. MALT located in the gastrointestinal tract is also called GALT[1]. MALT in this area also contains a large number of immune cells, which alone are larger than any other set of bone marrow, thymus, spleen, and lymph node cells. Mucosal lymph tissue is mainly composed of intraepithelial lymphocytes (IELs), lamina propria lymphocytes, IgA-producing plasma cells and macrophage antigen-presenting cells, dendritic cells, neutrophils, eosinophils, and mast cells. In certain areas of the mucosa, there are lymphoid follicles that contain T lymphocytes, B lymphocytes, etc. In general, it can be said that the intestine prevents the entry of bacteria and infectious agents in three ways, the first is through the mucosal layer that prevents the penetration of bacteria from the epithelium. The second barrier is the production and secretion of antimicrobial peptides in the intestinal lumen and killing them within the lumen. The third method of inhibition is the production of IgA from the plasma of lamina propria, which neutralizes pathogens within the intestinal lumen [3, 4].

2. The role and structure of mucosal lymph tissues

Mucous lymphatic tissues can be classified according to their structure and function. Structurally, mucosal lymph nodes are divided into two categories: organized or O-MALT[2] and diffuse or D-MALT[3]. Functionally, O-MALT is known as the site of induction of the immune response and D-MALT is the site of the immune response. In other words, immune responses are formed in O-MALT and perform their executive function in D-MALT. O-MALT is a place for antigen processing and production of effector and memory cells, after which the produced cells migrate to other mucosal diffuse lymph tissues such as D-MALT, leading to the protection of body surfaces. However, it has recently been shown that both types of lymph tissue play an important role in the production and differentiation of mucosal lymphocytes and mucosal immunity. Epithelial cells also play a role in the differentiation and production of cytotoxic T cells. It seems that intestinal mucosa and other mucosal surfaces affect bone marrow progenitor cells (T and B cells) and are effective in

[1] Gut Associated Lymphoid Tissue.

[2] Organized Mucosal Associated Lymphoid Tissue.

[3] Diffuse Mucosal Associated Lymphoid Tissue.

gene rearrangement of immunoglobulins and T cell receptors. The activation of the enzymatic machine required for the genetic synthesis of progenitor cells in the gut supports this theory. T cells also regulate the activity of epithelial cells. For example, intercellular permeability and ion secretion (by these cells) are affected by IFN-γ. Crypt cell proliferation in the small intestine and mucosal morphology are also regulated by T cell cytokines. O-MALT is called the afferent lymphoid region, which is the site of antigen entry and the formation of immune responses. While D MALT is an efferent lymphoid region and acts as a site of antigen interaction with differentiated cells (leading to antibody secretion and the activity of helper and cytotoxic lymphocytes) [1, 4, 5].

2.1 Organized mucosal associated lymphoid tissue (O-MALT)

O-MALT in the gastrointestinal tract includes Peyer's patches and isolated lymph follicles (ILF). The number and location of mucosal follicles vary greatly between species and in an individual also changes over time and exposure to antigens. Most of these centers are isolated and scattered throughout the airways and gastrointestinal tract, but their extent increases to the colon and rectum. Some of these lymphatic tissues together form large complexes such as the palatine, lingual, and pharyngeal tonsils called the Waldeyer's ring, mucosal follicles in the appendix, and Peyer's patches in the small intestine. Peyer's patches are more in the ileum (the last third of the small intestine) and less in the jejunum (not seen in the colon). Mucosal lymphoid follicles in both single form (ILF) and complex (Peyer's patches) are covered by a specific epithelium. The general structure of the lymph plaques of Peyer's patches is shown in **Figure 1**. Each Peyer's patches contain more than 100 lymphoid follicles, each with a dark border and a relatively lighter circular center. O-MALT in gastrointestinal lymphatic tissues includes Peyer's patches (in the ileum) and ILFs (in the colon).

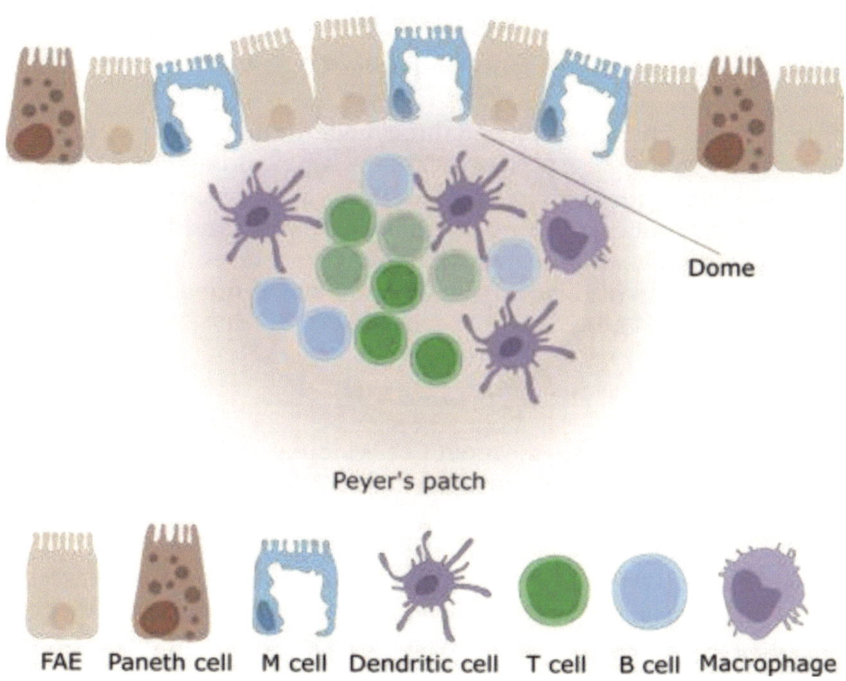

Figure 1.
The general structure of Peyer's patche lymph follicles. FAE, Follicule associated epithelium.

The follicles are separated from the mucosal epithelium by intercellular spaces and a dome-shaped area filled with lymphocytes called the corona. The mucosal surface above the corona of the follicle is free of villi on the surface of the epithelium of other areas and contains antigen-carrying cells or M cells (found only in this area). High endothelial venules (HEV) where lymphocytes leave the artery are located in the interfollicular section [1, 4, 5].

2.1.1 Lymphocytes in O-MALT

Lymphocytes in O-MALT and follicle associated Epithelium (FAE) has been studied in several species [6–8]. The follicles are the site of accumulation of B lymphocytes, dendritic cells, and macrophages. However, T lymphocytes are mainly predominant in the internal and parafollicular parts [6, 9]. Most of the parafollicular B lymphocytes and located in the corona are IgM^+ and the B cells in the germinal centers are IgA^+. CD4 + T lymphocytes are mostly found in the corona, below the epithelium of the dome area, and the parafollicular regions, and CD8 + T cells are often found in the interfollicular regions.

2.1.2 Antigen-presenting cells

Antigen-presenting cells in O-MALT (such as Peyer's patches) include follicular dendritic cells within the germinal center, interdigitating cells near lymphocytes of parafollicular regions, macrophages, and B cells. Macrophages are mostly concentrated in the coronal and B lymphocytes are often found in the follicular regions [7, 10, 11]. Antigen-presenting cells trap antigens of extracellular origin in endosomes. In these phagosomes, antigens are digested and processed by specific proteolytic enzymes, and finally the peptides are presented to T lymphocytes by MHC II. Cells isolated from Peyer Patch mice can be stimulated with antigen in vitro, resulting in a primary and secondary immune response, leading to the production of IgM class antibodies and IgG and IgA class antibodies, respectively [12].

2.2 Diffuse mucosal associated lymphoid tissue (D-MALT)

Diffuse lymphoid tissue is scattered throughout the mucosal surface and includes lymphocytes, diffuse plasma cells in the lamina propria, mucosal connective tissue, and intraepithelial lymphocytes (IELs). Some of these cells are derived from O-MALT and contain effector and memory lymphocytes. These cells are caused by antigen stimulation in areas such as Peyer's patches. In a regular process, antigen-stimulated cells begin to migrate from the site of stimulation and settle in other mucosal tissues [13, 14].

2.2.1 Intraepithelial lymphocytes (IELs)

Intraepithelial lymphocytes are often T cells located in the epithelial layer. About 15 to 20% of the population make up epithelial cells. These cells are considered guarding cells in the immune system and react with antigens earlier than others, and therefore show memory phenotype ($CD45RO^+$).

IELs are found in two types, Tαβ and Tγδ. The main function of these cells is to establish tolerance against symbiotic bacteria and to protect against pathogenesis. In humans, about 90% of IELs are Tαβ and only 10% are Tγδ. In mice, the percentage of Tγδ cells reaches 50%.

Most IEL cells are $CD8^+$ and are divided into two categories in terms of origin. Some of these are conventional Tαβ cells that have evolved in the thymus that can express both the $CD4^+$ marker and the $CD8^+$ marker. The other group is the unconventional or natural Tαβ cells and Tγδ, which have evolved in environments other than the thymus, such as the intestine. These lymphocytes have the power of self-renewal and are restricted to non-classical MHC molecules. These unconventional IELs usually show a specific CD8 consisting of α chain homodimer. Most intraepithelial Tγδ cells, as well as many Tαβ lymphocytes in the gut, express the CD8αα homodimer. For this reason, the expression of CD8αα has been considered an indicator of intraepithelial T cells in the intestine compared to peripheral blood T cells.

Few IELs are found with the $CD4^+CD8^+$ or $CD4^-CD8^-$ phenotype. Unlike conventional TCRs, which have a wide variety, TCRs in IELs have limited variability.

Most IELs are dormant under normal conditions but react as soon as they are exposed to the antigen due to a memory phenotype. $T\alpha\beta CD8^+$ and Tγδ cells show cytotoxic activity against infection. Production and storage of perforins and granzymes can be done in IEL.

Conventional T cells, unlike unconventional T cells, must be activated to play their executive role. Both abnormal Tαβ and Tγδ cells in the intestinal epithelium detect antigens at the level of non-classical MHC molecules such as CD1, which allows factors expressed on the surface of damaged epithelial cells to respond to stress. Thus, Tγδ cells can also be activated in response to foreign antigen peptides and host cell-derived danger signals.

Tγδ cells have a more limited gene repertoire of TCR and in the gut often express the Vδ1 chain, which is different from blood Tγδ. Vδ1-expressing Tγδ cells can detect non-classical MHCs induced by MICA and MICB stress. MICA and MICB are known as the damage-associated molecular pattern (DAMP) and increase in response to cellular stress. Tγδ can respond to tissue damage in the shortest possible time. By secreting IFN-γ, these cells increase the cytotoxic response against virus-infected cells and enhance the neutrophilic response against bacteria.

Tγδ lymphocytes in the gut play an important role in protecting mucosal surfaces from damage caused by immune responses. Tγδ lymphocytes also regulate immune responses by increasing TGFβ and limiting the migration of inflammatory leukocytes to the intestinal tract. In addition, these cells produce Insulin-like growth factor-1 (IGF-1) and keratinocyte growth factor (KGF).

The proportion of Tγδ cells is higher among IEL cells in infancy. As you age, the proportion of Tαβ cells increases, so Tγδ cells in infancy are likely to play an effective role in defending against pathogens [2, 5].

2.2.2 Lamina properia lymphocytes

Lamina Properia Lymphocytes include B cells (often transformed into plasma cells) and T lymphocytes. In mice, 40% of lamina properia lymphocytes are B cells that produce mainly IgA. 25% of the cell population are T lymphocytes (mainly with the CD4 + TH2 phenotype) [15–19]. Human lamina propria CD4 + T cells provide memory cell markers and do not proliferate in response to antigenic stimuli. Rather, they produce cytokines such as IFN-γ [20]. The predominant population of T lymphocytes in the lamina propria is CD4 + T (60–70%), the majority of which exhibit the TCRα/β phenotype. Most of these cells have the CD45RO (specific for memory cells) and are different from peripheral blood T lymphocytes in this respect. Lamina propria is an important center for IgA production. In these areas, O-MALT derived B lymphoblasts (such as Peyer's patches) are affected by cytokines such as IL-6 and undergo differentiation [21]. Lamina properia TH1 cells proliferate TH2 cells by secreting IL-2 and IFN-γ. On the other hand, TH2 cells, by producing IL-5 and IL-6, prepare for the differentiation of B cells into IgA-producing plasma cells [22].

The lymphocytes in the lamina propria are mainly in the late stages of differentiation and often turn into plasma cells. Furthermore, In the intestinal lamina propria cells such as macrophages, neutrophils, eosinophils. There are dendritic cells and mast cells. Lamina propria CD4 + T cells can react with these cells, enhancing their phagocytic and antimicrobial capacity. Macrophages may also be involved in the processing and delivery of antigens to T cells.

3. Innate lymphoid cells in intestinal mucosa

Innate Lymphoid Cells (ILCs) in the intestinal mucosa are involved in defense against pathogens, enhancing the function of the physical barrier, and tolerance to the microbial flora. There are two types of ILC2 and ILC3 in the mucosa, and ILC2 is involved in the defense against worms in the gut. Besides, in response to cytokines IL-33 and IL-25, they can secrete cytokines IL-5 and IL-13, the former of which is effective in activating eosinophils and the latter in increased mucus production and thus repelling worm parasites. ILC3 is also present in the gut and can produce the cytokines IL-17 and IL-22 in response to stimulation with IL-18 and IL-23 cytokines. The cytokines produced by these cells are involved in enhancing the physical function of the mucosa by stimulating the production of defensins and strengthening strong epithelial connections.

Other cells in the mucosa are Mucosal associated invariant T (MAIT), which are a subset of CD8 + T cells with invariant TCR Va7.2-Ja33. The main role of these cells is to defend against bacteria and fungi that cross the intestinal epithelial barrier and enter the bloodstream. Intestinal bacteria (normal flora or other bacteria) enter the liver through the portal vein and encounter the MAIT cells if they pass through the intestinal epithelium and enter the bloodstream. These cells detect fungal and bacterial metabolites through an MHC-like protein class 1 called MRI and, once activated, produce a cytotoxic role by producing inflammation-promoting cytokines. 50% of the population of T cells located in the liver belongs to this group [1, 4, 5].

3.1 Enterocytes and antigen-presenting

Mucosal epithelial cells (especially small intestinal enterocytes) act as antigen-presenting cells and present MHC II molecules [23–26]. Besides, CD1d (MHC I-like) molecules are present on the surface of these cells. Mature enterocytes from intestinal villi express class II molecules whereas crypt cell production may be affected by cytokines such as IFN-γ [27]. Enterocytes are able to present antigens to T cells in vitro. However, the T cell response is suppressive [28, 29] and this mechanism seems to be involved in mucosal tolerance.

4. Antigen penetration into O-MALT

4.1 Follicule associated epithelium (FAE)

The intestinal epithelium can be thought of as a complex of crypt-centered cells. In the small intestine, each crypt contains a large number of undifferentiated germ cells from which other cells are formed. Differentiated crypt cells then cover adjacent villi [30].

Goblet cells, enterochromaffin, and pIgR-containing enterocytes are located in the lateral wall of the villi. Cells that move from the crypt to the dome of the lymphoid follicles become pIgR-containing enterocytes and M cells [31].

The location of Peyer's patches and other parts of O-MALT in members of an animal species is known. Immature M cells remain even after lymphocyte depletion with radiotherapy [32, 33]. The formation of mucosal tissues is organized before birth [34]. However, the antigen transfer process causes the mucosal follicles to expand. In general, it can be said that the superficial components of epithelial cells together with local secretory products are involved in the formation of O-MALT.

4.2 M cells

The cytoplasm of M cells forms a thin membrane-like structure in the upper part of the cytoplasm that separates the inner space of the intestine from the space below the epithelium, hence it is also called the membrane epithelial cell. In other words, these cells have a large envelope in which many immune cells, such as antigen-supplying cells, are located in this envelope, closest to the intestinal tract (**Figure 2**).

An important role of M cells is the transfer of antigen to the O-MALT. These cells are not presenting of antigen, but only its transporter. These cells endocytose the antigen not specifically, but selectively, meaning that not every antigen can pass through M cells. M cells select and pass antigens based on molecular load, hydrophobicity, and viability.

Since the transfer of antigen by M cells can play an important role in the first stage of the immune response, the factors that affect this transfer are very important in choosing a mucosal immunization strategy. M cells make up between 10% in humans and animals and up to 50% in rabbits around the follicular epithelial cells (FAE) [35]. Areas specific to endocytosis are present between irregular or shallow short microvilli on the upper surface of the M cell [36]. These cells lack some of the digestive enzymes present on the anterior membrane of enterocytes. However, M cell membranes contain many glycoconjugates compounds that can be suitable binding sites for lectin-like microbial surface molecules [36–38]. These cells endocytose and transmit microorganisms, particles, and lectins that selectively attach to their apical membrane with high efficiency [36], in other words, substances that bind to mucosal surfaces elicit a strong secretory response. For example, oral administration of lectin leads to the production of anti-lectin-specific IgA. While

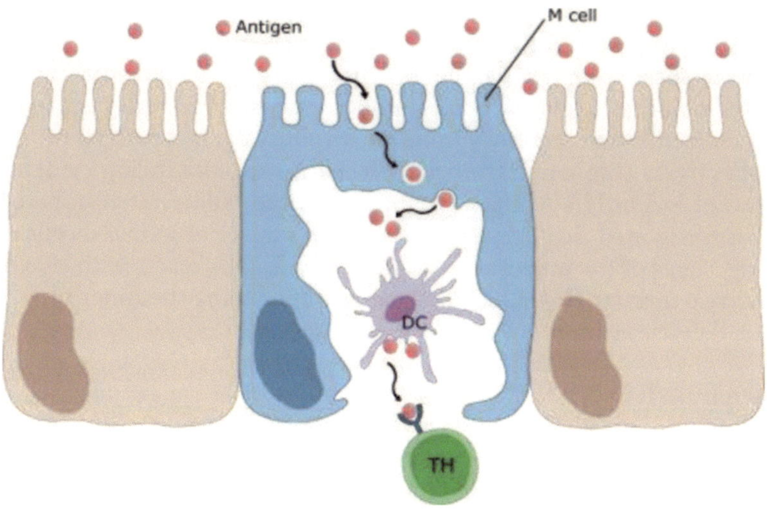

Figure 2.
M cell. The basement membrane of the M cell begins to form an intracellular envelope. M cells first transfer antigens from the airways and gastrointestinal tract to the envelope and then to the defense cells located beneath the epithelium.

the administration of the same amount of another immunogen that does not have adhesion and binding properties is ineffective [39].

The reason for the lack of adverse responses to food antigens and the normal intestinal flora should be sought in the inability of M cells to transmit soluble luminal antigens and nonadherent particles [40]. It seems that the introduction of small but frequent oral or inhaled amounts of soluble immunogens leads to tolerance [41].

Some viruses, bacteria, and protozoa, such as Cryptosporidium, selectively attach to M cells and transmit well. Among these viruses, only reovirus type I, poliovirus, and HIV 1 bind specifically to the upper membrane of M cells. These viruses do not attach to cell surfaces in the FAE or the epithelium of the villi.

In reovirus type I, one of the outer capsid proteins (δ1 or μ1), after being activated by the proteolytic process in the gastrointestinal tract, causes the virus to contact the M cell.

In animals, large numbers of gram-negative pathogens and *Streptococcus pyogenes* bind selectively or preferably to M cells. Some viruses (such as rotaviruses and transmissible gastroenteritis viruses), as well as bacteria such as *Escherichia coli* [42], Yersinia pseudo-tuberculosis, *Vibrio cholerae* [43–45], Shigella [46], *Yersinia enterocolitica* [47], and *Campylobacter jejuni* [48], have proliferated in M cells after infiltration and they cause local infection and inflammation. M cells use a carbohydrate-lectin detection system with multiple receptors to identify a variety of pathogenic microorganisms in the gut.

The cell surface of M is increased due to the presence of accessible membrane regions and specific binding regions of large ligands and is therefore different from other epithelial cells.

In the gut, immunoglobulins also bind specifically to M cells [49], so that for the first time in suckling rabbits, accumulation of milk slgA was observed on M cells of Peyer's patches.

Both Fc and Fab IgG fragments attach to the M cell. Lectins present on the surface of M cells identify abundant oligosaccharides present on immunoglobulins. Specific binding and transport of immunoglobulins by M cells may be involved in the regulation of immune responses. slgA usually prevents antigens and microorganisms from coming into contact with mucosal surfaces. The Fc Domain IgA molecule is hydrophilic (hydrophilic and hair-phosphatic) and binds IgA (attached to microorganisms) to epithelial cells. The Fc properties of the IgA molecule prevent the colonization of pathogens (without causing inflammation).

Antigens of these complexes are reabsorbed and evaluated by macrophages and lymphocytes inside or below the epithelium (containing Fcα receptors) [50–52]. This event intensifies the secretory immune response against pathogens that have not been effectively eliminated from the gut. However, convincing evidence of the ultimate fate of IgA or IgA-Antigen complexes is not available after uptake by M cells but it is speculated that Fcα receptors on the surface of mucosal cells may play a role in other stages of the mucosal immune response. IgA reacts with lactoferrin and lactoperoxidase through the FC region, thereby enhancing the function of these nonspecific defense elements.

4.3 Antigen transfer

M cells absorb adhesive molecules such as lectins and ferritin through membrane clathrin vesicles and discharge them into vesicular or tubular structures similar to the cytoplasmic apex endosomes (above the epithelial pocket) [36]. In this part of the cell structure, vesicular endosomes are rarely found and no structures are containing acid phosphatase [53]. During transfers, endocytic materials do not decompose extensively. However, the presence of endosomal hydrolase in M cell transport vesicles has not been ruled out. The apical vesicles of M cells are acidic [54].

Proteins and microbes that have entered the M cell vesicles are discharged out of the epithelial cell by the exocytosis membrane up to 10 minutes after vertebral endocytosis [36, 55].

Exocytic vesicles originate from endosomal intermediate components and structures. Lysosomes are present in the pericardial Golgi of M cells, but endocytic materials of the apical membrane have not been observed in these areas.

M cells shorten their transport path by lifting the lateral membrane toward the apex and shortening the lateral endosomes directly to specific regions of the lateral base (**Figure 2**). The intraepithelial membrane of M cells is different from the lateral membrane (which attaches to the adjacent cell) and the basement membrane (which attaches to the basal lamina).

For example, it has been shown that Na/K ATPase pumps are concentrated in the lateral part (not in the envelope membrane of M cells. It is said that the presence of a specific population of lymphocytes in the M cell envelope indicates the presence of specific lymphocyte receptors in the envelope membrane (**Figure 2**). The mechanism of distribution of specific lymphoid cells in this area is still unknown The pattern of glycosylation determines the specificity of M cells. The structure of LPS in *salmonella typhi* morium fimbriae plays a role in binding to M cells.

M cells, make up a small population of epithelial cells. However, their ability to transmit intestinal adhesive particles is remarkable.

4.4 M cells, areas of infiltration of pathogenic microorganisms

M cells have developed their non-specific mechanisms for binding and absorption of intestinal material so that the mucosal immune system can access a variety of microorganisms and particles. The ability of M cells to bind to bacteria such as *Vibrio cholerae* allows the immune system to sample these non-invasive pathogens well and to organize the appropriate secretory immune response. The secretion of sIgA anti-cholera toxin (CT) plays an important role in limiting the course of the disease and preventing the recurrence of infection [56–58].

Many pathogenic bacteria and viruses that attach to M cells use this intraepithelial transport pathway as an invasion pathway. For example, reoviruses and polioviruses reach the Peyer's patches by selectively binding to the apex of the M cells [59, 60]. *Salmonella typhimurium* in mice and *Salmonella typhi* in humans are gram-negative pathogens that transmit to M cells attached to Peyer's patches and cause disease [45]. An effective mucosal immune response against Salmonella cannot prevent the organism from spreading to the liver and spleen. Therefore, with intestinal infiltration into the host, the systemic spread of the disease will occur. In addition, early transport of *Shigella flexneri* [46] and *Yersinia enterocolitica* [47] causes these organisms to enter the lamina propria by invading the lateral basal surfaces of epithelial cells and infecting mucosal macrophages.

O-MALT contains IgA-producing plasma cell precursors and is the center of the mucosal IgA response. After being transfected by M cells, the antigens first encounter the antigen-presenting cells and the lymphocytes in the cell's inner envelope [7]. In the dome area below the FAE, $IgM^{+}B$ cells, CD4 + T cells, dendritic cells, and macrophages form a cellular network by which antigens are absorbed, processed, and delivered to lymphocytes. After activation, the process of maturation and differentiation of B cells occurs in O-MALT.

5. Dendritic cells in the gastrointestinal tract

In mucosal tissues, dendritic cells are known to be the main controllers of immune responses These cells act as a protective system and, by identifying pathogens, can stimulate naive T and B cells. Both O-MALT and D-MALT tissues contain dendritic cells. There are several subgroups of DCs in the mucosa, each with unique properties. DCs in the Peyer's patches are often located in the M cell envelope and the subepithelial dome (SED) and are $CD11b^+$, $CD8\alpha^-$, $CCR1^+$, and $CCR6^+$. CCR1 and CCR6 receptors bind to CCL9 (MIP-1γ) and CCL20 (MIP-3α) chemokines, respectively.

CCL9 and CCL20 are continuously secreted from FAE cells and are located by the CCR1 and CCR6 receptors, causing these DCs to be located in the Peyer's patches epithelium.

DCs of Peyer's patches secrete 10-IL in the absence of infection in response to the uptake of dietary antigens or microbiome, which inhibits the inflammatory response to these antigens. When exposed to pathogens, these DCs are rapidly recalled below the FAE by increasing CCL20 secretion from the epithelium. Microbial products cause the expression of co-stimulatory molecules on the surface of DCs, and excited DCs lead to the activation and differentiation of naive T cells into effector cells. In Peyer's patches, in addition to the above-mentioned DCs, there is another DC subclass, which, unlike the first type, is $CD11b^-$, $CD8a^+$ and $CCR6^-$. These cells are found in T cell-rich areas in Peyer's patches and produce IL-12 inflammatory cytokines.

A major route of antigen transport to Peyer's patches (O-MALT) is M cells. Other ways to transport antigens to the O-MALT region include the entry of food and soluble antigens through the epithelium. Moreover, the presence of FcRn on the surface of enterocytes enables these cells to detect IgA-coated antigens. The binding of FcRn to the antigen and antibody complex can trigger the entry of immune complexes from the luminal surface to the basal surface of enterocytes by transcytosis. When apoptosis kills pathogen-infected enterocytes, antigens can penetrate the subepithelial layer. More specifically, DCs uptake apoptotic cell debris and associated antigens (**Figure 3**).

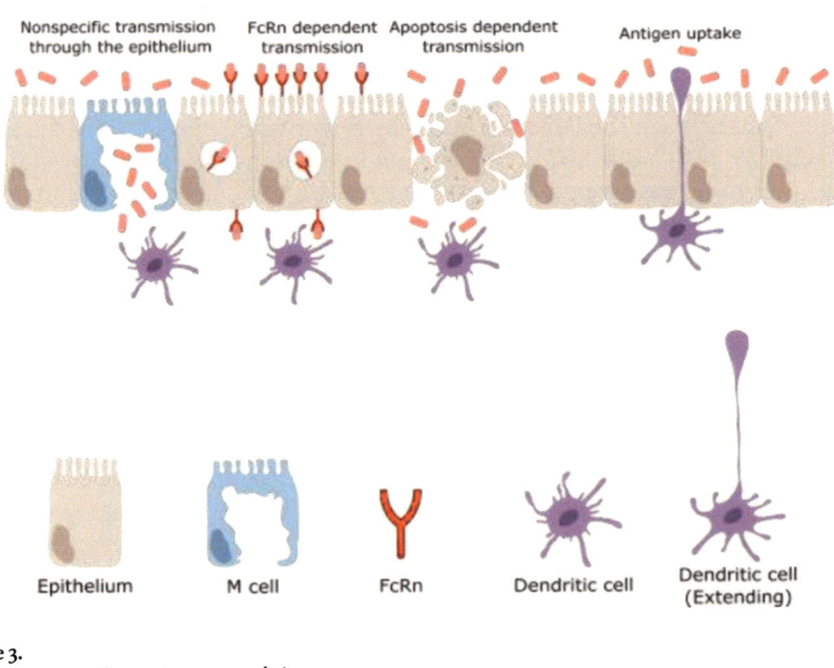

Figure 3.
Different ways antigen enters mucosal tissues.

Another way to pick up antigens in the gastrointestinal tract is through DCs and macrophages, can send their appendages into the intestinal lumen without disrupting the integrity of the epithelial cells and actively sampling the antigens in the lumen, thereby transporting the antigen to the Transmit lamina propria.

Lamina propria dendritic cells (LPDCs) that pick up antigens in ways other than M cells play an important role in maintaining tolerance to non-pathogenic intestinal antigens.

LPDCs express the CD103 index (integrin α_E: B7) at their surface and can migrate to T-cell-rich regions of the mesenteric lymph nodes through afferent lymphatics. In the mesenteric lymph nodes, LPDCs can react with naive T cells and activate them, inducing intestinal homing characteristics in these cells. As a result, active T cells can return to the gut and differentiate into effector cells. The migration of $CD103^+$DCs to the lymph nodes is dependent on CCR7 expression. CCR7 is constantly expressed on the surface of these DCs, but its expression increases during infection. When there is no infectious agent, about 5 to 10 percent of mucosal DCs migrate to the mesenteric lymph nodes.

$CD103^+$ dendritic cells produce the non-protein retinoic acid (RA) molecule that is involved in cell signaling. RA is the product of the effect of retinal dehydrogenase enzyme on vitamin A. RA production from these DCs induces CCR9 and integrin $\alpha 4$: $\beta 7$ markers on the surface of B and T cells, which is effective in implanting these cells in the intestine. LPDCs respond poorly to inflammatory stimuli such as TLR ligands and produce more IL-10. For this reason, the migration of $CD103^+$ DCs into the mesenteric lymph nodes in the absence of an infectious agent causes differentiation into Treg $FoxP3^+$ (iTreg) cells. RA secreted from DCs and TGFβ plays an important role in differentiating these Treg. TGFβ is abundantly produced by intestinal cells. In addition, intestinal DCs produce a substance called Indoleamine 2, 3-Dioxygenase (IDO). This enzyme catalyzes tryptophan and leads to the differentiation and induction of Treg cells in the intestine.

$CD103^+$ DCs in the small intestinal mucosa are effective in combating inflammation. Factors such as RA, TGFβ, PGE2, and TSLP[4] are effective in perpetuating this anti-inflammatory response. TSLP, RA, and TGFβ are made by intestinal epithelial cells.

Macrophages located in mucosal tissue naturally produce IL-10. This cytokine deactivates DCs and preserves mucosal Tregs.

Studies have indicated that $DC103^+$DCs, located in the large intestine, play a role in maintaining tolerance and the immune response to symbiotic bacteria and are rarely seen in Peyer's patches. In addition to $CD103^+$ DCs, other myeloid cells are found in the lamina propria, which stimulate inflammatory responses. These cells produce cytokines such as IL 6, IL 23, TNF a, and nitric oxide (NO), which are involved in differentiation into executive TH17 cells and class switching to IgA in B lymphocytes. These $CD103^-$ DCs are stimulated by TLR5 and express the CX3CR1 index, which is the receptor, and chemokine fractalkine. The aforementioned cells cannot migrate to the lymph nodes and are not able to present antigen to the naive T cell and produce RA. Furthermore, in addition, they are not classified as classical DCs, are more like macrophages, and are involved in the production of inflammatory cytokines.

6. Adaptive immunity in the gastrointestinal tract

Humoral immunity and mucosal IgA production are the main forms of acquired immunity in the gastrointestinal tract. Secretory IgA dimer into the lumen, IgG and

[4] Thymic Stromal Lymphopoietin.

IgM participate in the defense against pathogens. The role of cellular immunity in the gastrointestinal tract is to control responses in the gut with the help of Treg and TH17 cells.

After capturing the antigen, dendritic cells migrate to the mesenteric lymph nodes and Peyer's patches, and acquired intestinal immune responses are formed[5]. Active T and B lymphocytes enter the bloodstream through the lymph flow at the site of the thoracic duct. They then settle in the mucosal tissues through the appearance of implanted surface molecules in the intestinal mucosa [1, 4].

6.1 Mucosal B lymphocytes and IgA production

In Peyer's patches, most B cells in the corona and dark zone of the follicular germinal centers are IgM^+/ IgD^+, while in the light zone the germinal centers cells are more than 90% IgA^+ cells. IgA cells in the germinal centers leave the O-MALT, enter the mesenteric lymphatic ducts, and then the blood flows from there to the mucosal and glandular areas of different parts of D-MALT and become IgA-producing plasma cells. IgA cells in the germinal centers are called immune cells. Unlike villi capillaries, which allow the release of serum proteins into lamina propria, capillaries in Peyer's patches have no pores and are impermeable to serum proteins. Therefore, it can be said that immune response interactions such as antibody response, cell accumulation, and secretion of cytokines against intestinal O-MALT antigens are not affected by systemic processes. Based on this, it can be acknowledged that circulating IgA is unable to prevent viral invasion of Peyer's patches and the proliferation of infectious agents in the mucosa. Class switching to IgA occurs in O-MALT. The predominant class of antibodies in the gastrointestinal mucosa is the IgA dimer. In humans, two IgA subclasses are encoded in the genome by two separate and distant sequences. Class switching is associated with the removal of genes upstream of the CH fragment.

In the intestinal mucosa, by two mechanisms dependent or independent of T cells, the class is selectively switched to lgA. Cytokines are extremely important in any phenomenon of class change. In the gut, TGFβ also plays an important role in switching classes to IgA. If class switching is T-dependent, IgA is produced with a higher affinity for the antigen. The DCs capture the antigen, move it to the interfollicular zone (in Peyer's patches) or the mesenteric lymph nodes, and deliver it to the naive CD4 + T. CD4 + T cells are then activated and differentiated into TFH (follicular helper T cells). Then, they react with B IgM^+/ IgD^+ cells and induce class switching to IgA. The prerequisite for this is TGFβ and CD40L binding of T cell surface to CD40 expressed in B cell. NO production from dendritic cells can increase the expression of TGFβ receptor on B cells. In T-cell-independent switching, active dendritic cells produce cytokines such as APRIL[6], BAFF[7], and TGFβ, leading to the induction of class switching in B IgM^+ / IgD^+ cells (especially B1 cells). In this case, IgA is produced with less binding affinity than in the T cell-dependent state.

In the process of differentiating $BIgA^+$ cells into IgA-producing plasma cells, the cell secretory system is fully developed, α-CH fusion occurs at the mRNA level, and a J chain is produced. IL-2 is involved in regulating J chain production in B lymphocytes and plasma cells. In vitro, B cells committed to producing IgA of O-MALT origin undergo 6-IL differentiation in the final stages of differentiation. But in vivo studies do not confirm this finding. Therefore, it can be concluded that there are no

[5] Inductive Sites.

[6] A proliferation-inducing ligand.

[7] B-cell activating factor of the TNF family.

factors required for IgA differentiation and secretion. By migrating these lymphocytes to D-MALT regions and effector sites, the conditions for differentiation into end-cell cells are provided [1, 4, 5].

6.2 The role of secretory IgA in the regulation of immune responses

IgA B cells do not differentiate in O-MALT and therefore IgA concentration is low in these areas. Serum immunoglobulin concentrations are also very low in these areas [61]. However, sIgA located in the lamina propria and glandular secretions enter the O-MALT by binding to the apical membrane of M cells in the FAE [62].

T cells containing the Fc receptor in Peyer's patches act as helper cells and increase BIgA + cells. Fcα receptor T and B cells are involved in the specific regulation of the isotype of the mucosal immune system [63].

Antigen-IgA complexes are also transported to O-MALT by M cells [62], so it can be said that the Fcα receptor of B cells or macrophages enhances the immune response by increasing antigen uptake and processing. In conclusion, IgA reabsorption by M cells and reaction with Fcα receptors are involved in modulating the immune response [64].

Also, in mucous secretions and glands, anti-idiotypes can enhance the immune response by such a mechanism. This clarifies the reason for the reaction of breastfed infants (sIgA absorption) to oral and injectable vaccines [65].

6.3 Lymphocyte migration and homing

Lymphocyte and monocyte migration and implantation play an important role in the mucosal immune response. This process causes a set of specific cells to migrate to areas such as the Peyer's patches where antigens are present, and the widespread effector and memory cells to different parts of the mucosal surface provide comprehensive protection for the body.

Numerous molecules and receptors are involved in the lymphocytes homing into the intestinal mucosa, including homing receptors, cell adhesion molecules (integrins) of chemokines, and chemokine receptors.

Naive lymphocytes enter the mesenteric lymph node and O-MALT (Peyer's patches) through HEV. Lymphatic tissues facilitate the entry of naive lymphocytes expressing CCR7 and L-selectin by secreting CCL19 and CCL21. If in O-MALT and lymph nodes, these lymphocytes are exposed to specific antigens presented at the APC, the incidence of CCR7 and L-selectin is reduced. Once the cells are activated, they leave the mesenteric lymph nodes through the lymph and Peyer's patches and enter the bloodstream through the thoracic duct. Dendritic cells in the mucosa can induce specific molecules to localize activated lymphocytes in the gastrointestinal tract. Activated lymphocytes increase the expression of α4: β7 integrins that bind to MadCAM1 on their surface. MadCAM1 is expressed on the endothelial surface lining the blood vessels of the intestine and its associated lymphatic tissues. Due to this interaction, it provides the conditions for the adhesion of active lymphocytes to the endothelial vessels of the gastrointestinal tract. Activated T and B cells express the CCR9 chemokine receptor on their surface after initial exposure to antigen in the small intestine. This receptor binds to TECK (CCL25) at the epithelial surface of the small intestine, leading to the re-implantation of these cells in this area. Primary activation of lymphocytes in the colon leads to the development of the chemokine receptor CCR10, which binds to the MEG (CCL28) surface of the colon epithelial cells. Furthermore, CCL28 can be secreted by the mammary and salivary glands [1, 2].

Lymphocytes that have first been exposed to the antigen and have detected it on the surface of intestinal mucosal DCs have identified implantation molecules and can implant in the gastrointestinal mucosa. For this reason, it seems that vaccination against intestinal infections requires the administration of the vaccine in the mucosa because DCs in the mucosa will have the power to induce specific implantation molecules [4].

With the passage of active lymphocytes through the vascular endothelium, the expression of $\alpha4$: $\beta7$ integrins stops on their surface, and instead another integrin called α_E: $\beta7$ appears on their surface. α_E: $\beta7$ can attach to the cadmium E molecule on the surface of intestinal mucosal epithelial cells. In this way, the lymphocytes are kept in the vicinity of the epithelial cells after entering the lamina propria (**Figure 4**).

6.4 Secretory IgA

In an adult human, more than 3 grams of IgA is secreted daily in the mucosa and glands. Secretory IgA is made up of two interconnected molecules (each containing four immunoglobulin chains).

In mice, rats, and rabbits there is only one IgA isotype, but in humans, there are two isotopes IgA1 and IgA2 encoded by two separate genes [66].

IgA2 is often made by mucosal plasma cells, and the lack of 13 specific amino acids in the $\alpha2$ chain makes IgA2 resistant to specific anti-IgA1 proteases produced by purulent bacteria.

dimeric IgA also contains the J chain and the secretory component (SC). The carboxylic part of Fc is the two IgA molecules next to each other and their Fab is outward. In humans, mice, and rabbits, the penultimate cysteine of the two α chains binds to the cysteine J chain through disulfide bonding.

The J chain has an Ig-like domain and the SC has five Ig-like domains. A complete slgA molecule consists of two IgA monomeric molecules of a J chain and a secretory component. The secretory component covers areas sensitive to proteolytic digestion and the IgA hinge, and the secretory variants of this immunoglobulin are highly resistant to proteases [1, 4].

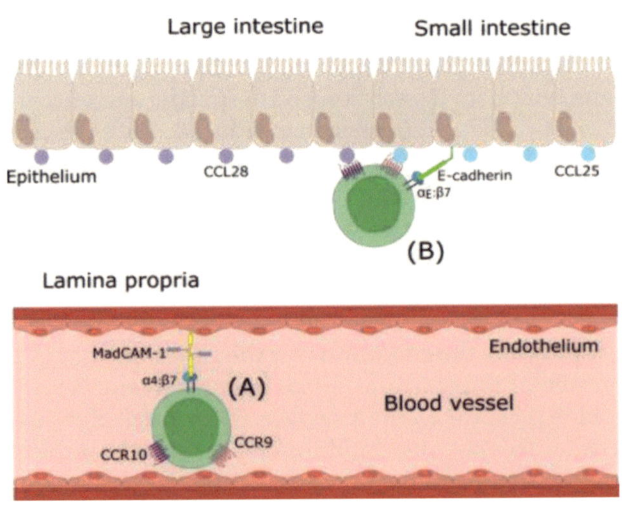

Figure 4.
Homing in gastrointestinal mucosa. Effector T lymphocytes attach to MadCAM-1 surface endothelial cells for homing in the gut (A). Intestinal epithelial cells express specific chemokines for T cells that intend to home in the gut (B).

7. Intraepithelial IgA transport

7.1 Poly immunoglobulin receptor (pIgR)

The transfer of IgA from the production site in the mucosal and glandular tissue areas to the secretions takes place in an active process with the involvement of membrane polymer receptors (**Figure 5**).

The pIgR receptor is a membrane glycoprotein consisting of five Ig-like domains (reinforced with disulfide bounds) at the cell surface, an intramembrane fragment, and a 100-amino acid sequence within the cytoplasm.

The human immunoglobulin polymer receptor gene is located on chromosome 1. The genes of these receptors in epithelial cells are affected by cytokines such as IFN-γ in vitro and are expressed on the surface of these cells. Therefore, it can be said that mucosal inflammation has an aggravating role in the transfer of slgA to secretions [1, 66].

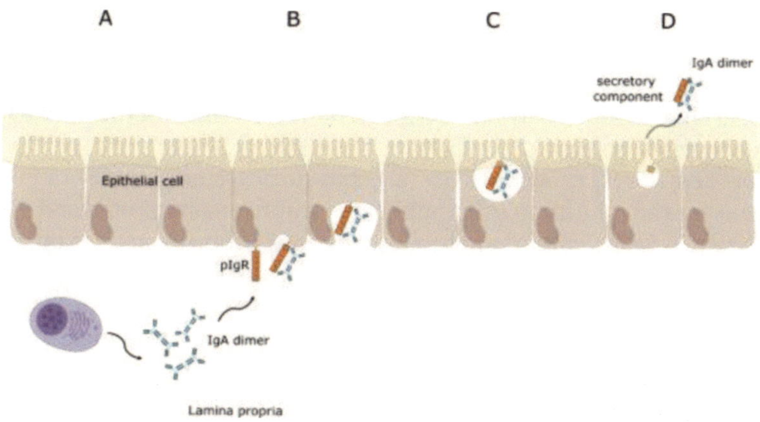

Figure 5.
Mechanism of IgA dimer production in lamina propria and its transmission by epithelial cells. Lamina propria plasma cells produce IgA dimers (A). These antibodies are transported into the epithelial cells via pIgR at the basal surface (B). Following the release of IgA from the luminal surface of these cells by the mechanism of transcytosis (C), due to proteolytic cleavage, part of the receptor remains attached to the IgA dimer, which is the secretory component or SC (D).

7.2 Binding of IgA to the immunoglobulin receptor

IgA binds to the first Immunoglobulin-like domain of the Poly-Ig receptor. Following the separation of pIgR from the epithelial cell, a disulfide bond is established between the cysteine of the fifth SC region and the Fc portion of one of the IgA monomer monomers. Domains 2, 3, and 4 of the secretory component do not participate in the binding but are necessary for the establishment of the two cysteine roots [66].

8. Mechanisms of secretory IgA protection

8.1 Immune exclusion

Secretory IgA dimer is responsible for binding to microorganisms in the intestine and mucosal surfaces of the gastrointestinal tract, respiratory tract, and genital tract [67, 68].

The slgA-antigen complex can be easily trapped in mucus, excreted by bowel movements, and the beat of cilia of the respiratory tract. Also, the sIgA can directly block the microbial binding sites to epithelial cells [69].

The basic way of protection by sIgA is the same as immune exclusion. Therefore, the presence of appropriate levels of specific sIgA can only cause protection (even in the absence of other immunological mechanisms) [2].

9. Respiratory mucosa

The airways are an important route for the entry of pathogen antigens, allergens, and airborne particles. The upper respiratory tract mucosa contains the nasal lymphatic tissue (NALT), the bronchial lymphatic tissue (BALT), and the airway lymph nodes, and the lower respiratory tract mucosa contains the smaller airway lymph nodes and alveoli.

The immune system is present in the airways like other mucous membranes and plays an important role in regulating homeostasis and preventing harmful immune responses to harmless antigens. The respiratory system also contains specialized and organized mucosal tissues such as the palatine, lingual, pharyngeal, and adenoids, which form a ring-like structure called the "Waldeyer's ring" in the pathway of air and food antigens (**Figure 6**).

The extensive vascular network of the respiratory system provides a favorable environment for the migration of lymphocytes and the passage of blood vessels to the lung tissue. Leukocytes do not follow the conventional method of homing in lymphoid tissues and do not have processes such as rolling and attaching to the endothelium and passing through the HEV.

One of the defense mechanisms in the mucosa is physical and mechanical defense, which is seen in the respiratory system as a mechanism of clearance of the ciliary mucosa (mucociliary). The most abundant cells in the upper airways are ciliated epithelial cells that form the physical barrier [2, 5].

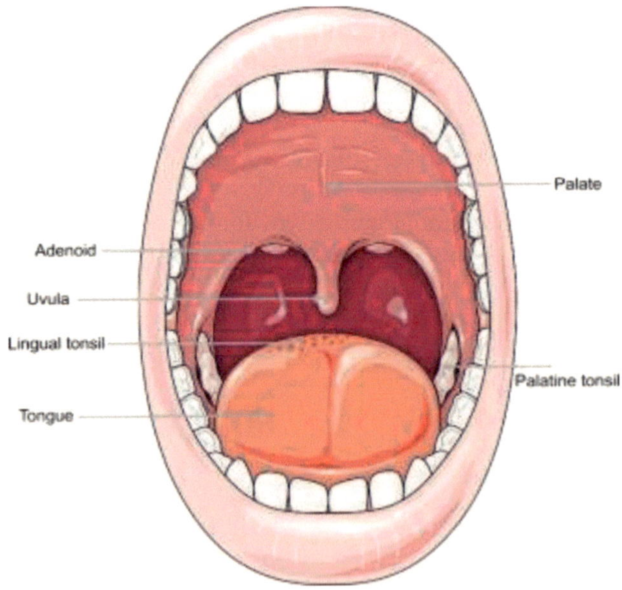

Figure 6.
Waldeyer's ring. The tonsils and adenoids form a ring of lymphatic tissue in the gastrointestinal tract and airways called the Waldeyer's ring.

Goblet cells are present in the margins of ciliated epithelial cells and are responsible for secreting mucus.

The mucus layer is directed to the upper respiratory tract by the movement of the cilium, so that suspended particles and pathogens are excreted or swallowed through sneezing and coughing which is called mucociliary clearance. Various cells in the respiratory tract, such as ciliated epithelial cells, alveoli, and immune cells located subepithelial, can produce and secrete antimicrobial peptides such as defensins, cathelicidins, collectins, and protease inhibitors [5].

9.1 Waldeyer's ring

The tonsils and adenoids are a great place to trap antigens from the mouth and nose. In humans, the Waldeyer's ring forms a network of lymphatic tissue in the nasopharyngeal mucosa, which is the structure of NALT. The epithelial surface of the tonsils and adenoids is the site of antigen entry due to its proximity to the external environment.

The palatine tonsils are two oval masses of secondary lymphatic tissue that are located in pairs behind the oral cavity and at the beginning of the oropharynx and are the entry point for respiratory and gastrointestinal antigens. The tonsils have several depressions called crypts. The presence of crypts increases the surface of the tonsils and the ability to remove antigens. The outer layer of each crypt is composed of epithelial cells, which have M-like cells present and perform the function of antigen uptake and transport through the epithelium. Below the epithelium of each crypt is one or more secondary lymph follicles.

Most cell populations of NALT lymphatic structures are composed of T and B lymphocytes and to a lesser extent dendritic cells and macrophages. NALT is structurally similar to MALT and has FAE-containing cells similar to M goblet and IELs. Lymphatic follicles are also seen in the subepithelial layer. Most tonsils located in the tonsils are B cells that turn into antibody-producing plasma cells (often IgA). The number of CD4 + T cells in this area is very low and IEL lymphocytes CD8 + T is found as CD8 + αβT or in the unusual phenotypes CD8αα + αβ T and CD8αα + γδ T.

Lymphatic tissues along the airways form the BALT structure. The upper airways have more organized lymphatic structures than the lower airways. In the lungs, active immune cells migrate mainly to the mediastinal and cervical lymph nodes, which enlarge in the face of infectious agents. In the BALT structure, the number of M and IEL cells in the overlying epithelium is very rare and there are no goblet cells in this area. In BALT, similar to MALT, lymph follicles are seen. B cells located inside the follicles usually have a memory phenotype and are mostly IgA^+. In the absence of infection, BALT is difficult to detect. Therefore, BALT is considered a secondary structure in cases of infection [4, 5].

9.2 Regulation of immune responses by airway epithelial cells

Airway epithelial cells specialize in regulating immune responses in the respiratory tract. While these cells can detect pathogenic microbes, they do not respond to harmless antigens and cause respiratory homeostasis These cells produce antimicrobial peptides, inflammatory cytokines, and chemokines, and express much lower levels of TLRs than the gastrointestinal epithelium, However, the expression of these TLRs is strongly influenced by TNF-α and IFN-γ [5].

9.3 Dendritic cells in the respiratory mucosa

BALT and NALT have a large number of DCs. These cells help maintain homeostasis by detecting and differentiating between pathogenic and harmless antigens and by inducing tolerance to their antigens. Airway DCs are often of the myeloid class, but plasmacytoid DCs are rarely seen.

There is also a population of positive langerin DCs in the upper airways that are somewhat similar to cutaneous Langerhans cells and are involved in immune surveillance. In the lower airways and lung tissue, there are lung parenchymal dendritic cells (LPDCs) or interstitial DCs that are scattered in the alveolar epithelium and the alveolar space or the connective tissue between the epithelium and the arteries. LPDCs are often $CD11b^+$ and belong to the myeloid class.

DCs in the respiratory tract are considered strong cells in antigen uptake but have weak power in stimulating T lymphocytes. Airway DCs mainly direct the response to T2 and Treg, and by producing TGFβ lead to the switching of B cell class to IgA-producing plasma cells. In other words, airway dendritic cells regulate and modulate the immune response. Similar to MALT, dendritic cells meet and stimulate T cells by moving to the lymph nodes in the lungs. The lymph cells, then activated by lymph flow and then blood flow, return to the position of the lungs and participate in the immune response [4].

9.4 Lymphocyte homing in the respiratory mucosa

Integrins play an important role, especially α4 (α4: β7 and α4:β1) in the process of lymphocyte homing in the respiratory mucosa. E-cadherins are prominent in lung and intestinal cells and bind to αE:β7 integrins and are involved in the establishment of lymphocytes. Active T lymphocytes attach to CCL5 (RANTES) by expressing the CCR5 chemokine receptor at their surface and are located in the parenchyma of lung tissue. CCL5 is a chemotactic agent that is naturally secreted from lung tissue and increases during inflammation. In the airways, IgA-producing plasma blast implant by binding to the CCR10 chemokine receptor on its surface and the CCL28 chemokine secreted from the respiratory epithelium [1, 5].

10. Mucosal vaccination

By administering one or more oral doses of mucosal vaccine, in addition to producing sIgA on mucosal surfaces, it also stimulates cellular and systemic immune responses. With the entry of pathogens into O-MALT, the process of production and maintenance of memory lymphocyte population is established. In addition to the characteristics of injectable vaccines, oral vaccines must be able to pass through the stomach, intestines, and be resistant to bacterial enzymes and low pH.

Also, oral vaccines must be able to escape clearance mechanisms such as being trapped in mucus and be able to reach specific areas of the FAE-covered mucosa.

Furthermore, in addition, these vaccines need to compete by binding to the inner membrane to penetrate M cell vesicles. Immunological epitopes should be able to maintain their immunogenicity after crossing the epithelial barrier and penetrating the vesicles and be available to antigen-presenting cells for processing [2].

10.1 How vaccines get access to O-MALT

10.1.1 Inert particulate carriers

Vaccine access to Peyer's patches depends on the ability of M cells to transmit adherent multivalent macromolecules. One of the strongest products that have been proven to be effective in the form of systemic vaccines is the Immune stimulating complex (ISCOM).

ISCOMs are particles 35 nm in diameter that are formed by the accumulation of protein antigens, such as the surface proteins of viruses, in a specific pattern. It should be noted that this form of immunogen was created for the proper and immunological present of viral surface proteins [70].

Immunization by ISCOMs leads to IgG production and cellular immune response against other viruses such as measles as well as inhibition of TH cells [70]. Intranasal immunization with ISCOM and influenza hemagglutinin leads to a local increase in anti-influenza cytotoxicity [71]. As a result, ISCOMs, as mucosal antigens, can be thought to produce IgA. In other words, ISCOMs are useful for mucosal use and are resistant to salt and bile acids.

Oral immunization in multiple doses with ISCOM containing ovalbumin or bacterial proteins results in the production of sIgA, systemic IgA, and cellular immunity [72].

They can also be used to immunize viral proteins that are naturally resistant to digestive proteases. Because they may not be resistant in the gut unless they are inside the capsule. Today, with the help of small hydroxyapatite crystals, effective solutions for particle penetration have been developed.

Crystals of 0.1 to 0.5 microns attach to M1 cells and are efficiently transported to intraepithelial envelopes. Because hydroxyapatite is a non-immunogenic and non-toxic component of bone structure, these antigen-coated crystals can be consumed in large quantities. These compounds should be used in capsule coatings [2].

10.1.2 Live vaccine vectors

The best way to stimulate mucosal immunity is to insert antigens into living microorganisms that can attach to M cells and settle and multiply in Peyer's patches and mucous membranes. Because living microorganisms elicit a strong and long-lasting immune response, a large number of viral and bacterial carriers are considered for this purpose. Given that living carriers can produce antigens for a long time and cause the production of antibodies as well as the development of cellular immune responses, the possibility of their use as a vaccine is being strongly considered.

The vaccinia virus recombinant has been tested as an oral vaccine [73]. But the mechanism of its absorption and transfer to Peyer's patches is still unknown. This method can probably be a safe and effective method of mucosal immunization. Because infection of mucosal cells with the recombinant virus can cause the presence of antigens on the cell surface. The vaccinia virus recombinant is used as a mucosal vaccine to enhance the capacity of bacterial carriers for foreign DNA [74]. Because viral carriers have limited replication and are unable to germinate the virus, the infection may be transient, with limited antigen present and the carrier cannot spread well in the mucosa of Peyer's patches.

Different species of bacteria can settle in Peyer's patches, including the live Attenuated strains of Salmonella and BCG [75, 76]. BCG is an effective adjuvant whose systemic immunization is safe. Once given at the time of birth, this vaccine provides long-term safety. BCG is also considered an oral vaccine [77] and is effective in transmitting O-MALT through M cells [78].

By orally administering recombinant Salmonella, laboratory animals have been vaccinated against a range of foreign antigens, including the heat-stable *E. Coli* enterotoxin [79], the streptococcal adhesin [80], and the malaria circumsporozoite protein [81]. In general, Salmonella is considered a strong mucosal immunogen. However, this limits the use of these carriers for repeated immunizations. Because the anti-secretory immune response prevents re-absorption of oral doses of the carrier that deliver this antigen or other recombinant antigens.

IgA secretion of the superficial salmonella typhoid epitope of Morium can favorably prevent the penetration of these microorganisms into the mucosa [82].

However, applying effective methods to various events, such as immunogen retention in the gut, the ability of immunogen to bind to the surface of M cells, effective interaction with antigen-supplying cells, or facilitating its detection by M cells, can enhance mucosal immunity.

Acknowledgements

This work has been financed by Intechopen publications and I would like to thank Dr. Elena Franco-Robles and Ms. Karmen Daleta as well as Ms. Mia Miskulin for closed cooperation and sincere support.

Conflict of interest

The authors declare no conflict of interest.

Thanks

I am grateful to my family, Dr. Farideh Talebi, Dr. Tooba Ghazanfari, MSc. Davood Jamali, Dr. Sara Ghaffarpour, Dr. Ensieh Sadat Mirsharif, Dr. Ali Mohammad Mohseni Majd, Dr. Mohammad Saber Zamani from Islamic Azad University Science and Research Branch, Dr. Amirhossein Gaeini from Iran University, Dr. Alireza Mafi from Isfahan University as well as MSc. Zahra Hosseinpur Yektaei from Shahed University and MSc. Abdolkarim Talebi Taheri from Shahid Beheshti University.

Author details

Saeed Sepehrnia
Shahed University Medical of Science, Tehran, Iran

*Address all correspondence to: sepehrniasaeed@gmail.com

References

[1] Abbas, A.K., A.H. Lichtman, and S. Pillai, Cellular and Molecular Immunology E-Book. 2017: Elsevier Health Sciences.

[2] Kraehenbuhl, J.P. and M.R. Neutra, Molecular and cellular basis of immune protection of mucosal surfaces. Physiol Rev, 1992. 72(4): p. 853-879.

[3] Howard L., Weiner M., Oral Tolerance For The Treatment Of Autoimmune Diseases. Annual Review of Medicine, 1997. 48(1): p. 341-351.

[4] Murphy, K. and C. Weaver, Janeway's Immunobiology. , 2016. W.W. Norton.

[5] Williams, A.E., Immunology: Mucosal and Body Surface Defences. , 2011. Wiley.

[6] Bjerke, K., P. Brandtzaeg, and O. Fausa, T cell distribution is different in follicle-associated epithelium of human Peyer's patches and villous epithelium. Clin Exp Immunol, 1988. 74(2): p. 270-275.

[7] Ermak, T.H. and R.L. Owen, Differential distribution of lymphocytes and accessory cells in mouse Peyer's patches. Anat Rec, 1986. 215(2): p. 144-152.

[8] Ermak, T.H., H.J. Steger, and J. Pappo, Phenotypically distinct subpopulations of T cells in domes and M-cell pockets of rabbit gut-associated lymphoid tissues. Immunology, 1990. 71(4): p. 530-537.

[9] Butcher, E.C., et al., Surface phenotype and migratory capability of Peyer's patch germinal center cells. Adv Exp Med Biol, 1982. 149: p. 765-772.

[10] Mayrhofer, G., C.W. Pugh, and A.N. Barclay, The distribution, ontogeny and origin in the rat of Ia-positive cells with dendritic morphology and of Ia antigen in epithelia, with special reference to the intestine. Eur J Immunol, 1983. 13(2): p. 112-122.

[11] Spalding, D.M., et al., Accessory cells in murine Peyer's patch. I. Identification and enrichment of a functional dendritic cell. J Exp Med, 1983. 157(5): p. 1646-1659.

[12] Kiyono, H., et al., In vivo immune response to a T-cell-dependent antigen by cultures of disassociated murine Peyer's patch. Proc Natl Acad Sci U S A, 1982. 79(2): p. 596-600.

[13] Dunkley, M.L. and A.J. Husband, Distribution and functional characteristics of antigen-specific helper T cells arising after Peyer's patch immunization. Immunology, 1987. 61(4): p. 475-482.

[14] Guy-Grand, D., C. Griscelli, and P. Vassalli, The mouse gut T lymphocyte, a novel type of T cell. Nature, origin, and traffic in mice in normal and graft-versus-host conditions. J Exp Med, 1978. 148(6): p. 1661-1677.

[15] Brandtzaeg, P., et al., Lymphoepithelial interactions in the mucosal immune system. Gut, 1988. 29(8): p. 1116-1130.

[16] Ernst, P.B., A. Dean Befus, and J. Bienenstock, Leukocytes in the intestinal epithelium: an unusual immunological compartment. Immunology Today, 1985. 6(2): p. 50-55.

[17] Hirata, I., et al., Immunohistological characterization of intraepithelial and lamina propria lymphocytes in control ileum and colon and in inflammatory bowel disease. Dig Dis Sci, 1986. 31(6): p. 593-603.

[18] Selby, W.S., et al., Lymphocyte subpopulations in the human small intestine. The findings in normal

mucosa and in the mucosa of patients with adult coeliac disease. Clin Exp Immunol, 1983. 52(1): p. 219-228.

[19] Taguchi, T., et al., Analysis of Th1 and Th2 cells in murine gut-associated tissues. Frequencies of CD4+ and CD8+ T cells that secrete IFN-gamma and IL-5. J Immunol, 1990. 145(1): p. 68-77.

[20] Kanof, M.E., et al., CD4 positive Leu-8 negative helper-inducer T cells predominate in the human intestinal lamina propria. J Immunol, 1988. 141(9): p. 3029-3036.

[21] Beagley, K.W., et al., Peyer's patch B cells with memory cell characteristics undergo terminal differentiation within 24 hours in response to interleukin-6. Cytokine, 1991. 3(2): p. 107-116.

[22] Matsumoto, R., et al., Interleukin-5 induces maturation but not class switching of surface IgA-positive B cells into IgA-secreting cells. Immunology, 1989. 66(1): p. 32-38.

[23] Bland, P.W., Antigen Presentation by Gut Epithelial Cells: Secretion by Rat Enterocytes of a Factor with IL-1-Like Activity, in Recent Advances in Mucosal Immunology: Part A: Cellular Interactions, J. Mestecky, et al., Editors. 1987, Springer US, Boston, MAp. 219-225.

[24] Brandtzaeg, P., et al., Interactions of lymphoid cells with the epithelial environment. Monogr Allergy, 1988. 24: p. 51-59.

[25] Spencer, J., T. Finn, and P.G. Isaacson, Expression of HLA-DR antigens on epithelium associated with lymphoid tissue in the human gastrointestinal tract. Gut, 1986. 27(2): p. 153-157.

[26] Vidal, K., D. Kaiserlian, and J.P. Revillard, Heterogeneity of murine gut epithelium: three subsets defined by expression of dendritic cell markers. Reg Immunol, 1989. 2(6): p. 360-365.

[27] Bland, P., MHC class II expression by the gut epithelium. Immunol Today, 1988. 9(6): p. 174-178.

[28] Bland, P.W. and L.G. Warren, Antigen presentation by epithelial cells of the rat small intestine. I. Kinetics, antigen specificity and blocking by anti-Ia antisera. Immunology, 1986. 58(1): p. 1-7.

[29] Bland, P.W. and L.G. Warren, Antigen presentation by epithelial cells of the rat small intestine. II. Selective induction of suppressor T cells. Immunology, 1986. 58(1): p. 9-14.

[30] Schmidt, G.H., M.M. Wilkinson, and B.A. Ponder, Cell migration pathway in the intestinal epithelium: an in situ marker system using mouse aggregation chimeras. Cell, 1985. 40(2): p. 425-429.

[31] Pappo, J. and R.L. Owen, Absence of secretory component expression by epithelial cells overlying rabbit gut-associated lymphoid tissue. Gastroenterology, 1988. 95(5): p. 1173-1177.

[32] Ermak, T.H., et al., M cells and granular mononuclear cells in Peyer's patch domes of mice depleted of their lymphocytes by total lymphoid irradiation. Am J Pathol, 1989. 134(3): p. 529-537.

[33] Owen, R.L. and T.H. Ermak, Structural specializations for antigen uptake and processing in the digestive tract. Springer Semin Immunopathol, 1990. 12(2-3): p. 139-152.

[34] Spencer, J., et al., The development of gut associated lymphoid tissue in the terminal ileum of fetal human intestine. Clin Exp Immunol, 1986. 64(3): p. 536-543.

[35] Pappo, J., H.J. Steger, and R.L. Owen, Differential adherence of epithelium overlying gut-associated lymphoid tissue. An ultrastructural study. Lab Invest, 1988. 58(6): p. 692-697.

[36] Neutra, M.R., et al., Transport of membrane-bound macromolecules by M cells in follicle-associated epithelium of rabbit Peyer's patch. Cell and Tissue Research, 1987. 247(3): p. 537-546.

[37] Bye, W.A., C.H. Allan, and J.S. Trier, Structure, distribution, and origin of M cells in Peyer's patches of mouse ileum. Gastroenterology, 1984. 86(5 Pt 1): p. 789-801.

[38] Owen, R.L. and D.K. Bhalla, Cytochemical analysis of alkaline phosphatase and esterase activities and of lectin-binding and anionic sites in rat and mouse Peyer's patch M cells. Am J Anat, 1983. 168(2): p. 199-212.

[39] de Aizpurua, H.J. and G.J. Russell-Jones, Oral vaccination. Identification of classes of proteins that provoke an immune response upon oral feeding. J Exp Med, 1988. 167(2): p. 440-451.

[40] Stokes, C.R., Induction and control of intestinal immune responses, in Local immune responses of the gut. 2019, CRC Press. p. 97-142.

[41] Mowat, A.M., The regulation of immune responses to dietary protein antigens. Immunol Today, 1987. 8(3): p. 93-98.

[42] Inman, L.R. and J.R. Cantey, Specific adherence of Escherichia coli (strain RDEC-1) to membranous (M) cells of the Peyer's patch in Escherichia coli diarrhea in the rabbit. J Clin Invest, 1983. 71(1): p. 1-8.

[43] Owen, R.L., et al., M cell transport of Vibrio cholerae from the intestinal lumen into Peyer's patches: a mechanism for antigen sampling and for microbial transepithelial migration. J Infect Dis, 1986. 153(6): p. 1108-1118.

[44] Winner, L., 3rd, et al., New model for analysis of mucosal immunity: intestinal secretion of specific monoclonal immunoglobulin A from hybridoma tumors protects against Vibrio cholerae infection. Infect Immun, 1991. 59(3): p. 977-982.

[45] Kohbata, S., H. Yokoyama, and E. Yabuuchi, Cytopathogenic effect of Salmonella typhi GIFU 10007 on M cells of murine ileal Peyer's patches in ligated ileal loops: an ultrastructural study. Microbiol Immunol, 1986. 30(12): p. 1225-1237.

[46] Wassef, J.S., D.F. Keren, and J.L. Mailloux, Role of M cells in initial antigen uptake and in ulcer formation in the rabbit intestinal loop model of shigellosis. Infect Immun, 1989. 57(3): p. 858-863.

[47] Grützkau, A., et al., Involvement of M cells in the bacterial invasion of Peyer's patches: a common mechanism shared by Yersinia enterocolitica and other enteroinvasive bacteria. Gut, 1990. 31(9): p. 1011-1015.

[48] Walker, R.I., et al., Selective association and transport of Campylobacter jejuni through M cells of rabbit Peyer's patches. Can J Microbiol, 1988. 34(10): p. 1142-1147.

[49] Roy, M.J. and M. Varvayanis, Development of dome epithelium in gut-associated lymphoid tissues: association of IgA with M cells. Cell Tissue Res, 1987. 248(3): p. 645-651.

[50] Moța, G., et al., The Fc receptor for IgA expression and affinity on lymphocytes and macrophages. Mol Immunol, 1988. 25(2): p. 95-101.

[51] Stafford, H.A., K.L. Knight, and M.W. Fanger, Receptors for IgA on rabbit lymphocytes. II.

Characterization of their binding parameters for IgA. J Immunol, 1982. 128(5): p. 2201-5.

[52] Yodoi, J., M. Adachi, and N. Noro, IgA binding factors and Fc receptors for IgA: comparative studies between IgA and IgE Fc receptor systems. Int Rev Immunol, 1987. 2(2): p. 117-141.

[53] Owen, R.L., R.T. Apple, and D.K. Bhalla, Morphometric and cytochemical analysis of lysosomes in rat Peyer's patch follicle epithelium: their reduction in volume fraction and acid phosphatase content in M cells compared to adjacent enterocytes. Anat Rec, 1986. 216(4): p. 521-527.

[54] Allan, C.H., D.L. Mendrick, and J.S. Trier, Rat intestinal M cells contain acidic endosomal-lysosomal compartments and express class II major histocompatibility complex determinants. Gastroenterology, 1993. 104(3): p. 698-708.

[55] Owen, R.L., Sequential uptake of horseradish peroxidase by lymphoid follicle epithelium of Peyer's patches in the normal unobstructed mouse intestine: an ultrastructural study. Gastroenterology, 1977. 72(3): p. 440-451.

[56] Cash, R.A., et al., Response of man to infection with Vibrio cholerae. I. Clinical, serologic, and bacteriologic responses to a known inoculum. J Infect Dis, 1974. 129(1): p. 45-52.

[57] Jertborn, M., A.M. Svennerholm, and J. Holmgren, Saliva, breast milk, and serum antibody responses as indirect measures of intestinal immunity after oral cholera vaccination or natural disease. J Clin Microbiol, 1986. 24(2): p. 203-209.

[58] Svennerholm, A.M., et al., Mucosal antitoxic and antibacterial immunity after cholera disease and after immunization with a combined B subunit-whole cell vaccine. J Infect Dis, 1984. 149(6): p. 884-893.

[59] Siciński, P., et al., Poliovirus type 1 enters the human host through intestinal M cells. Gastroenterology, 1990. 98(1): p. 56-58.

[60] Wolf, J.L., et al., Intestinal M cells: a pathway for entry of reovirus into the host. Science, 1981. 212(4493): p. 471-472.

[61] Allan, C.H. and J.S. Trier, Structure and permeability differ in subepithelial villus and Peyer's patch follicle capillaries. Gastroenterology, 1991. 100(5 Pt 1): p. 1172-1179.

[62] Weltzin, R., et al., Binding and transepithelial transport of immunoglobulins by intestinal M cells: demonstration using monoclonal IgA antibodies against enteric viral proteins. J Cell Biol, 1989. 108(5): p. 1673-1685.

[63] Maliszewski, C.R., et al., Expression cloning of a human Fc receptor for IgA. J Exp Med, 1990. 172(6): p. 1665-1672.

[64] Mellman, I., et al., Structure and function of Fc receptors on macrophages and lymphocytes. J Cell Sci Suppl, 1988. 9: p. 45-65.

[65] Hanson, L.A., et al., Antibody-mediated immunity in the neonate. Padiatr Padol, 1990. 25(5): p. 371-376.

[66] Kraehenbuhl, J.P. and M.R. Neutra, Transepithelial transport and mucosal defence II: secretion of IgA. Trends Cell Biol, 1992. 2(6): p. 170-174.

[67] Tomasi, T.B., Mechanisms of Immune Regulation at Mucosal Surfaces. Reviews of Infectious Diseases, 1983. 5: p. S784-S792.

[68] Underdown, B.J. and J.M. Schiff, Immunoglobulin A: strategic defense initiative at the mucosal surface. Annu Rev Immunol, 1986. 4: p. 389-417.

[69] Williams, R.C. and R.J. Gibbons, Inhibition of bacterial adherence by secretory immunoglobulin A: a mechanism of antigen disposal. Science, 1972. 177(4050): p. 697-699.

[70] Morein, B., et al., Iscom, a novel structure for antigenic presentation of membrane proteins from enveloped viruses. Nature, 1984. 308(5958): p. 457-460.

[71] Jones, P.D., et al., Cellular immune responses in the murine lung to local immunization with influenza A virus glycoproteins in micelles and immunostimulatory complexes (iscoms). Scand J Immunol, 1988. 27(6): p. 645-652.

[72] Mowat, A.M. and A.M. Donachie, ISCOMS--a novel strategy for mucosal immunization? Immunol Today, 1991. 12(11): p. 383-385.

[73] Mackett, M., G.L. Smith, and B. Moss, General method for production and selection of infectious vaccinia virus recombinants expressing foreign genes. J Virol, 1984. 49(3): p. 857-864.

[74] Moss, B., et al., Live recombinant vaccinia virus protects chimpanzees against hepatitis B. Nature, 1984. 311(5981): p. 67-69.

[75] Curtiss, R., 3rd, et al., Stable recombinant avirulent Salmonella vaccine strains. Adv Exp Med Biol, 1989. 251: p. 33-47.

[76] Aldovini, A. and R.A. Young, Humoral and cell-mediated immune responses to live recombinant BCG-HIV vaccines. Nature, 1991. 351(6326): p. 479-482.

[77] Stover, C.K., et al., New use of BCG for recombinant vaccines. Nature, 1991. 351(6326): p. 456-460.

[78] Fujimura, Y., Functional morphology of microfold cells (M cells) in Peyer's patches. Gastroenterologia Japonica, 1986. 21(4): p. 325-334.

[79] Clements, J.D., et al., Oral immunization of mice with attenuated Salmonella enteritidis containing a recombinant plasmid which codes for production of the B subunit of heat-labile Escherichia coli enterotoxin. Infect Immun, 1986. 53(3): p. 685-692.

[80] Barletta, R.G., S.M. Michalek, and R. Curtiss, 3rd, Analysis of the virulence of Streptococcus mutans serotype c gtfA mutants in the rat model system. Infect Immun, 1988. 56(2): p. 322-330.

[81] Sadoff, J.C., et al., Oral Salmonella typhimurium Vaccine Expressing Circumsporozoite Protein Protects against Malaria. Science, 1988. 240(4850): p. 336-338.

[82] Michetti, P., et al., Monoclonal secretory immunoglobulin A protects mice against oral challenge with the invasive pathogen Salmonella typhimurium. Infect Immun, 1992. 60(5): p. 1786-1792.

Chapter 2

Probiotic: An Uprising Human Health Concept

Amishi Bhatt, Dhyey Kothari, Charmy Kothari and Ramesh Kothari

Abstract

Most of our gut microbiota live with us in a mutually beneficial life-long relationship. The gut microbiota plays a vital role in the host's overall health through its metabolic activities. Human microbiota might be supported by consuming friendly bacteria (probiotics) and consuming foods to improve the microbiota (prebiotics). During the last two decades, probiotics' interest has increased with rising scientific shreds of evidence of benefits on human health. Hence, they have been exploited as various food products, mainly fermented foods. Probiotics as a treatment modality may restore normal microbiota and functioning of the gastro-intestinal (GI) tract. Strong scientific evidence is associating these bacteria with the prevention and therapy of various GI disorders. (In light of the ongoing trend of probiotics, further research is needed to obtain the perspective of potential applications for better health. Probiotic applications have been extended from health applications to food and agricultural applications. The benefits of probiotics led to its applications in probiotic 'health food' industries and agricultural sectors.

Keywords: Probiotics, Prebiotics, Food products, Gut microbiome, Benefits

1. Introduction

The human body exists in close relation with numerous structurally and functionally diverse microbes inhabiting different parts of the body. The mouth, the gastrointestinal tract (GIT), and the vagina are most heavily populated. This composition is known as microbiota which is acquired soon after birth [1]. The microbiota that is exclusively found in GIT is referred to as 'Gut microbiota.' Gut microbiota is primarily non-pathogenic and plays a vital role in conferring health benefits to the host [2]. Through metabolic activities and physiological regulation such as resistance to pathogens, improvement of intestinal barrier function, promotion of nutrient absorption, formation of bioactive compounds [2]. It may also influence the physiology, biochemistry of the host [3].

The idea that bacteria can confer health benefits to humans was postulated 100 years ago by Elie Metchnikoff. The 'probiotic' word is derived from the Greek word, meaning "for life" and has had several different meanings over the years [4]. The increase in evidence of the benefits of probiotics and prebiotics, especially in health improvement, led to its applications in various food industries. This book chapter highlights the significance of gut microbiota and the emergence of probiotic concepts to benefit human health. In this chapter, we have made a little attempt to introduce the concept of probiotics and prebiotics, their benefits to humans' health, and their probability of being applicable in various fields.

2. Gut microbiota

The human body harbors a complex ecosystem that includes more than 1000 various microorganisms [5, 6]. It means the number of bacteria within the gut is about ten times that of eukaryotic cells in the human body. In a healthy animal, the internal tissues such as blood, brain, muscle, etc. in a healthy animal are usually free of microorganisms. However, the surface tissues, such as skin and mucous membranes, are constantly in contact with environmental organisms and become readily colonized by various microbial species. The microbiota extends from mouth to anus and into the vaginal tract of women. In the healthy host, enteric bacteria colonize the alimentary tract soon after birth, and the composition of the intestinal microbiota remains relatively constant [7]. The normal flora of humans consists of a few eukaryotic fungi and protists, but bacteria are the most numerous and obvious microbial components of the normal flora. The total genomic content of microbiota is referred to as a microbiome that inhabits a specific anatomical site of the body [8]. The mixture of organisms regularly found at any anatomical site is referred to as the "normal flora". However, researchers in the field who prefer the term "indigenous microbiota," which includes resident microbiota, transient microbiota, and opportunistic microbiota.

The gut microbiome exhibits various interactions with the human body. It may be mutualistic or pathogenic. The interactions between the gut microbiome and host have evolved into symbiotic relations. It confers various benefits to the human body, significantly strengthens the host's immune system, and protects against various diseases caused by harmful pathogens. Hence, it is helpful to study the symbiotic relationship of the gut microbiome with the host and its influence on the host's overall health.

2.1 Composition of gut microbiota

The gut microbiota is composed of four main phyla: Firmicutes, Bacteroidetes, Actinobacteria, and Proteobacteria. Predominantly, anaerobic bacteria colonize the Gastrointestinal tract (GIT) [9].

GI tract consists of the stomach, small intestine, and large intestine. Various parts of the GI tract differ in their environmental characteristics, chemical compositions, and physiological properties. Therefore types and numbers of microbiota vary in different parts. In general, microorganisms increase in numbers from the stomach to the small intestine to the large intestine.

2.1.1 Microbiota of stomach

The microbes in the stomach are primarily of similar types that are present in the mouth and throat. Generally, aerobic microbes inhabit the stomach, and that too in a lesser amount than the population of mouth and stomach. The stomach receives many microbes from the mouth through food and water, but most of them are killed due to hydrochloric acid (HCl). Thus, few microorganisms that can tolerate high pH can form normal resident flora of the stomach.

Organisms generally found in the stomach are – *Lactobacillus, Enterococcus, Streptococcus, Staphylococcus, Peptostreptococcus, Candida, Helicobacter pylori,* etc. [10, 11]. Some of them are hazardous to health, such as *Helicobacter pylori, which* can cause chronic gastritis and peptic ulcers.

2.1.2 Microbiota of small intestine

The small intestine is a tube about 6 meters long-running from the stomach to the large intestine. The small intestine usually has three sections: duodenum, jejunum, and ileum. Each section reflects slightly different functions. The microbiota of the small bowel is the least well understood due to its inaccessibility for study.

Duodenum is adjacent to the stomach, and it is slightly acidic. The duodenum includes similar types of organisms that are found in the stomach. It mainly acquires acid-resistant organisms such as Lactobacillus and Enterococcus. The intestine becomes less acidic from the duodenum to the ileum; hence, the microbial population increases. In the jejunum, prominently, lactobacillus, Enterococci, *Candida albicans*, etc., are found. In ileum microbial population resembles that of the large intestine. It mainly includes obligate anaerobes such as *Clostridium perfringes*, anaerobic *E. coli*., Bacilli, Streptococcaceae. Actinomycinaeae and Corynebacteriaceae are abundant in the duodenum, jejunum, or ileum [12, 13].

2.1.3 Microbiota of large intestine

The large intestine follows on from the small intestine. The large intestine receives remains of food that enzymes have not digested. The chyme, on entering the large intestine, is referred to as feces. The large intestine is divided into three distinct parts: caecum, colon, and rectum. About 1100 different species of microbes are present in the large intestine [14].

The large intestine harbors obligate anaerobes and facultative anaerobes. The more common genera include Bacteroides, *Clostridium*, *Eubacterium*, *Roseburia*, *Faecalibacterium*, and *Ruminococcus* [15, 16]. The large bowel includes increased Lachnospiraceae (Firmicutes) proportions, and Bacteroidetes are found in the colon [13]. It also inhibits *E.coli, Lactobacillus, Bifidobacterium, Enterococcus* in smaller numbers.

2.2 Benefits of gut microbiota

Earlier, the gut microbiota was thought to be commensals whose only benefit was controlling the abundance of pathogenic bacteria. However, as the knowledge about these symbionts increased, their essential roles, such as aiding digestion and various metabolites, were also known to improve the immune system [17, 18]. The gut microbiota plays a crucial role in immunomodulation and the nervous system and intestinal mucosal system development. In addition, gut microbiota plays a crucial role in synthesizing essential vitamins such as vitamin B12, vitamin K, nicotinic acid, pyridoxine, thiamine [19]. The gut microbiota generates short-chain fatty acids (SCFAs) by fermenting complex carbohydrates. These SCFAs play a significant role in inflammatory response and regulation of immune response. The gut microbiota also influences epithelial homeostasis [19].

There are pieces of evidence that gut microbiota provides extra nutrition. It could be due to the digestion by enzymes of the resident microbiota. Another benefit of gut microbiota is a defense against a range of pathogens, including *Listeria cytogenes, Clostridium botulinum*, and *Cryptosporidium parvum*. The gut microbiota provides a hostile environment, produces antimicrobial substances, and strengthens the human body's defenses to defend against pathogens. It also stimulates peristalsis, so gut contents are moved more quickly, making it more difficult for newly-arrived pathogens to be established.

2.3 Disturbance of gut microbiota

The composition of gut microbiota may vary between individuals though some key bacterial species are typically present in most. Diet is thought to explain over 50% of these microbial structural variations in mice and 20% in humans, signaling the potential for dietary strategies in disease management through gut microbiota modulation [20]. The gut microbiota shows drastic changes in infants with lactation followed by an introduction to solid food. The mode of intake, medication dosage may influence the gut microbiota. Gut microbes are regularly purged and have the ability to double in specific time intervals. The short-term and long-term dietary changes and modification in micronutrient intake can significantly change gut microbiota composition. The experiment conducted by Wu et al. showed a dramatic shift in the fecal microbiota of the participants due to high fat/low fiber and low fat/high fiber. Fiber content and type were thought to be primer determinants of the composition of the microbiota of the gut.

Through antibiotics, improvement in human health is achieved through the drugs have negative consequences also. Antibiotic drugs control the infections caused by pathogens, but other beneficial bacteria are also harmed. A disturbed microbiota may not function well against infections caused by new pathogens, resulting in the overgrowth of pathogens such as *Clostridium difficile* [21]. Several factors may influence the disturbance of gut microbiota caused by antibiotics: (i) the dose and duration of the drug (ii) the range of microbes affected by antibiotics (e.g., broad-spectrum or narrow-spectrum) (iii) the proportion of antibiotic that is being absorbed into the body or resides in the intestine.

Most antibiotics are taken orally, and some are given intravenously. The latter type has a significant influence to disturb microbiota. Different antibiotics have different effects, e.g., penicillin has minor effects on the gut microbiota, while ampicillin causes significant disturbance to the gut microbiota. Thus, there is a need to develop an alternative that is safer and effective for use. Increasing knowledge of probiotics and their efficacy against pathogens can aid the recovery of gut microbiota. Probiotics may be suitable to take after or simultaneously as antibiotics to reduce the risk of disease from disturbance of microbiota.

3. Probiotics

Probiotics are live organisms which when administered in an adequate amount, confers health benefits to the host (FAO and WHO, 2002). The characteristics of effective probiotics are their ability to survive the passage through the digestive tract and utilize the nutrients and substrates in a normal diet. Probiotics are healthy gut flora and thereby improve digestion. Several criteria have been used to prove any strain as novel probiotic strains, categorized into two groups: safety and functionality. The concept of probiotics deals with the constant introduction of the new microbes beneficial to the human host as an attempt to change the indigenous microbial population equilibrium to increase overall health [22].

3.1 History of Probiotics

The concept of using microbes to improve health is a hundred years old. During the twentieth century, probiotics gained much interest due to an increase in scientific evidence proving the beneficial effects of probiotics. The idea that bacteria could benefit human health was postulated almost 100 years ago by Elie Metchnikoff while working at the Pasteur Institute in Paris. Metchnikoff's adoption of an idea to use beneficial bacteria to improve the bacterial population of the intestine arose from his inquiries into how old age could be delayed and life prolonged. Metchnikoff concluded that fermented milk drank by peasants of Bulgaria has a key role (Metchnikoff 1907) [21] in their longevity. He found a bacterium from peasant's milk and named it *Bacillus bulgaricus.* He explained that the production of lactic acid by a bacterium reduces the harmful effects of other microorganisms. It is not sure which bacterium was found by Metchnikoff. It may be *Lactobacillus bulgaricus,* a strain that is commonly used in yogurt.

The term probiotic literally means 'for life is derived from the Greek language. Lilly and Stillwell first coined this term in 1965 to describe "substances secreted by one microorganism which stimulates the growth of another" and thus was contrasted with the term antibiotic [23]. Parker modified this definition to "organisms which contribute to intestinal microbial balance" [24]. The concept of probiotics became weak after the early death of Metchnikoff and the development of antibiotic drugs. Though, interest in the general public did not fall entirely. One of the factors that gained the popularity of probiotics towards the end of the century is the rise of resistant strains of pathogens against different antibiotics.

3.2 Mechanism and action of probiotics

The mechanisms of probiotic action are diverse. The activities of these strains can influence other factors such as the presence of other bacteria in the intestinal environment or even the disease setting in which the strain is being used [25]. The characteristics of effective probiotics are their ability to survive the passage through the digestive tract and utilize the nutrients and substrates in a normal diet. However, some mechanisms have been reported for most of the probiotic strains, which include: colonization resistance, antimicrobial activity, antimutagenic effects, antigenotoxic effects, influence on enzyme activity, etc.

The probiotic bacteria have antagonistic effects on different microorganisms and competitive adherence to mucosa and epithelium. These characteristics also work as antimicrobial activity. By decreasing luminal pH, they are inhibiting other bacterial adherence, translocation, and secretion of antimicrobial substances such as antimicrobial peptides (e.g., bacteriocin), organic acids (lactic and acetic acid), hydrogen peroxide (in environments in which oxygen is present), diacetyl, β-hydroxypropionaldehyde [26–30]. The probiotics are also capable to modulate cell proliferation and apoptosis. Polysaccharide fermentation by probiotic strains increases the availability of short-chain fatty acids (SCFAs), which felicitate repair of epithelial damage. Some strains also produce mucus excessively, which enhances the intestinal barrier. It can separate bacteria from the lumen and prevent the colonization of the epithelium [31]. Probiotics can exert control over epithelial cells, dendritic cells, monocytes, macrophages, lymphocytes, IgA through different mechanisms for the stimulation of the human immune system; increased IgA decreases the number of pathogens, thus improving gut health [32, 33]. **Figure 1** shows various mechanisms by which probiotics benefits health of host.

3.3 Types of probiotic microbes

There is a growing number of microorganisms described as probiotics. Among the various types of microbes, bacteria are used as probiotics mainly. The potential of intestinal and dairy species Lactobacilli and Bifidobacteria as probiotics was postulated over a hundred years ago. At that time, the yearning to understand the microbial ecology of these groups in the human intestine was linked to the aspiration to manage and maintain human health. The link between Lactobacilli and human health was first proposed in the late 1800s by Metchnikoff [34].

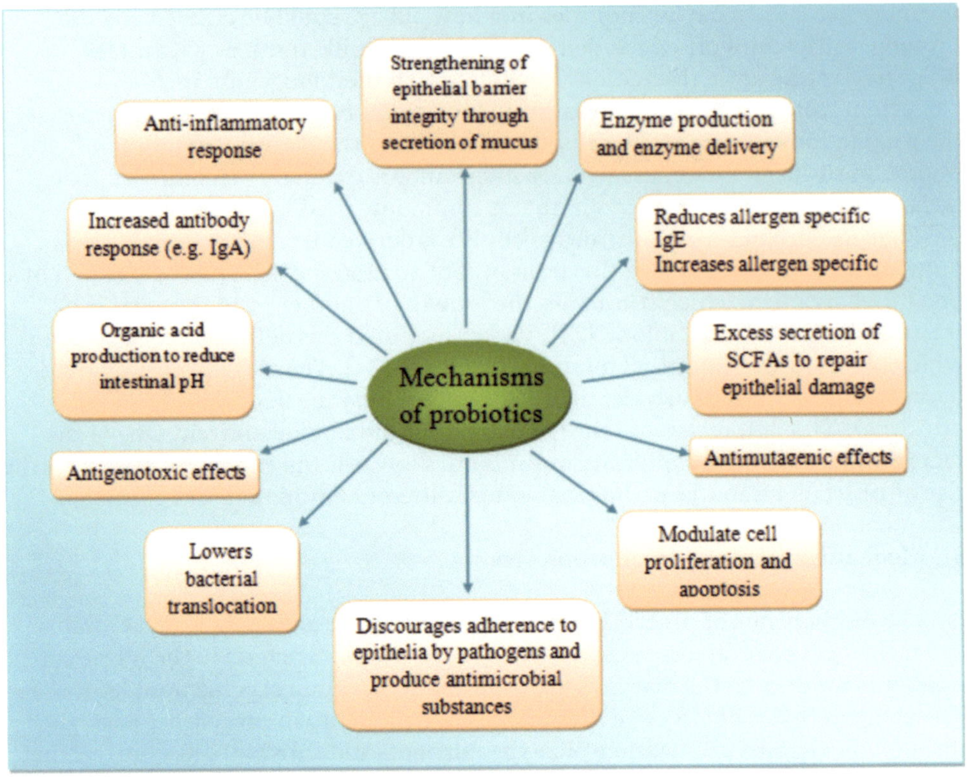

Figure 1.
Mechanism of probiotics.

The majority of the different species included in probiotics belong to the genus *Lactobacillus*. Metchnikoff favored this bacterium. They are normal flora of the small bowel as there is a wide range of food in that part of the small intestine. There are fewer lactobacilli present in the large bowel also. Lactobacilli are easy to grow, which aid as an essential factor in using probiotics at a commercial scale. Other characteristics of lactobacilli are resistance to gastric stress and the ability to grow in a microaerophilic environment that makes them well-suited to live in the gastrointestinal tract. Lactobacilli are heterofermentative and require many micronutrients to grow. The species most commonly used in probiotics are *L. acidophilus, L. casei, L. crispatus, L. johnsonii, L. plantarum, L. reuteri, L. rhamnosus, L. salivarius.* The probiotic effect of lactobacilli is as follow:

- Secretion of lactic acid lowers the pH of GIT and eliminates harmful bacteria. Some lactobacilli produce acetic acid, which gives a more substantial effect than lactic acid against pathogens.

- Lactobacilli produce antibiotic-like compounds referred to as bacteriocins, which restrict the growth of pathogens. Some of them also produce hydrogen, which exerts antibacterial effects.

- Lactobacilli tend to attach to mucosa and form colonies, which is the primary requirement of good probiotics. They block the attachment of pathogens and may also influence the immune cells in the gut wall. Some lactobacilli also produce mucus in excess to discourage attachment of pathogens.

Probiotic Lactic acid bacteria	
Lactobacillus spp.	*Bifidobacterium spp.*
Lactobacillus rhamnosus	*Bifidobacterium lactis*
Lactobacillus plantarum	*Bifidobacterium bifidum*
Lactobacillusreuteri	*Bifidobacterium animalis*
Lactobacillus acidophilus	*Bifidobacterium breve*
Lactobacillus casei	*Bifidobacterium infantis*
	Bifidobacterium longum
Other lactic acid bacteria	**Non-lactic acid bacteria and yeast**
Lactococcus lactis	*Propionibacterium freudenreichii*
Streptococcus thermophilus	*Saccharomyces cerevisiae*

Table 1.
List of probiotic microorganisms [21, 37–39].

There are other genera of lactic acid-secreting bacteria. One of them is *Enterococcus, which* has species such as *E. faecium* that are used as probiotics. The mechanism is similar to those of lactobacilli.

Bifidobacteria are the second most commonly used type of bacteria in probiotic products. One of the reasons for their less popularity could be their incapability to grow and process commercially. Henry Tissier identified the unusually shaped *Bifidobacterium* from the stool of the baby. A large number of these bacteria in the intestine of the baby reassured that they are probably beneficial. Bifidobacteria reduce lactose intolerance, cholesterol levels, improve the gut immune system, and prevent gut infection in infants. Some of the species frequently used in probiotics are *Bif. adolescentis, Bif. animals, Bif. bifidium, Bif. breve, Bif. longum, and Bif. infantis.*

Like lactobacilli and bifidobacteria, other organisms such as *E. coli, Bacillus subtilis, Saccharomyces cerevisiae, S. boulardii*. Most *E. coli* are benign commensals, but some are opportunistic pathogens. *E. coli* Nissle 1971 (EcN) is the best known *E. coli* probiotic [35, 36]. Nissle bacteria are protected from stomach acid by added enteric coating. The coating won't dissolve until it reaches the ileum and caecum. EcN strengthens the barrier function of epithelial cells against pathogens. EcN has been used as an anti-diarrhoeal and to treat constipation and ulcerative colitis [21]. *Bacillus subtilis* is a spore-forming bacterium; the spores protect the cells from gastric acid. Some of the spores germinate in the intestine and influence the gut immune system and stimulate lactobacilli's growth. Some other *Bacillus* species are used as probiotics, such as *B. coagulance, B. licheniformis, B. pumilus,* and *B. clausii. Saccharomyces boulardii,* a sub-species of *S. cerevisiae* is used as probiotics. *S. boulardii*is not normal flora of the gut, but it can live there temporarily and gives anti-diarrhoeal effects. Some probiotic organisms with Generally Regarded As Safe (GRAS) status are listed in **Table 1**.

4. Benefits of probiotics

There are certain diseases related to the disturbance of microbiota of the gastrointestinal tract. Some of them are infectious diarrhea, irritable bowel syndrome (IBS), inflammatory bowel disease (IBD), lactose intolerance, antibiotic-associated diarrhea, constipation, gastritis, and stomach ulcers. There are evidences available showing influence of probiotics to treat such diseases. Other body parts may benefit from probiotics as microbiota is present in other body parts, not just the intestine. Furthermore, the immune system is connected to all parts of the body, so by influencing one part of the immune system, probiotics may influence others.

4.1 Effect of probiotics on diarrhea

Infectious diarrhea, traveler's diarrhea (TD), antibiotic-associated diarrhea are various types of diarrhea caused by different conditions. Infectious diarrhea is generally caused by pathogenic microbes such as viruses, bacteria, yeast, or protozoan. Generally, normal bowel movements return after about three days, but they may not in children with acute diarrhea. In infants, rotavirus is the most common microbe responsible for diarrhea. Probiotics have been tried in many clinical studies as a supplement for rehydration therapy to treat infectious diarrhea in infants. The results have been positive and consistent [40]. In young children, the probiotics were also found to be effective in preventing the development of infectious diarrhea. The types of probiotic microbes used are lactobacilli, bifidobacteria, *S. boulardii* (yeast).

The traveler's diarrhea may be caused by the water supply being contaminated with fecal matter, contaminated food. In the case of traveler's diarrhea, the use of probiotics is more likely to be considered by adults. Though, the use of probiotics in TD has given a mixed response as the cause of TD differs depending on the local situation [41].

The use of antibiotics has revolutionized the treatment of bacterial infections. However, it promotes the rise of resistant bacteria and disturbs gut microbiota's composition, which makes us vulnerable to pathogenic infection. Such infection of the intestine leads to diarrhea, referred to as 'antibiotic-associated diarrhea (AAD)'. When the gut microbiota is disturbed, *Clostridium difficile* increases to infection level; this bacterium causes about one-fifth of AAD. In several studies, probiotic yeast *S. boulardii* was effective against *C. difficile* when given along with antibiotics [42]. In a number of cases, probiotic microbes such as LAB, *S. boulardii, Clostridium butyricum* prevented such diarrhea, although not all studies have shown probiotics to be effective [42–45].

4.2 Effect of probiotics in Irritable Bowel Syndrome (IBS)

The irritable bowel syndrome is a common gastrointestinal disorder. In IBS an abnormal condition of gut contractions (motility) and increased gut sensations (visceral hypersensitivity) characterized by abdominal pain/discomfort, gas, bloating, mucous in stools, and irregular bowel habits with constipation or diarrhea. Several studies show the effect of probiotics on this disease; however, the mechanism by which probiotic organisms affect this condition is still unknown. A review and meta-analysis by Ford et al. concluded the beneficial effects of probiotics as a treatment on IBS symptoms, including RCTs published between 1939 and 2013, and it was emphasized that multi-strain probiotics had a more distinct effect on IBS symptoms [46, 47]. However, *Lactobacillaceae* and *Bifidobacteriaceae* (genus: *Lactobacillus* and *Bifidobacterium*) were the two most common families used in multi-strain probiotic supplements [47].

4.3 Effect of probiotics in inflammatory bowel disease (IBD)

Inflammatory bowel disease is a group of the chronic intestinal disease characterized by inflammation of the large or small intestine. Crohn's disease (CD) and ulcerative colitis (UC) are the most common types of IBD. UC only affects the large bowel, and the inflammation is usually found in the rectum and the sigmoid colon but can be found anywhere along with the large bowel. CD can affect any part of the digestive tube from mouth to the anus but is most often found in the area of the junction of the ileum and caecum. The evidence of benefit from probiotics in UC is strong, while the evidence in Crohn's is weak. There have been eight controlled trials involving people with UC in one study, and seven of them showed significant benefit from probiotics. Use of probiotics extended periods of remission or reduced active disease [48]. Some studies have been conducted with *E. coli* Nissle (EcN), *Saccharomyces boulardii*. These microbes have been reported to have some beneficial effects in IBD [41, 49]. *E. coli* probiotic was found to be as effective as a standard drug used in UC to prevent relapse. In comparison, only a small number of trials showed the benefit of probiotic yeast *S. boulardii* in Crohn's disease.

4.4 Effect of probiotics in lactose intolerance

The inability of some adults to digest the sugar lactose, which is present in milk, is referred to as 'lactose intolerance. The lactose is hydrolyzed by the enzyme lactase, which is also known as lactose- galactosehydrolase (EC 3.2.1.108). The lactose is digested into glucose and galactose, which is taken up by intestinal cells and transported to the bloodstream. The remaining lactose, which is not hydrolyzed, passes to the colon [36]. The person with lactose intolerance produces less lactase, which is inefficient in digesting much of the milk sugar. The undigested lactose causes intestinal difficulties. When lactose intolerant people consume milk, they may suffer from excess gas, diarrhea, cramps, bloating, abdominal rumblings, and flatulence. One of the reasons for excess gas could be the fermentation of glucose by gut microbiota. As lactose is an active osmotic compound, it causes osmotic pressure, leading to high water content in the feces, causing clinical symptoms as diarrhea [36]. Probiotics have gained attention as an alternative to compensate for the low level of lactase [41, 50]. Probiotic can affect at two levels: (i) By increasing hydrolytic activity in the small intestine (ii) By increasing colonic fermentation [51]. Several studies have shown the effect of probiotic yogurt in better lactose digestion in lactose-intolerant people. The probiotic bacteria used in yogurt (*Lactobacillus bulgaricus* and *Streptococcus thermophilus)* produce a significant amount of their own lactase. Evidence suggests that probiotic organisms can digest lactose in yogurt products and continue digestion in the small intestine when consumed [52]. They prevent excess gas production and reduce or eliminate diarrhea. The yogurt allows more time for lactase to digest lactose as yogurt has a thicker consistency; it takes a longer time to pass through the intestine. There is some evidence showing that Russian fermented milk- kefir or variants of kefir (sugary kefirs, kefir grains) effectively alleviate lactose intolerance [53]. There are probiotic products available in capsule, tablet, or powder form (e.g., *Lactobacillus* and *Bifidobacterium* species used in non-milk products); however, they do not appear to be as effective as yogurt.

4.5 Effect of probiotics in gastritis and stomach ulcers

A bacterium, *Helicobacter pylori,* causes inflammation of the mucosal barrier of the stomach. As well as frequent long-term use of nonsteroidal anti-inflammatory drugs is the major factor involved in gastric ulcer development [53]. Gastric mucosal damage is common; if not treated adequately, it may lead to gastric cancer. To eradicate *H. pylori*, three drugs are used simultaneously: two antibiotics and a proton pump inhibitor [54]. However, this treatment fails in most of the cases due to antibiotic-resistant strains of *H. pylori*; thus, a fourth antibiotic is added to standard triple therapy used previously. The therapy may cause side effects such as diarrhea, taste disturbance, and nausea.

The growing interest in probiotics to prevent or treat gastrointestinal diseases has attracted the attention of many researchers to explore the role of probiotics in the prevention and treatment of gastric ulcers [50]. Some studies have found out that when probiotics are used in conjunction with standard drugs, the rate of eradication was higher than drug therapy or probiotics alone [55]. However, side effects caused by drug therapy were reduced by probiotics. Most of the studies have used lactobacilli, but not all strains showed effects against *H. pylori*. Probiotic yeasts *S. boulardii* also showed potential therapeutic effects in gastric ulcers. *S. boulardii* acquires neuraminidase activity which removes sialic acid, which results in the prevention of binding of *H. pylori* to epithelial cells [53].

4.6 Effect of probiotic in vaginal infections

In a healthy woman, the vagina has a resident microbial population. These resident microbiota live on the lining of the vagina wall. Most of them are lactobacilli. The vaginal lactobacilli have a protective influence against urogenital infections [50]. The vaginal infections are referred to as vaginitis. In which pathogenic infections cause inflammation of the vaginal lining. If a bacterium causes vaginitis, it is known as bacterial vaginosis (BV). If vaginitis is caused by a fungus (generally *Candida- a* type of fungus), it is known as vaginal candidiasis (VC). Both types of vaginitis symptoms are similar, such as burning sensation during urination, itching in the vaginal area, and greyish or white discharge. Antibiotics or antifungals treat the infection. There is evidence that some women have H_2O_2 – secreting lactobacilli in their intestine, which lowers the risk of BV. This suggests that the rectum act as a reservoir supplement vaginal microbiota when it becomes disturbed. This information leads to the development of probiotics to protect the female reproductive system [56, 57]. Though studies have shown mixed responses. In the case of VC, a small number of clinical studies have been undertaken of probiotics against *Candida*. In most of the studies, probiotics didn't show any significant effect. However, when probiotics were taken along with antifungal drugs, they improved the effectiveness of antifungal significantly [58].

4.7 Effect of probiotics in upper respiratory infections

The upper respiratory tract (URT) consists of the nose, throat, and windpipe. The nose and throat have microbiota, and the upper part of the windpipe has a changing microbial population as cilia move mucus upward to the throat. The various diseases associated with URT are common cold, sore throat, pharyngitis, epiglottitis, laryngitis, and diphtheria [29]. Most commonly, viruses such as rhinoviruses, coronaviruses, parainfluenza, and influenza viruses and bacteria such as streptococci, *Mycoplasma pneumoniae, Chlamydia pneumoniae, Corynebacterium diphtheria, Staphylococcus aureus, Haemophilus influenzae* type b, *Streptococcus pyrogens*, and *Streptococcus pneumonia* are associated with URT infection [59, 60]. Infection of URT may spread to the lungs, causing bronchitis and pneumonia. Some studies have shown that probiotics may reduce the severity and duration of the condition. Some probiotic bacteria such as *Lactobacillus rhamnosus, Streptococcus thermophilus, Bifidobacterium animals* were beneficial to reduce and prevent URT risks in children and adults [29]. Probiotics may also improve the effectiveness of influenza vaccination in the elderly. This improved immune reaction may enhance protection against acquiring influenza, although it is yet to be confirmed.

4.8 Effect of probiotics in constipation

Constipation is quite a common condition that can be acute or chronic. Constipation causes a general feeling of abdominal discomfort. To pass the stool straining may put pressure on the tissues and structures of the anal area with adverse consequences such as hemorrhoids (piles). Other diseases associated with constipation are irritable bowel syndrome and cancer of the large bowel. Several studies have been conducted using *Lactobacillus rhamnosus, Lactobacillus casei, Bifidobacterium animalis,* and probiotic *E. coli.* [61, 62]. Prebiotics also may be effective against constipation as FOS, GOS, and lactulose have mild laxative effects [63]. These laxative effects can be due to osmosis as prebiotics are soluble fibers. Prebiotics also boost bifidobacteria and lactobacilli, and these probiotic bacteria accelerate the transit of large bowel content. However, meta-analyses also indicate that groups of probiotics and synbiotics have more efficiency than individual probiotics [64].

4.9 Other benefits

The list of benefits of probiotics is not limited to the ones mentioned above. However, it includes a range of benefits that need to be explored for further human studies. Some evidences suggest that probiotics may influence cancer incidence [50]. As well as researchers are exploring various alternatives of drugs from probiotics that can be used to treat a disease like cancer and with lesser or no side effects. (i.e., L-asparaginase that is used in cancer treatment from *L. casei, L. reuteri,* etc. is being explored) [43, 65]. Furthermore, evidences suggests that food products with probiotic organisms may reduce serum cholesterol levels and control blood pressure. Probiotics may also prevent coronary heart disease [66, 67]. Several studies examined the effect of probiotics and *pre*biotics to treat allergic conditions. However, studies to prevent allergic conditions like asthma and allergic rhinitis did not show a positive response. However, studies examined that when pregnant women have probiotic intake, it improves the functioning of the mother's immune system and indirectly improves the immature immune system of the infant, reducing the risk of allergies such as eczema and dermatitis [68]. But there are insufficient evidences to recommend probiotics as standard therapy to prevent allergies [44]. There is a close relationship between microbiota and the immune system of the skin. Consumption of probiotics has provided some protection against ultraviolet radiation from the sun. *Vitreoscilla filiformis* showed a beneficial effect on a patient with seborrhoeic dermatitis and atopic eczema [69]. As described earlier, LAB, especially lactobacilli and bifidobacteria, exert a beneficial effect in infants with atopic eczema. A *pre*biotic cream has been developed with encouraging results in controlling acne-associated organism *Propionibacterium acne.* However, much more exploration and research are needed to use probiotics routinely for the skin.

5. Application of probiotics

Due to the health benefits exerted by probiotic organisms, they have a wide range of applications in clinical uses and various industries such as food industries and agriculture industries. Most species of lactobacilli and bifidobacteria are used commercially. Among them *L. rhamnosus, L. plantarum, L. casei, L.paracasei, B. animalis* are widely used. With that in some products organism such as *S. thermophilus* is used.

5.1 Application of probiotics in the food industry

Increasing knowledge of probiotic benefits leads to the development of functional foods. Functional foods, also known as "nutraceuticals" or "designer foods," are ingredients that offer health benefits that extend beyond their nutritional value. Some types contain supplements or other additional ingredients designed to improve health, and they are slowly emerging as 'health food' on supermarket shelves worldwide [70]. A wide variety of dairy products such as milk, yogurt, cheese, ice cream, chocolate mousse, quark, etc., include probiotic organisms to improve their nutrition characteristics [70–74]. Furthermore, whey-based and fortified dairy beverages are also available, including probiotic and *pre*biotic. *L. rhamnosus* GG is widely used in such beverages [75, 76]. The development of non-dairy-based products has gained attention in developed countries as a population

Food product	Probiotic organism used	References
Acidophilus milk	*Lactobacillus acidophilus*	[79]
Yogurt, bio-yogurts	*Streptococcus thermophilus* *Lactobacillus bulgaricus* *Bifidobacterium bifidum*	[76, 80, 81]
Cheese	*Lactobacillus acidophilus* *Lactobacillus paracasei* *Lactobacillus reuteri* *Bifidobacterium infantis*	[81, 82]
Kefir (Fermented milk beverage)	*Lactobacillus kefir* *Lactobacillus paracasei* *Lactobacillus parabuchneri* *Lactobacillus casei* *Lactobacillus lactis* *Lactococcus lactis* *Acetobacter lovaniensis* *Saccharomyces cerevisiae*	[80]
Yosa (oat-bran pudding)	*Lactobacillus acidophilus*	[80]
Uji	*Lactobacillus paracasei*	[80]
Sorghum	*Lactobacillus acidophilus*	[80]
Sauerkraut	*Leuconostocmesenteroides* *Lactobacillus Brevis,* *Pediococcuspentosaceus, Lactobacillus Plantarum* *Lactobacillus sakei*	[80, 83]
Kombucha (Fermented tea beverage)	*Saccharomyces cerevisiae*	[80]
Kimchi (Fermented vegetable dish)	*Lactobacillus sakei, Lactobacillus Plantarum,* *Lactobacillus curvatus,*	[80]
Natto	*Bacillus subtilis*	[84]
Miso	*Aspergillus oryzae* *Saccharomyces cerevisiae*	[80, 83]
Sourdough	*Lactobacillus sanfransiscensis,* *Saccharomyces cerevisiae*	[80, 85]
Bulgarian boza	*Lactobacillus coryniformis*	[35]
Hardline (Grapes)	*Lactobacillus Plantarum,* *Lactobacillus paracasei,* *Lactobacillus casei*	[35]

Table 2.
List of probiotic food products.

with vegetarianism and lactose intolerance is higher [77]. Non-dairy based product includes fermented vegetable and fruit-based probiotics. Other non-dairy products such as cereal, soy, and meat-based probiotics such as fermented oats, sourdoughs, sausages, fish are available [78]. Probiotic organisms and substances secreted by them are used to preserve and enhance the quality of food. Various probiotic food products are listed in **Table 2**.

5.2 Application of probiotics in agriculture

Other than human, probiotics application is extended to agriculture as well. One of them is probiotic farming, which is referred to as bio-intensive agriculture that combines various organic farming techniques to make soil healthier. It introduces beneficial microorganisms into the growing environment. The use of probiotics increases crop yield, limits the need for harmful fertilizers and pesticides and depletes damages caused by them. Probiotics also amplify plant's resistance to pests and diseases. Due to antagonistic effects exhibited by probiotic bacteria by 'induced systemic resistance,' plants are protected from pathogenic microorganisms. *Bacillus* spp., LAB, *Actinomycetous,* etc. Protect plants from cropping hazards. Furthermore, plant probiotic microorganisms (PPM) can influence the synthesis of phytohormones and their balance in plants. Some commercial plant products that use probiotic cultures are Kodiak (*Bacillus subtilis* GB03), YiedShield (*B. pumilis* GB34), Rotex (*Phlebiopsisgigantea*) [21]. Probiotics used in animal feed supplements advantageously alter gastrointestinal flora and improve host animals' health and productivity. Probiotic solely or in combination with prebiotic improves the pattern of microbial population in GIT and benefits host's health [86]. Probiotic is generously applied in poultry and aquaculture. Some feed additives can modulate the intestinal milieu and exert beneficial substances in the intestine [87]. Probiotics gained attention to use as an alternative to antibiotics in poultry to get the product with quality and safety [88]. It also reduces their mortality rate and increases bone quality. In ruminants, probiotics increase forage intake, increasing fiber digestion rate, which results in improved weight gain, milk yield, and milk fat content [86]. Probiotic also decreases the prevalence of coliform infection in pre-ruminant calves. The use of probiotics in aquaculture prevents the adhesion of pathogens from fishing intestinal mucus.

5.3 Application of probiotics in clinical use

As described earlier, probiotics prevent or mitigate various diseases and severe symptoms by various mechanisms, but it is advisable to take care when used in immune-compromised patients. Encouraging evidences are emerging for probiotics' efficiency in the management of pouchitis and pediatric atopic diseases. Probiotics are also helpful in preventing postoperative infections [89]. There is strong evidence that some bacterial strains are efficient in enhancing immune function. Probiotics are also beneficial in mental disorders and reduce carcinogenic activity, cholesterol level, and blood pressure [35]. The significance of probiotics in preventing traveler's diarrhea, sepsis-associated with severe pancreatitis, ulcerative colitis, and reduction of hyper cholesterol is unproven [89, 90]. The chemotherapeutic drugs such as L-asparaginase with fewer side effects from probiotic bacteria are still being explored. A study reported the use of kimchi to treat cancer [21]. Furthermore, the development of alternative antibiotics such as lantibiotics, antimicrobial peptides (AMPs) from probiotic bacteria are being explored to reduce side effects caused by traditional drug therapies and as a next-generation drug system against resistant pathogens. LAB bacteriocin- Nisin is commercially used as a food preservative [35]. It also has biomedical applications as it exhibits anti-microbial activity against resistant pathogens and anti-biofilm properties to use in combination with therapeutic drugs [91]. Although probiotics have shown encouraging evidence of efficacy in various diseases, there is much exploration needed for standard clinical practice in humans.

6. Conclusion

Exploration of gut microbiota indicates that beneficial gut microbiota plays a crucial and constructive role in maintaining the health of host (human). The symbiotic relation of gut microbiota with host and benefits exhibited by them leads to the development of probiotics and prebiotics. Studies on various mechanisms of probiotics have shown their abilities to prevent or treat various diseases in human. Due to this efficiency, probiotics and prebiotics and their applications in various fields have shown a substantial increase in the last two decades. Probiotics are mainly applied in the food industry to develop functional foods and supplements to benefit consumers. The applications of probiotics are also extended to the agriculture industry to boost the productivity and quality of crops and animals. The emergence of encouraging evidence has given a sight to use probiotics in clinical practices with minimum side effects. However, clinical use of probiotics as standard practice is under the umbrella of research yet.

Author details

Amishi Bhatt[1], Dhyey Kothari[2], Charmy Kothari[3] and Ramesh Kothari[1*]

1 Department of Biosciences, Saurashtra University, Rajkot, Gujarat, India

2 Government Medical College, Bhavnagar, Gujarat, India

3 Department of Biotechnology, Christ College, Affiliated to Saurashtra University, Rajkot, Gujarat, India

*Address all correspondence to: kothari1971@gmail.com

References

[1] Lebeer S, Vanderleyden J, De Keersmaecker SC. Genes and molecules of lactobacilli supporting probiotic action. Microbiology and Molecular Biology Reviews. 2008 Dec 1;72(4):728-64.

[2] Grimoud J, Durand H, Courtin C, Monsan P, Ouarné F, Theodorou V, Roques C. In vitro screening of probiotic lactic acid bacteria and prebiotic glucooligosaccharides to select effective synbiotics. Anaerobe. 2010 Oct 1;16(5):493-500.

[3] Ghoshal UC, Park H, Gwee KA. Bugs and irritable bowel syndrome: the good, the bad and the ugly. Journal of gastroenterology and hepatology. 2010 Feb;25(2):244-51.

[4] Fuller R. History and development of probiotics. InProbiotics 1992 (pp. 1-8). Springer, Dordrecht.

[5] Ridlon JM, Kang DJ, Hylemon PB, Bajaj JS. Bile acids and the gut microbiome. Current opinion in gastroenterology. 2014 May;30(3):332.

[6] Van den Abbeele P, Van de Wiele T, Verstraete W, Possemiers S. The host selects mucosal and luminal associations of coevolved gut microorganisms: a novel concept. FEMS microbiology reviews. 2011 Jul 1;35(4):681-704.

[7] Arnold JW, Roach J, Azcarate-Peril MA. Emerging technologies for gut microbiome research. Trends in microbiology. 2016 Nov 1;24(11):887-901.

[8] Bhattarai Y, Si J, Pu M, Ross OA, McLean PJ, Till L, Moor W, Grover M, Kandimalla KK, Margolis KG, Farrugia G. Role of gut microbiota in regulating gastrointestinal dysfunction and motor symptoms in a mouse model of Parkinson's disease. Gut Microbes. 2021 Jan 1;13(1):1866974.

[9] Ogunrinola GA, Oyewale JO, Oshamika OO, Olasehinde GI. The human microbiome and its impacts on health. International Journal of Microbiology. 2020 Jun 12;2020.

[10] Cresci GA, Izzo K. Gut Microbiome. InAdult Short Bowel Syndrome 2019 Jan 1 (pp. 45-54). Academic Press.

[11] Simon GL, Gorbach SL. The human intestinal microflora. Digestive diseases and sciences. 1986 Sep 1;31(9):147-62.

[12] Hsiao WW, Metz C, Singh DP, Roth J. The microbes of the intestine: an introduction to their metabolic and signaling capabilities. Endocrinology and metabolism clinics of North America. 2008 Dec 1;37(4):857-71.

[13] Dieterich W, Schink M, Zopf Y. Microbiota in the gastrointestinal tract. Medical Sciences. 2018 Dec;6(4):116.

[14] Qin J, Li R, Raes J, Arumugam M, Burgdorf KS, Manichanh C, Nielsen T, Pons N, Levenez F, Yamada T, Mende DR. A human gut microbial gene catalogue established by metagenomic sequencing. nature. 2010 Mar;464(7285):59-65.

[15] Kho ZY, Lal SK. The human gut microbiome–a potential controller of wellness and disease. Frontiers in microbiology. 2018 Aug 14;9:1835.

[16] Tap J, Mondot S, Levenez F, Pelletier E, Caron C, Furet JP, Ugarte E, Muñoz-Tamayo R, Paslier DL, Nalin R, Dore J. Towards the human intestinal microbiota phylogenetic core. Environmental microbiology. 2009 Oct;11(10):2574-84.

[17] Anwar H, Irfan S, Hussain G, Faisal MN, Muzaffar H, Mustafa I, Mukhtar I, Malik S, Ullah MI. Gut microbiome: A new organ system in body. InParasitology and Microbiology

Research 2019 Nov 5 (pp. 1-20). IntechOpen.

[18] Ghaisas S, Maher J, Kanthasamy A. Gut microbiome in health and disease: Linking the microbiome–gut–brain axis and environmental factors in the pathogenesis of systemic and neurodegenerative diseases. Pharmacology & therapeutics. 2016 Feb 1;158:52-62.

[19] Thursby E, Juge N. Introduction to the human gut microbiota. Biochemical Journal. 2017 Jun 1;474(11):1823-36.

[20] Leeming ER, Johnson AJ, Spector TD, Le Roy CI. Effect of diet on the gut microbiota: rethinking intervention duration. Nutrients. 2019 Dec;11(12):2862.

[21] Yadav R, Shukla P. Probiotics for human health: current progress and applications. Recent advances in applied microbiology. 2017:133-47.

[22] 13A Claesson MJ, Van Sinderen D, O'Toole PW. The genus Lactobacillus—a genomic basis for understanding its diversity. FEMS microbiology letters. 2007 Apr 1;269(1):22-8.

[23] Lilly DM, Stillwell RH. Probiotics: growth-promoting factors produced by microorganisms. Science. 1965 Feb 12;147(3659):747-8.

[24] Faust K, Sathirapongsasuti JF, Izard J, Segata N, Gevers D, Raes J, Huttenhower C. Microbial co-occurrence relationships in the human microbiome. PLoScomput biol. 2012 Jul 12;8(7):e1002606.

[25] Prisciandaro L, Geier M, Butler R, Cummins A, Howarth G. Probiotics and their derivatives as treatments for inflammatory bowel disease. Inflammatory bowel diseases. 2009 Dec 1;15(12):1906-14.

[26] Walsh MC, Gardiner GE, Hart OM, Lawlor PG, Daly M, Lynch B, Richert BT, Radcliffe S, Giblin L, Hill C, Fitzgerald GF. Predominance of a bacteriocin-producing Lactobacillus salivarius component of a five-strain probiotic in the porcine ileum and effects on host immune phenotype. FEMS microbiology ecology. 2008 May 1;64(2):317-27.

[27] Ng SC, Hart AL, Kamm MA, Stagg AJ, Knight SC. Mechanisms of action of probiotics: recent advances. Inflammatory bowel diseases. 2009 Feb 1;15(2):300-10.

[28] Karpiński TM, Szkaradkiewicz AK. Characteristic of bacteriocines and their application. Pol J Microbiol. 2013 Jan 1;62(3):223-35.

[29] Laforest-Lapointe I, Becker AB, Mandhane PJ, Turvey SE, Moraes TJ, Sears MR, Subbarao P, Sycuro LK, Azad MB, Arrieta MC. Maternal consumption of artificially sweetened beverages during pregnancy is associated with infant gut microbiota and metabolic modifications and increased infant body mass index. Gut Microbes. 2021 Jan 1;13(1):1-5.

[30] Ljungh A, Wadstrom T. Lactic acid bacteria as probiotics. Current issues in intestinal microbiology. 2006 Sep 1;7(2):73-90.

[31] Martens EC, Neumann M, Desai MS. Interactions of commensal and pathogenic microorganisms with the intestinal mucosal barrier. Nature Reviews Microbiology. 2018 Aug;16(8):457-70.

[32] Macia L, Thorburn AN, Binge LC, Marino E, Rogers KE, Maslowski KM, Vieira AT, Kranich J, Mackay CR. Microbial influences on epithelial integrity and immune function as a basis for inflammatory diseases. Immunological reviews. 2012 Jan;245(1):164-76.

[33] Yadav et al., 2017] Yadav R, Shukla P. An overview of advanced

technologies for selection of probiotics and their expediency: a review. Critical reviews in food science and nutrition. 2017 Oct 13;57(15):3233-42.

[34] Kleerebezem M, Vaughan EE. Probiotic and gut lactobacilli and bifidobacteria: molecular approaches to study diversity and activity. Annual review of microbiology. 2009 Oct 13;63:269-90.

[35] Yadav M, Mandeep, Shukla P. Probiotics of diverse origin and their therapeutic applications: a review. Journal of the American College of Nutrition. 2020 Jul 3;39(5):469-79.

[36] Guo S, Chen S, Ma J, Ma Y, Zhu J, Ma Y, Liu Y, Wang P, Pan Y. Escherichia coli Nissle 1917 protects intestinal barrier function by inhibiting NF-κB-mediated activation of the MLCK-P-MLC signaling pathway. Mediators of inflammation. 2019 Jul 3;2019.

[37] Kechagia M, Basoulis D, Konstantopoulou S, Dimitriadi D, Gyftopoulou K, Skarmoutsou N, Fakiri EM. Health benefits of probiotics: a review. International Scholarly Research Notices. 2013;2013.

[38] Özer BH, Kirmaci HA. Functional milks and dairy beverages. International Journal of Dairy Technology. 2010 Feb;63(1):1-5.

[39] Żukiewicz-Sobczak W, Wróblewska P, Adamczuk P, Silny W. Probiotic lactic acid bacteria and their potential in the prevention and treatment of allergic diseases. Central-European journal of immunology. 2014;39(1):104.

[40] Floch MH, Montrose DC. Use of probiotics in humans: an analysis of the literature. Gastroenterology Clinics. 2005 Sep 1;34(3):547-70.

[41] Syngai GG, Gopi R, Bharali R, Dey S, Lakshmanan GA, Ahmed G. Probiotics-the versatile functional food ingredients. Journal of food science and technology. 2016 Feb 1;53(2):921-33.

[42] Blaabjerg S, Artzi DM, Aabenhus R. Probiotics for the prevention of antibiotic-associated diarrhea in outpatients—a systematic review and meta-analysis. Antibiotics. 2017 Dec;6(4):21.

[43] Rivas-Jimenez L, Ramírez-Ortiz K, González-Córdova AF, Vallejo-Cordoba B, Garcia HS, Hernandez-Mendoza A. Evaluation of acrylamide-removing properties of two Lactobacillus strains under simulated gastrointestinal conditions using a dynamic system. Microbiological research. 2016 Sep 1;190:19-26.

[44] Tang RB, Chang JK, Chen HL. Can probiotics be used to treat allergic diseases?. Journal of the Chinese Medical Association. 2015 Mar 1;78(3):154-7.

[45] Casem EA. Saccharomyces boulardii in prevention of antibiotic-associated diarrhea in children: a randomized controlled trial. PIDSP Journal. 2013;13(2):70-6.

[46] Ford AC, Quigley EM, Lacy BE, Lembo AJ, Saito YA, Schiller LR, Soffer EE, Spiegel BM, Moayyedi P. Efficacy of prebiotics, probiotics, and synbiotics in irritable bowel syndrome and chronic idiopathic constipation: systematic review and meta-analysis. American journal of gastroenterology. 2014 Oct 1;109(10):1547-61.

[47] Dale HF, Rasmussen SH, Asiller ÖÖ, Lied GA. Probiotics in irritable bowel syndrome: an up-to-date systematic review. Nutrients. 2019 Sep;11(9):2048.

[48] Rioux KP, Fedorak RN. Probiotics in the treatment of inflammatory bowel disease. Journal of clinical gastroenterology. 2006 Mar 1;40(3):260-3.

[49] Jia K, Tong X, Wang R, Song X. The clinical effects of probiotics for inflammatory bowel disease: A meta-analysis. Medicine. 2018 Dec;97(51).

[50] Lin DC. Probiotics as functional foods. Nutrition in Clinical Practice. 2003 Dec;18(6):497-506.

[51] Oak SJ, Jha R. The effects of probiotics in lactose intolerance: a systematic review. Critical reviews in food science and nutrition. 2019 Jun 17;59(11):1675-83.

[52] Doron S, Gorbach SL. Probiotics: their role in the treatment and prevention of disease. Expert review of anti-infective therapy. 2006 Apr 1;4(2):261-75.

[53] Acik M, ÇAKIROĞLU FP, Altan M, BAYBO T. Alternative source of probiotics for lactose intolerance and vegan individuals: sugary kefir. Food Science and Technology. 2020 Sep;40(3):523-31.

[54] Lionetti E, Indrio F, Pavone L, Borrelli G, Cavallo L, Francavilla R. Role of probiotics in pediatric patients with Helicobacter pylori infection: a comprehensive review of the literature. Helicobacter. 2010 Apr;15(2):79-87.

[55] Franceschi F, Cazzato A, Nista EC, Scarpellini E, Roccarina D, Gigante G, Gasbarrini G, Gasbarrini A. Role of probiotics in patients with Helicobacter pylori infection. Helicobacter. 2007 Nov;12:59-63.

[56] Santos CM, Pires MC, Leao TL, Hernández ZP, Rodriguez ML, Martins AK, Miranda LS, Martins FS, Nicoli JR. Selection of Lactobacillus strains as potential probiotics for vaginitis treatment. Microbiology. 2016 Jul 1;162(7):1195-207.

[57] Reid G. Probiotics for urogenital health. Nutrition in Clinical Care. 2002 Jan;5(1):3-8.

[58] Kajander K, Myllyluoma E, Rajilić-Stojanović M, Kyrönpalo S, Rasmussen M, Järvenpää S, Zoetendal EG, De Vos WM, Vapaatalo H, Korpela R. Clinical trial: multispecies probiotic supplementation alleviates the symptoms of irritable bowel syndrome and stabilizes intestinal microbiota. Alimentary pharmacology & therapeutics. 2008 Jan;27(1):48-57.

[59] Dasaraju PV, Liu C. Chapter 93: infections of the respiratory system. Medical Microbiology. 4th ed. Galveston: University of Texas Medical Branch at Galveston. 1996.

[60] Thomas M, Bomar PA. Upper respiratory tract infection. StatPearls [Internet]. 2020 Oct 28.

[61] Fernàndez-Banares F. Nutritional care of the patient with constipation. Best Practice & Research Clinical Gastroenterology. 2006 Jan 1;20(3):575-87.

[62] Xinias I, Mavroudi A. Constipation in Childhood. An update on evaluation and management. Hippokratia. 2015 Jan;19(1):11.

[63] Macfarlane GT, Steed H, Macfarlane S. Bacterial metabolism and health-related effects of galacto-oligosaccharides and other prebiotics. Journal of applied microbiology. 2008 Feb;104(2):305-44.

[64] Kamiński M, Skonieczna-Żydecka K, Łoniewski I, Koulaouzidis A, Marlicz W. Are probiotics useful in the treatment of chronic idiopathic constipation in adults? A review of existing systematic reviews, meta-analyses, and recommendations. Przegladgastroenterologiczny. 2020;15(2):103.

[65] Aishwarya SS, Selvarajan E, Iyappan S, Rajnish KN. Recombinant l-Asparaginase II from Lactobacillus

casei subsp. casei ATCC 393 and Its Anticancer Activity. Indian journal of microbiology. 2019 Sep;59(3):313-20.

[66] Wang L, Guo MJ, Gao Q, Yang JF, Yang L, Pang XL, Jiang XJ. The effects of probiotics on total cholesterol: A meta-analysis of randomized controlled trials. Medicine. 2018 Feb;97(5).

[67] Kechagia M, Basoulis D, Konstantopoulou S, Dimitriadi D, Gyftopoulou K, Skarmoutsou N, Fakiri EM. Health benefits of probiotics: a review. International Scholarly Research Notices. 2013;2013.

[68] Dotterud CK, Storrø O, Johnsen R, Øien T. Probiotics in pregnant women to prevent allergic disease: a randomized, double-blind trial. British Journal of Dermatology. 2010 Sep;163(3):616-23.

[69] Nakatsuji T, Gallo RL. Dermatological therapy by topical application of non-pathogenic bacteria. Journal of Investigative Dermatology. 2014 Jan 1;134(1):11-4.

[70] Lang T. Functional foods.

[71] Heller KJ, Bockelmann W, Schrezenmeir J, deVrese M. Cheese and its potential as a probiotic food. Handbook of fermented functional foods. 2003 Mar 26:203-25.

[72] Đurić MS, Iličić MD, Milanović SD, Carić MĐ, Tekić MN. Nutritive characteristics of probiotic quark as influenced by type of starter. Acta periodicatechnologica. 2007(38):11-9.

[73] Aragon-Alegro LC, Alegro JH, Cardarelli HR, Chiu MC, Saad SM. Potentially probiotic and synbiotic chocolate mousse. LWT-Food Science and technology. 2007 May 1;40(4):669-75.

[74] Cruz AG, Antunes AE, Sousa AL, Faria JA, Saad SM. Ice-cream as a probiotic food carrier. Food Research International. 2009 Nov 1;42(9):1233-9.

[75] Succi M, Tremonte P, Reale A, Sorrentino E, Grazia L, Pacifico S, Coppola R. Bile salt and acid tolerance of *Lactobacillus rhamnosus* strains isolated from Parmigiano Reggiano cheese. FEMS microbiology letters. 2005 Mar 1;244(1):129-37.

[76] Ong L, Henriksson A, Shah NP. Chemical analysis and sensory evaluation of Cheddar cheese produced with Lactobacillus acidophilus, Lb. casei, Lb. paracasei or Bifidobacterium sp. International Dairy Journal. 2007 Aug 1;17(8):937-45.

[77] Granato D, Branco GF, Nazzaro F, Cruz AG, Faria JA. Functional foods and nondairy probiotic food development: trends, concepts, and products. Comprehensive reviews in food science and food safety. 2010 May;9(3):292-302.

[78] Charalampopoulos D, Wang R, Pandiella SS, Webb C. Application of cereals and cereal components in functional foods: a review. International journal of food microbiology. 2002 Nov 15;79(1-2):131-41.

[79] Farag MA, El Hawary EA, Elmassry MM. Rediscovering acidophilus milk, its quality characteristics, manufacturing methods, flavor chemistry and nutritional value. Critical reviews in food science and nutrition. 2020 Oct 10;60(18):3024-41.

[80] Plengvidhya V, Breidt F, Lu Z, Fleming HP. DNA fingerprinting of lactic acid bacteria in sauerkraut fermentations. Applied and Environmental Microbiology. 2007 Dec 1;73(23):7697-702.

[81] Stanton C, Gardiner G, Meehan H, Collins K, Fitzgerald G, Lynch PB, Ross RP. Market potential for probiotics. The American journal of clinical nutrition. 2001 Feb 1;73(2):476s-83s.

[82] Ross RP, Fitzgerald G, Collins K, Stanton C. Cheese delivering

biocultures--probiotic cheese. Australian Journal of Dairy Technology. 2002 Jul 1;57(2):71.

[83] Nielsen ES, Garnås E, Jensen KJ, Hansen LH, Olsen PS, Ritz C, Krych L, Nielsen DS. Lacto-fermented sauerkraut improves symptoms in IBS patients independent of product pasteurisation–a pilot study. Food & function. 2018;9(10):5323-35.

[84] Sun P, Wang JQ, Zhang HT. Effects of Bacillus subtilis natto on performance and immune function of preweaning calves. Journal of Dairy Science. 2010 Dec 1;93(12):5851-5.

[85] Bartkiene E, Lele V, Ruzauskas M, Domig KJ, Starkute V, Zavistanaviciute P, Bartkevics V, Pugajeva I, Klupsaite D, Juodeikiene G, Mickiene R. Lactic acid bacteria isolation from spontaneous sourdough and their characterization including antimicrobial and antifungal properties evaluation. Microorganisms. 2020 Jan;8(1):64.

[86] Yirga H. The use of probiotics in animal nutrition. J. Prob. Health. 2015;3(2):1-0.

[87] Kabir SM. The role of probiotics in the poultry industry. International Journal of Molecular Sciences. 2009 Aug;10(8):3531-46.

[88] Langhout P. New additives for broiler chickens. World poultry. 2000;16(3):22-7.

[89] Gill HS, Guarner F. Probiotics and human health: a clinical perspective. Postgraduate Medical Journal. 2004 Sep 1;80(947):516-26.

[90] Tanriover MD, Aksoy DY, Unal S. Use of probiotics in various diseases: Evidence and promises. Pol Arch Med Wewn. 2012 Jan 1;122(Suppl 1):S72-7.

[91] Shin JM, Gwak JW, Kamarajan P, Fenno JC, Rickard AH, Kapila YL. Biomedical applications of nisin. Journal of applied microbiology. 2016 Jun;120(6):1449-65.

Chapter 3

The Immunomodulatory Role of Probiotics

Faisal Siddique, Kashif Akram, Etab Saleh Alghamdi, Qandeel Arshad and Ayesha Siddique

Abstract

Probiotics are particularly beneficial living microorganisms that help improve human health. Although probiotics have long been used as nutritional supplements in various cultures around the world, new research has investigated their antimicrobial and immune boosting effects in individuals. Lactobacillus and Bifidobacterium are popular probiotics used worldwide that benefit human health by acting as antibacterial, antiviral, and antifungal agents, reducing pathogen binding to the host receptor and thus capturing pathogenic microorganisms. Probiotics have been shown to be beneficial in a variety of bacterial and viral diseases worldwide. The regulation of the host's immune response is one of the most important mechanisms of probiotic action. Immunomodulatory effects of probiotic-derived compounds have been characterized using genomic and proteomic analysis. These compounds have the ability to regulate and initiate mucosal immunity against various diseases. Probiotics produce many bactericidal compounds, which inhibit the growth of pathogenic microorganisms and their toxins, promoting the sustainability and structural integrity of enterocytes. This chapter focused on recent scientific research findings that help us better understand how probiotics regulate the host immune response and how they can be used to prevent and treat disease and there beneficial role to improve the health status of individuals.

Keywords: Immunomodulatory, Antibacterial, Antiviral, Probiotics, Lactobacillus

1. Introduction

The human body is prone to many virulent microbes and their oxidative metabolic substances. The human body is shielded from potentially pathogenic microbes by the immune system [1]. The gastrointestinal tract, which is approximately 7.5 meters long, is the largest area of the immune system. Furthermore, trillions of bacteria reside in the gut, particularly in the colon, which served as the main reservoir for these mutualistic species. Most of the time, it is said that the number of human cells in the body is ten times less than that of bacterial cells, while this proportion has been revamped to about 1:1 [2]. Normal vaginal and fecal microorganisms were injected at birth to study the host microbe's relationship with the newborn. This inoculum contains aerobic, anaerobic, gram-positive, and gram-negative bacteria belonging to dominant species such as Sneathia spp., Lactobacillus spp., and Prevotella spp. [3]. It has been studied that how gestational stage, environment, type of delivery, attitude, and breastfeeding habits influenced the proliferation and stability of the infant's microbiome [4].

The host-microbe relationship is critical for the growth of the gastrointestinal immunity within the first weeks after giving birth. The proliferation and growth of gut microorganisms continues until about the age of two years, at which point the intestinal immune system is said to be mature [5]. The intestinal environment of gut microorganisms is generally stable, particularly at the species and genus levels. Besides that, irrational antibiotic use, pathogenic parasites, malnutrition, or cold and hot stress all have an impact on the structural composition of gut microbiota [6].

Antimicrobial drugs, as well as human-targeted medicines, have been attributed to changes in gut microbial composition. More than a thousand antimicrobial drugs have been evaluated against forty different intestinal bacteria around the world. They discover 24 drugs that inhibit the growth of one or even more bacterial strains in vitro [7]. The defensive mechanism is triggered by innate immunity when an individual's body is exposed to a foreign particle or sustains tissue damage. Innate immunity protects cells physiology by signaling adaptive immune responses to persistent threats and stimulating inflammatory response. Inconsistent innate and adaptive responses, on the other hand, result in highly inflammatory reactions, tissue damage, and disease. The host mucosal immune response induced by gut microbiota is important for maintaining intestinal homeostasis and developing a systemic defense response. Manipulation of the intestinal microbiota can thus be a viable alternative route to improving health and to prevent and/or cure illness [8].

Probiotics were described as 'live microorganisms that impart benefits to the host health when taken in sufficient quantities as component of food". Saccharomyces, Lactobacillus, and Bifidobacterium are three important probiotic Genus that have been extensively researched and used in animal and human feed [9]. Recent research indicates that probiotics have a number of beneficial effects on the host's gastrointestinal tract protection mechanism. They produce bactericidal substances by which they counteract pathogenic microorganisms' consequences and bind to the intestinal epithelium by interacting with pathogenic microorganisms and their toxins. Probiotics facilitate the longevity of epithelial cells, improve the immune barrier, and improve the immune response to intestinal epithelium, all of which lead to gastric mucosal homeostasis [10]. Most notably, immune system regulation is among the most potential factors behind probiotics' beneficial health effects. Probiotics strengthen innate and adaptive immunity and suppress bacterial infection through toll-like receptor-regulated signal transduction pathways. Probiotic bacteria have been seen to enhance intrinsic host immune mechanisms. The use of probiotic microbes has significant effects on people's immune systems, such as stabilizing the non-immunological or innate immune response triggered by gut microbes, improving adaptive intestinal immune response, and regulating non-specific inflammatory and hypersensitivity reactions [11].

2. Historical background of probiotics

The concept of probiotics therapy emerged after the discovery of gut microbiome that is an inherent part of the intestinal epithelial cells. A probiotic is represented as a live microorganism's dietary supplement that benefits the individual by boosting the intestinal microbiome in the gastrointestinal tract. The probiotic definition is incomplete for the aim of human health and nutrition. In response, the European Commission and the International Institute of Life Sciences collaborated to reframe the concept of probiotics as a live microbial food item which is beneficial to human health [12].

In 1953, German researcher Werner Kollath coined the term probiotic, which is comes from the Latin terms pro, which means for, and biotic, which means "bios" or "life." Probiotics were defined by Lilly and Stillwell in 1965 as substances produced naturally by one microorganism that promotes the growth of another. In 1992, Fuller described probiotics as "live microorganisms added as a supplement in feed that benefits the host by improving its intestinal microbial balance" Probiotics have a modern history dating back to the early 1900s, when future Nobel laureate Elie Metchnikoff, a Russian scientist working at the Pasteur Institute in Paris, performed groundbreaking research [13].

Louis Pasteur established the microbes required for the fermentation process, while Metchnikoff first sought to determine the potential impact of the microbiota on public health. He attributed Bulgarian village peoples' long life spans to their regular consumption of yoghurt, which are fermented dairy products. He related this to Stamen Grigorov, a physician who found the Bulgarian bacillus, and further proposed that lactobacilli could mitigate the decaying impact of digestive fermentation, that led to illness and aging. Furthermore, Socrates said over two thousand years ago that "death lies in the guts" and that "poor absorption is the root of all evil." Metchnikoff also reported that toxins generated by microbial decomposition in the gastrointestinal tract and then discharged into to the bloodstream trigger aging [14]. Such microbes were originally referred to as decomposing microbes, but they are now known as proteolytic clostridia. Metchnikoff also noted that "the gastrointestinal microbiota' reliance on food allows us to take steps to change the microbiome in our gastrointestinal tract and exchange pathogenic microorganisms with good bacteria." Metchnikoff scientific theory of probiotics was the foundation for the first dairy industry in France [15].

Modern techniques have selected probiotics strains that manufacture fortified milk with strong nutritional and organoleptic features more than anyone else. Yoghurt was the first functional fermented food based to historical evidence [16]. However, since probiotics are usually associated to the consumption of fermented foods, they have a long and distinguished history. In ancient Indian Vedic literature, milk and milk products are associated to a reliable and comfortable life. According to legend, the first kefir grain was distributed by Prophet Muhammad (SAW) to the descendants of Caucasian mountaineers as a reward. Kefir is a fermented milk drink that contains a lot of lactic acid bacteria and probiotics. Cheese and yoghurt have been used by Hippocrates, Marco Polo, Galeno, and Chinese people throughout history [17].

3. Probiotics stimulate innate immune system

The most distinguished cells of natural immunity in probiotic research are the dendritic and epithelial cells. These are the first cells to interact with the gut microbiota and its toxic metabolites. Gut associated lymphoid tissue (GALT) and intestinal mucosa is the reservoir of intestinal dendritic cells. Dendritic cells are also known as detector cells because they have unique receptors that attach to specific sites on pathogen surfaces. Dendritic cells also act as a catalyst for various forms of signaling pathways that modify phenotypes and secreted cytokines such as Toll-like receptors and c-type lectin receptors [18].

Bifidobacterium infantis 35624 is a probiotic strain that can regulate dendritic cells activity, leading to a rise in cDC1 (CD103+ DC) in the basal lamina. It has many advantages for human health because it decreases the incidence of Dextran sulphate sodium-induced colitis, which is caused by a retinoid acid-dependent process [19]. Furthermore, oral administration of B. infantis 14.518 to Albino

BALB/C mice stimulates the growth, development, and maturation of dendritic cells in GALT, which is responsible for the regulation of T cells and the inhibition of Th2-biased responses through a process known as differentiation [20]. Additionally, other *B. longum*, *B. infantis*, *L. rhamnosus*, and *L. casei* enhance CCR7, CD40, and CD80 production in both juvenile and old Dendritic cells donors, whereas only old donors can boost IFN-γ and TGF- expression. The oral administration of *B. longum bv. infantis* CCUG increased IL-10 output [21].

The use of probiotic strain *L. rhamnosus* JB-1 has many advantages to regulate the dendritic cells by production of haemoxygense, stimulation of DC-SIGN and TLR-2 pattern recognition receptors (PRRs). *L. rhamnosus* JB-1 helps reduce inflammation via inhibiting the expression of co-stimulatory molecules, production and maturation of cytokines and TH1/TH17 through stimulations of the human monocyte derived dendritic cells. The immunomodulatory activity of *L. rhamnosus* JB-1, which expresses Foxp3 and induces IL-10 development, has been documented. Probiotic bacterial strain cell wall components also regulate the immunomodulation of DCs. When capsular polysaccharide binds with TLR-2 receptors on dendritic cells, it stimulates the development of IL-10 from T helper cells, which reduces the inflammatory response caused by colitis [22]. Similarly, exo-polysaccharides derived from *Bacillus subtilis* are useful in the treatment of intestinal infections because they protect against *Citrobacter rodentiumin* toxicity. Probiotics, on the other hand, control the microbial populations in the intestine after modifying dendritic cells activation [23].

The absorptive role of intestinal epithelium is well described. Epithelial cells produce a mucosal barrier to safeguard the individual from harmful microbes and toxicants. The intestinal mucosa barrier has a powerful connection with the intrinsic immune system of the Peyer's patches and lamina propria [24]. Probiotics are well-known for preserving the integrity of the intestinal barrier through a variety of mechanisms, including starvation of infectious agents as they compete for nutrients, detachment of bacteria from intestinal epithelium, which prevents pathogen invasion, immune response regulation, and aiding in regulatory T cell responses. Most of these are probiotics' positive effects on the host's internal health [25]. The use of *B. infantis* prevents Salmonella infection by reducing the induction of Peyer's patch macrophage inflammatory protein-1 (MIP)-1 and MIP-1 through a Treg-dependent pathway [26]. Human-defensin-2 is a probiotic-produced antimicrobial peptide that strengthens the mucosal barrier against pathogenic microbes. Defensins are wide ranging anti-microbial peptides released by macrophages, epithelial cells, neutrophils and, Paneth cells as part of a natural immune reaction [27]. *Shirota strain (L. casei)* increases defensin mRNA transcription in Caco-2 colonic intestinal cells by increasing hBD-2 [28].

Multiple probiotic strains of the genus Bifidobacterium, such as *B. infantis, B. adolescentis, B. bifidum, and B. longum*, could be modulate the apoptosis process in intestinal epithelial cells. They can also enhance mucin secretion, which serves as the first line of protection against infectious agents in the intestine [29]. *L. rhamnosus* GG3 induces mucin production in intestinal epithelial cells by activating the Muc2 and p40 genes expression. When an antigen attaches to enterocytes, pro-inflammatory neurotransmitters, chemokine's, and some tumor necrosis factor are secreted, triggering an efficient immune response [30]. *L. casei* and *L. rhamnosus* reduce the production of proinflammatory cytokines in enterocytes after infection with *Clostridium difficile*. *B. polyfermenticus*, *Bifidobacterium lactus*, *B. animalis ssp. lactis Lactobacillus casei*, *L. paracasei* ssp. *paracasei*, and *L. plantarum* stimulate the production of natural killer cells after infection [31].

4. Probiotics stimulate humoral immune system

Probiotics are used to sensitize the host's immune system to potentially dangerous pathogens. Oral administration of B. bifidum increased humoral immune response to egg albumin, whereas *B. breve* increased IgA exposure to cholera toxin [32]. Oral administration of *L. rhamnosus* triggered antibody IgA secreted B-cells in children with rotavirus infection in control studies [33]. Lactobacilli were given orally to suckling rats that had been sensitized with cow milk, and the number of cells secreting antibodies β-lactoglobulin increased. Human babies develop atopic dermatitis after consuming cow milk. Probiotic therapy, on the other hand, has been scientifically proven to minimize atopic dermatitis infection in humans. Food antigens are processed in the intestine with the aid of the gut microbiota. Low-molecular-weight peptides produced by bacteria collected from of the gastric microbiota can stimulate the immune reaction [34].

Probiotic derived proteases have been shown to digest cow milk casein and produce peptides that inhibit inflammatory cytokines in healthy people. A study was conducted to see whether caseins digested by probiotic bacteria producing proteases might induce the production of cytokine and anti-CD3 immunoglobulin mononuclear cells in atopic dermatitis in infants with cow milk allergies. Casein from cow's milk stimulates the synthesis of IL-4, which causes hypersensitivity [35]. Oral administration of *L. rhamnosus* GG, on the other hand, breaks down casein and inhibits IL-4 synthesis. These results indicate that probiotics in diet change the composition of potentially toxic pathogens, thus altering their immunogenicity function [36].

The ability of probiotics to increase the number of T-regulated lymphocytic cells contributes for their anti-inflammatory and anti-colitis properties. *B. longum* has helped in the treatment of colorectal colitis in mice by upregulating T-regulated lymphocytic cells. As a result, IL-10 and IL-12 levels in the blood have risen, while inflammatory cytokines including IL-23, IL-12, and IL-27 have decreased [37]. In healthy people, *B. infantis* induces Foxp3 T-cells to become activated, which decreases the levels of inflammatory cytokines in psoriasis patients [38].

Probiotics strain produced short chain fatty acids molecules such as propionate, isobutyrate, acetate, butyrate etc., which directly or indirectly regulate the homeostasis of T-cells. Butyrate activates Foxp3+ cells and Treg cell production outside of the hypothalamus. Propionate regulated the production of T-cell by inhibiting histone deacetylase. Probiotics e.g. *L. acidophilu, B. breve, L. gasseri, B. longum, B. longum subsp. infantis* prevented the development of Th17 inflammatory cells, which are responsible for the pathogenesis and progression of different inflammatory diseases such as irritable bowel syndrome [39]. Further to that, *L. rhamnosus* GG and *B. breve* inhibit IL-17 and IL-23, which are necessary for Th17 growth, stability, and stimulation. INFγ and TNF-α was produced by various Lactobacillus and Bifidobacterium species, which inhibited the expansion of Th17 inflammatory cells. *B. longum* (JCM) increased IL-27 development, which has been linked to a reduction in the amount of IL-17 stimulating Th-17 cells [40].

Probiotics have the ability to shift the immune response from Th2 to Th1. L. casei can stimulate IL-12 development, polarizing the Th1 response and mitigating Th2 linked illnesses. *L. rhamnosus* curtails Th2 as well as Th17 cells and improves clinical symptoms of seasonal allergies, atopic dermatitis and psoriatic arthritis. Probiotic fermented dairy milk modified the allergic process triggered by ovoalbumin in rats, polarizing a Th1 instead of a Th2 pattern reaction and leading throughout the production of IgG rather than IgE, with increased concentration of IFN-γ and IL- 10 accountable immunomodulation [41].

Probiotics have a direct effect on the cells of the lamina propria and payers patches, resulting in an increase in IgA production cells. IgA plays an important function in the prevention of mucosal pathogens. Toxins are neutralized by IgA, which prevents pathogens bacteria from binding to intestinal epithelial cells. *L. gasseri* (SBT2055) has been shown in mice to activate the TLR2 signal pathway, which triggers IgA generating cells in the mucosa and payers patches of the small intestine. While B lymphocytes are responsible for production of specific immunoglobulin and are the primary players in the adaptive immune response, they can also deprecating antibodies by manufacturing IL-10 through inflammatory and chronic diseases. The use of probiotics during combination with influenza vaccine increased an individual's total number of IgG and memory B-cells [42].

5. Role of probiotics as antibacterial

The oral cavity is a highly complex structure containing over 700 different types of bacteria. When there is a disturbance in this environment, abnormalities such as periodontal disease may occur, resulting in a reduction of indigenous microbial populations to the advantage of infectious agents. The causative agents of oral cavity disease are *S. mutans, A. viscosus, F. nucleatum* and *P. gingivalis*. Microbial resistance tends to be a safe way to battle against the establishing of bacterial pathogens with in oral ecosystem, and this fight might well be enabled by probiotic strains [43].

Anti-bacterial substances formed by probiotic strains included defensin, acetaldehydes, hydrogen peroxide, bacteriocins, organic acids, ethanol, and peptides. Peptides and bacteriocins, in general, are essential in increasing the vascular permeability of target cells that contributes to activation of the membrane permeability and, eventually, cell damage [44].

Probiotics have antibacterial effect, which is an essential feature. Bacteriocin synthesis may be one way to accomplish this antibacterial activity. Bacteriocins are produced by the industrial probiotic strains *L. casei* YIT 9029 and *L. johnsonii* LA1. The antimicrobial compound's existence can be deduced from its behavior, which includes a limited inhibiting range, lack of function if administered with proteinases, and relatively tiny molecular weights [45]. *L. amylovorus* (DCE 471), *L. johnsonii* (LA1), and *L. casei* (YIT 9029) all developed bacteriocins that prevented helicobacter pylori infection in humans. Regrettably, H. pylorus was not inhibited by a fourth bacteriocin induced by *L. acidophilus* (IBB 801). This suggests that certain bacteriocins formed by unique probiotic strains may help to inhibit this specific bacterium [46].

The most commonly used probiotic strains are from the Lactobacillus genus, which is recognized as safe. Some researchers have explained the function of probiotics in the buccal mucosa during the last few decades. Intake of lactic acid bacteria containing items has been shown to mitigate dental caries of mutant streptococci, but the studied species were ATCC strains rather than standard probiotic species such as *L. rhamnosus* GG. It has been demonstrated that probiotic strains with good antibacterial activity are needed to eliminate or stop harmful bacteria [47]. Lactobacilli have long been considered to be able to produce antimicrobial compounds. Lactobacilli may produce organic acid compounds as a result of carbohydrate fermentation, which can intervene with the function of neighboring microbes via depressing the pH of the environment. Some probiotic strains produce bacteriocins, which are well-known types of microbial animosity. *L. gasseri* was abundant in healthier people's oral mucosa and developed bacteriocin against pathogenic microbes. *L. reuteri* appears to be able to produce reuterin, a powerful antibacterial substance derived from glycerol fermentation [48].

6. Role of probiotics as antiviral

A number of microorganisms have been found in the human respiratory tract as the primary source of the respiratory virus. We may reduce the occurrence of disease development in humans by limiting the penetration of respiratory tract viruses into the membranes of mucosal epithelial cells. The human body contains a diverse community of mutually advantageous commensal bacteria known as microbiota [49]. Probiotics are microorganisms that have potential health benefits when eaten in a specific amount. There are two basic types of probiotics: Lactobacillus and Bifidobacterium and Both have a positive impact on human health since it acts as an antiviral agent, lowering the binding ability of viruses to the host receptor and thereby capturing the virus. Probiotics administering protects individuals from various respiratory viral infections like Respiratory syncytial virus, SARS-CoV-2, Influenza A virus. This antiviral activity was investigated by the strain's specificity as well as the host immune status [50].

L. casei shirota (LcS) is a lactobacillus probiotic strain isolated from the oral microbiota. It has been stated that when Lcs was presented to influenza (H1N1) infected mice, the viral titer declined. Furthermore, LcS stimulates the innate or nonspecific immune system by increasing the production of antiviral cytokines like IFN-α. Another study discovered immunomodulatory activity against Respiratory syncytial virus. LcS, on the other hand, has shown negligible findings into clinical trials, especially among older community, when compared to the control group [51]. Clinical trials were conducted on *L. Casei* (DN-114,001) demonstrated substantial antiviral activity in separate studies in infants, adults, and the elderly. It decreases the clinical signs and symptoms of respiratory tract infection in infants, adults, and the elderly [52].

L. fermentum is a bacteria present in both people and animals microbiota and is commonly used it as a probiotic in people. This probiotic was tested in clinical studies, specifically in children and young adults, as well as lab animals to examine the process of viral prevention toward respiratory infections. The efficacy of *L. fermentum* CJL-112 and *L. fermentum*-1 have been studied against Influenza virus (H1N1) infected with mice and the findings indicate a marked decline in viral count, with significant stimulation of IL-12 and Immunoglobulin (IgA) development, allowing for an improvement in mouse longevity. The combined effect of probiotic (*L. fermentum* CECT5716) and prebiotic (galacto-oligosaccharides) had assessed in healthy infants, and this research showed a significant decrease in the incidence of urinary and respiratory tract illness [53].

L. acidophilus is a well-known lactic acid bacteria strain that is used in medicinal treatments. Since *L. acidophilus* is commonly used to treat gastrointestinal issues, just few researchers have examined into its antiviral activity. *L. acidophilus* L-92, retrieved from a healthy Japanese citizen, demonstrated antiviral activity against influenza virus through IFN-α and natural killer cell modulation. The antiviral activity of *L. brevis* KB-290 against H1NI was examined, and virus levels were found to be depleted as a result of IgA and IFN-α stimulation [54]. Bifidobacteria aids in digestion, immunity, and the prevention of almost all gastrointestinal infections. These strains have been used in several clinical studies against viral respiratory diseases to determine the mechanism of antiviral effect [55].

B. longum (BB536) demonstrated anti-H1N1 activity in mice after parenteral route for two weeks prior to disease, owing to a decrease in IL-6 and IFN production. Moreover, this probiotic strain exhibited the potential to dramatically reduce the clinical signs and symptom. The combination of *B. animalis ssp. Lactis and L. reuteri* indicated the strongest antiviral activity against respiratory system microbes.

L. rhamnosus GG is the most extensively researched probiotic, with substantial reductions in diarrhea length and rotavirus pathogenicity [56].

The COVID-19 disease affects the lungs and the gastrointestinal tract, inducing pro-inflammatory Th1-cells to release various cytokines such as TNF-alpha leading to the establishment of the cytokine storm. Dysregulation in the intestinal microbiome contributes to an imbalance of Th1 and Th2, which stimulates the formation of pro-inflammatory cytokines and, eventually, a cytokine storm in epithelial cells in the lungs [57]. Probiotics promote the proliferation of "beneficial bacteria" in the intestine, resulting in a change in the stability of Th1/Th2 cells, which lowers the cytokine storm and the severity of infections. It was recently found that using probiotic bacteria derived from Lactobacillus and Bifidobacterium improves the chance of healing from COVID-19 patients. *L. paracasei* and *L. coryniformis* has the ability to bind angiotensin converting enzyme type 2, which is a receptor needed by the SARS-CoV-2 virus for attachment, preventing its entrance into cell and thereby decrease the possibility of COVID-19 infection [58].

7. Role of probiotics as antifungal

The global fungal load is extremely high, and it is expected to rise even higher as the proportion of immunocompromised people rises. In contrast, the drugs used to treat fungal pollutions are extremely small, and some of them are extremely dangerous. *Candida gullemondii*, *C. auris, C. glabrata,* Aspergillus and Fusarium species are evolving as impervious and hazardous fungal pathogens. These species are responsible for 5–10% of global food spoilage [59].

Aflatoxin is an extremely hepatotoxic bioactive compound produced by fungi, which is a major global concern. A toxin-free feed is demanded by the existing agriculture and livestock production industries. Use of such microbes to food preservation has grown in popularity in recent years, owing to customer needs for less reliance on chemical preservatives. Lactic acid bacteria are widely regarded as a "beneficial organism," that is used to avoid contamination of food and feed, as well as to chemically store food. It is also intended to produce antimicrobial agents [60].

L. fermentum L23 and *L. rhamnosus* L60 produced bioactive compounds such as hydrolytic enzymes, organic acids, bacteriocins, and hydrogen peroxide and blocked the fungal growth of most all aflatoxigenic strains. L60 has decreased Aflatoxin B1 output by greater than 90 percent and L23 by up to 100 percent. As a result, L23 and L60 have been used to properly manage aflatoxigenic fungi in livestock feed [61].

Probiotics have been shown to decrease *C. albicans* infections in a variety of body organ systems and are widely regarded as important for good health. Probiotics, for example, can treat gastroenteritis, dairy allergy, and the signs and symptoms of irritable bowel syndrome. *C. albicans* has been assigned two virulent functions: filamentation and biofilm growth. We can minimize both of these virulent functions through using probiotics. The yeast form of candida is more readily phagocytized than the hyphal form, and probiotics help the host organism combat pathogens by preventing filamentation. However, the exact mechanisms by which fungal infections are prevented are unknown [62].

8. Conclusion

Nowadays, the discovery of the use of probiotic strains has improved our understanding of the relationship between diet and people's health. Probiotics boost innate and humoral immunity against pathogens. Probiotic bacteria bind to gut epithelial cells and release cytokines (IFN-γ) and interleukins (IL-10) that establish a microclimate in the tracheae, bronchi, and reproductive organs and gut lamina propria, triggering clonal proliferation of B cells to make IgA and activating Treg cells, thereby maintaining immune balance in the gastrointestinal tract. COVID-19 is a newly emerging virus that causes deadly disease all over the world. Probiotic strains, especially lactobacillus species therapy, may be critical in controlling COVID-19, and probiotic treatment may be considered as a choice for the reduction and mitigation of COVID-19 infection globally.

Conflict of interest

The authors declare no conflict of interest.

Author details

Faisal Siddique[1*], Kashif Akram[2], Etab Saleh Alghamdi[3], Qandeel Arshad[4] and Ayesha Siddique[5]

1 Department of Microbiology, Cholistan University of Veterinary and Animal Sciences, Bahawalpur, Pakistan

2 Department of Food Sciences, Cholistan University of Veterinary and Animal Sciences, Bahawalpur, Pakistan

3 Department of Food and Nutrition, King Abdul-Aziz University, Jeddah, Saudi Arabia

4 Riphah International University, Lahore, Pakistan

5 Department of Soil and Environmental Sciences, University of Agriculture, Faisalabad, Pakistan

*Address all correspondence to: faisalsiddique@cuvas.edu.pk

References

[1] Khanmohammadi S, Rezaei N. Role of Toll-like receptors in the pathogenesis of COVID-19. Journal of Medical Virology. 2021;93(5):2735-2739. DOI: 10.1002/jmv.26826

[2] Sender R, Fuchs S, Milo R. Are we really vastly outnumbered? Revisiting the ratio of bacterial to host cells in humans. Cell. 2016;164(3):337-340. DOI: 10.1016/j.cell.2016.01

[3] Dominguez-Bello MG, Costello EK, Contreras M, Magris M, Hidalgo G, Fierer N, Knight R. Delivery mode shapes the acquisition and structure of the initial microbiota across multiple body habitats in newborns. Proceedings of the National Academy of Sciences. 2010;107(26):11971-11975. DOI: org/10.1073/pnas.1002601107

[4] Moore RE, Townsend SD. Temporal development of the infant gut microbiome. Open biology. 9(9):190128. DOI: 10.1098/rsob.190128

[5] Azad MAK, Sarker M, Wan D. Immunomodulatory Effects of Probiotics on Cytokine Profiles. Biomedical Research International. 2018;8063647. DOI: 10.1155/2018/8063647.

[6] Dongarrà ML, Rizzello V, Muccio L, Fries W, Cascio A, Bonaccorsi I, Ferlazzo G. Mucosal immunology and probiotics. Current allergy and asthma reports. 2013;13(1):19-26. DOI: org/10.1007/s11882-012-0313-0

[7] Maier L, Pruteanu M, Kuhn M, Zeller G, Telzerow A, Anderson EE, Brochado AR, Fernandez KC, Dose H, Mori H, Patil KR. Extensive impact of non-antibiotic drugs on human gut bacteria. Nature. 2018;555(7698):623-628. DOI: 10.1038/nature25979

[8] Cheng HY, Ning MX, Chen DK, Ma WT. Interactions between the gut microbiota and the host innate immune response against pathogens. Frontiers in immunology. 2019;10:607-612. DOI: org/10.3389/fimmu.2019.00607

[9] Ezema C. Probiotics in animal production: A review. Journal of Veterinary Medicine and Animal Health. 2013;5(11):308-316. DOI: 10.12691/jaem-7-1-3.

[10] Vallianou N, Stratigou T, Christodoulatos GS, Tsigalou C, Dalamaga M. Probiotics, prebiotics, synbiotics, postbiotics, and obesity: current evidence, controversies, and perspectives. Current obesity reports. 2020;29:1-4. DOI: 10.1007/s13679-020-00379-w

[11] Markowiak P, Śliżewska K. Effects of Probiotics, Prebiotics, and Synbiotics on Human Health. Nutrients. 2017;9(9):1021. DOI: 10.3390/nu9091021.

[12] Vankerckhoven V, Huys G, Vancanneyt M, Vael C, Klare I, Romond MB, Entenza JM, Moreillon P, Wind RD, Knol J, Wiertz E. Biosafety assessment of probiotics used for human consumption: recommendations from the EU-PROSAFE project. Trends in Food Science & Technology. 2008;19(2):102-114. DOI: org/10.1016/j.tifs.2007.07.013

[13] Behnsen J, Deriu E, Sassone-Corsi M, Raffatellu M. Probiotics: properties, examples, and specific applications. Cold Spring Herbicide Perspective Medicine. 2013;3(3):a010074. DOI: 10.1101/cshperspect.a010074.

[14] Pande R, Bagad M, Dubey V, Ghosh AR. Prospectus of probiotics in modern age diseases. Asian Pacific Journal of Tropical Biomedicine. 2012;2(3):S1963-S1974. DOI: org/10.1016/S2221-1691(12)60526-7

[15] Raghuwanshi S, Misra S, Bisen PS. Indian perspective for probiotics: A

review. Indian Journal of Dairy Science. 2015;68(3):195-205. DOI: 10.5146/IJDS.V68I3.46442.G21253

[16] Maldonado Galdeano C, Novotny Nunez I, Carmuega E, de Moreno de LeBlanc A, Perdigon G. Role of probiotics and functional foods in health: gut immune stimulation by two probiotic strains and a potential probiotic yoghurt. Endocrine, Metabolic & Immune Disorders-Drug Targets. 2015;15(1):37-45. DOI: 10.2174/1871530314666141216121349.

[17] Gasbarrini G, Bonvicini F, Gramenzi A. Probiotics history. Journal of clinical gastroenterology. 2016;50:S116-S119. DOI: 10.1097/MCG.0000000000000697

[18] Mörbe UM, Jørgensen PB, Fenton TM, von Burg N, Riis LB, Spencer J, Agace WW. Human gut-associated lymphoid tissues (GALT); diversity, structure, and function. Mucosal Immunology. 2021:1-10. DOI: 10.1038/s41385-021-00389-4

[19] Konieczna P, Groeger D, Ziegler M, Frei R, Ferstl R, Shanahan F, Quigley EM, Kiely B, Akdis CA, O'Mahony L. Bifidobacterium infantis 35624 administration induces Foxp3 T regulatory cells in human peripheral blood: potential role for myeloid and plasmacytoid dendritic cells. Gut. 2012;61(3):354-366. DOI: 10.1136/gutjnl-2011-300936.

[20] Di Costanzo M, Carucci L, Berni Canani R, Biasucci G. Gut Microbiome Modulation for Preventing and Treating Pediatric Food Allergies. International Journal of Molecular Sciences. 2020; 21(15):5275. DOI: 10.3390/ijms21155275

[21] Yahfoufi N, Mallet JF, Graham E, Matar C. Role of probiotics and prebiotics in immunomodulation. Current Opinion in Food Science. 2018;20:82-91. DOI: org/10.1016/j.cofs.2018.04.006

[22] Liu Y, Mian MF, Neufeld KA, Forsythe P. CD4+ CD25+ T cells are essential for behavioral effects of Lactobacillus rhamnosus JB-1 in male BALB/c mice. Brain, behavior, and immunity. 2020;88:451-460. DOI: 10.1016/j.bbi.2020.04.014

[23] Turroni F, Ventura M, Buttó LF, Duranti S, O'Toole PW, Motherway MO, van Sinderen D. Molecular dialogue between the human gut microbiota and the host: a Lactobacillus and Bifido-bacterium perspective. Cellular and Molecular Life Sciences. 2014;71(2): 183-203. DOI: 10.1007/s00018-013-1318-0

[24] Galdeano CM, Cazorla SI, Dumit JM, Vélez E, Perdigón G. Beneficial effects of probiotic consumption on the immune system. Annals of Nutrition and Metabolism. 2019;74(2):115-124. DOI: 10.1159/000496426

[25] Chelakkot C, Ghim J, Ryu SH. Mechanism's regulating intestinal barrier integrity and its pathological implications. Experimental & molecular medicine. 2018;50(8):1-9. DOI: 10.1038/s12276-018-0126-x

[26] Yang GY, Yu J, Su JH, Jiao LG, Liu X, Zhu YH. Oral administration of Lactobacillus rhamnosus GG ameliorates Salmonella infantis-induced inflammation in a pig model via activation of the il-22bp/il-22/stat3 pathway. Frontiers in cellular and infection microbiology. 2017;7:323. DOI: 10.3389/fcimb.2017.00323

[27] Wan LY, Chen ZJ, Shah NP, El-Nezami H. Modulation of intestinal epithelial defense responses by probiotic bacteria. Critical reviews in food science and nutrition. 2016;56(16):2628-2641. DOI: 10.1080/10408398.2014.905450.

[28] Belguesmia Y, Domenger D, Caron J, Dhulster P, Ravallec R, Drider D, Cudennec B. Novel probiotic evidence of lactobacilli on immunomodulation

and regulation of satiety hormones release in intestinal cells. Journal of Functional Foods. 2016;24:276-286. DOI: org/10.1016/j.jff.2016.04.014

[29] Turroni F, Duranti S, Milani C, Lugli GA, van Sinderen D, Ventura M. Bifidobacterium bifidum: a key member of the early human gut microbiota. Microorganisms. 2019;7(11):544. DOI: 10.3390/microorganisms7110544

[30] Martín R, Chamignon C, Mhedbi-Hajri N, Chain F, Derrien M, Escribano-Vázquez U, Garault P, Cotillard A, Pham HP, Chervaux C, Bermúdez-Humarán LG. The potential probiotic Lactobacillus rhamnosus CNCM I-3690 strain protects the intestinal barrier by stimulating both mucus production and cytoprotective response. Scientific reports. 2019;9(1):1-4. DOI: org/10.1038/s41598-019-41738-5

[31] Valdés-Varela L, Gueimonde M, Ruas-Madiedo P. Probiotics for prevention and treatment of *Clostridium difficile* infection. Updates on *clostridium difficile* in Europe. 2018:161-176. DOI: 10.1007/978-3-319-72799-8-10.

[32] Abd El AE, El-Wardany I, Abu-Taleb AM, Wakwak MM, Ebeid TA, Saleh AA. Assessment of in ovo administration of Bifidobacterium bifidum and Bifidobacterium longum on performance, ileal histomorphometry, blood hematological, and biochemical parameters of broilers. Probiotics and Antimicrobial Proteins. 2020;12(2):439-450. DOI: 10.1007/s12602-019-09549-2

[33] Kandasamy S, Vlasova AN, Fischer D, Kumar A, Chattha KS, Rauf A, Shao L, Langel SN, Rajashekara G, Saif LJ. Differential effects of Escherichia coli Nissle and Lactobacillus rhamnosus strain GG on human rotavirus binding, infection, and B cell immunity. The Journal of Immunology. 2016;196(4):1780-1789. DOI: 10.4049/jimmunol.1501705.

[34] Salas-Jara MJ, Ilabaca A, Vega M, García A. Biofilm forming Lactobacillus: new challenges for the development of probiotics. Microorganisms. 2016;4(3):35. DOI: 10.3390/microorganisms4030035

[35] Wróblewska B, Kaliszewska-Suchodoła A, Fuc E, Markiewicz LH, Ogrodowczyk AM, Złotkowska D, Wasilewska E. Effect of Low-Immunogenic Yogurt Drinks and Probiotic Bacteria on Immunoreactivity of Cow's Milk Proteins and Tolerance Induction In Vitro and In Vivo Studies. Nutrients. 2020;12(11):3390. DOI: 10.3390/nu12113390.

[36] Lee KH, Song Y, Wu W, Yu K, Zhang G. The gut microbiota, environmental factors, and links to the development of food allergy. Clinical and Molecular Allergy. 2020;18:1-1. Doi: org/10.1186/s12948-020-00120-x

[37] Jang SE, Jeong JJ, Kim JK, Han MJ, Kim DH. Simultaneous amelioratation of colitis and liver injury in mice by Bifidobacterium longum LC67 and Lactobacillus plantarum LC27. Scientific reports. 2018;8(1):1-4. DOI: org/ 10.1038/s41598-018-25775-0

[38] Groeger D, O'Mahony L, Murphy EF, Bourke JF, Dinan TG, Kiely B, Shanahan F, Quigley EM. Bifidobacterium infantis 35624 modulates host inflammatory processes beyond the gut. Gut microbes. 2013;4(4):325-339. DOI: 10.4161/gmic.25487

[39] Wong CB, Odamaki T, Xiao JZ. Beneficial effects of Bifidobacterium longum subsp. longum BB536 on human health: Modulation of gut microbiome as the principal action. Journal of Functional Foods. 2019;54:506-519. DOI: j.jff.2019.02.002

[40] Ghadimi D, Helwig U, Schrezenmeir J, Heller KJ, de Vrese M. Epigenetic imprinting by commensal probiotics inhibits the IL-23/IL-17 axis in an in vitro model of the intestinal

mucosal immune system. Journal of leukocyte biology. 2012;92(4):895-911. DOI: 10.1189/jlb.0611286.

[41] Alonso VR, Guarner F. Linking the gut microbiota to human health. British Journal of Nutrition. 2013;109(S2): S21-S26. DOI: 10.1017/S00071145120 05235

[42] Hiramatsu Y, Hosono A, Konno T, Nakanishi Y, Muto M, Suyama A, Hachimura S, Sato R, Takahashi K, Kaminogawa S. Orally administered Bifidobacterium triggers immune responses following capture by CD11c+ cells in Peyer's patches and cecal patches. Cytotechnology. 2011;63(3):307-317. DOI: 10.1007/s10616-011-9349-6

[43] Patil S, Rao RS, Sanketh DS, Amrutha N. Microbial flora in oral diseases. The journal of contemporary dental practice. 2013;14(6):1202. DOI: 10.5005/jp-journals-10024-1477

[44] Sarao LK, Arora M. Probiotics, prebiotics, and microencapsulation: A review. Critical reviews in food science and nutrition. 2017;57(2):344-371. DOI: 10.1080/10408398.2014.887055.

[45] Prosekov AY, Dyshlyuk LS, Milentyeva IS, Sykhikh SA, Babich OO, Ivanova SA, Pavsky VA, Shishin MV, Matskova LV. Antioxidant and antimicrobial activity of bacteriocin-producing strains of lactic acid bacteria isolated from the human gastro-intestinal tract. Progress in Nutrition. 2017;19(1):67-80. DOI: 10.23751/pn.v19i1.5147

[46] Saracino IM, Pavoni M, Saccomanno L, Fiorini G, Pesci V, Foschi C, Piccirilli G, Bernardini G, Holton J, Figura N, Lazzarotto T. Antimicrobial efficacy of five probiotic strains against Helicobacter pylori. Antibiotics. 2020 May;9(5):244. DOI: 10.3390/antibiotics9050244

[47] Lin TH, Lin CH, Pan TM. The implication of probiotics in the prevention of dental caries. Applied microbiology and biotechnology. 2018;102(2):577-586. DOI: 10.1007/s00253-017-8664-z.

[48] Monika K, Malik T, Gehlot R, Rekha K, Kumari A, Sindhu R, Rohilla P. Antimicrobial Property of Probiotics. Environment Conservation Journal. 2021;22(SE):33-48. DOI: 10.36953/ECJ.2021.SE.2204

[49] Lu W, Fang Z, Liu X, Li L, Zhang P, Zhao J, Zhang H, Chen W. The Potential Role of Probiotics in Protection against Influenza a Virus Infection in Mice. Foods. 2021;10(4):902. DOI: 10.3390/foods10040902

[50] Mirzaei R, Attar A, Papizadeh S, Jeda AS, Hosseini-Fard SR, Jamasbi E, Kazemi S, Amerkani S, Talei GR, Moradi P, Jalalifar S. The emerging role of probiotics as a mitigation strategy against coronavirus disease 2019 (COVID-19). Archives of virology. 2021:1-22. DOI: 10.1007/s00705-021-05036-8.

[51] Kanauchi O, Andoh A, AbuBakar S, Yamamoto N. Probiotics and paraprobiotics in viral infection: clinical application and effects on the innate and acquired immune systems. Current pharmaceutical design. 2018;24(6):710-717. DOI: 10.2174/1381612824666180.

[52] Guillemard E, Tanguy J, Flavigny AL, de la Motte S, Schrezenmeir J. Effects of consumption of a fermented dairy product containing the probiotic Lactobacillus casei DN-114 001 on common respiratory and gastrointestinal infections in shift workers in a randomized controlled trial. Journal of the American College of Nutrition. 2010;29(5):455-468. DOI: 10.1080/07315724.2010.10719882.

[53] Jayashree S, Karthikeyan R, Nithyalakshmi S, Ranjani J, Gunasekaran P, Rajendhran J. Anti-adhesion property of the potential probiotic strain Lactobacillus fermentum

8711 against methicillin-resistant Staphylococcus aureus (MRSA). Frontiers in microbiology. 2018;9:411. DOI: 10.3389/fmicb.2018.00411.

[54] Inoue Y, Kambara T, Murata N, Komori-Yamaguchi J, Matsukura S, Takahashi Y, Ikezawa Z, Aihara M. Effects of oral administration of Lactobacillus acidophilus L-92 on the symptoms and serum cytokines of atopic dermatitis in Japanese adults: a double-blind, randomized, clinical trial. International archives of allergy and immunology. 2014;165(4):247-254. DOI: 10.1159/000369806

[55] Barba-Vidal E, Castillejos L, López-Colom P, Rivero Urgell M, Moreno Muñoz JA, Martín-Orúe SM. Evaluation of the probiotic strain Bifidobacterium longum subsp. infantis CECT 7210 capacities to improve health status and fight digestive pathogens in a piglet model. Frontiers in microbiology. 2017;8:533. DOI: 10.3389/fmicb.2017.00533

[56] Alegre I, Viñas I, Usall J, Anguera M, Abadias M. Microbiological and physicochemical quality of fresh-cut apple enriched with the probiotic strain Lactobacillus rhamnosus GG. Food Microbiology. 2011;28(1):59-66. DOI: 10.1016/j.fm.2010.08.006.

[57] Santacroce L, Inchingolo F, Topi S, Del Prete R, Di Cosola M, Charitos IA, Montagnani M. Potential beneficial role of probiotics on the outcome of COVID-19 patients: An evolving perspective. Diabetes & Metabolic Syndrome: Clinical Research & Reviews. 2021. DOI: 10.1016/j.dsx.2020.12.040.

[58] Siddique F, Abbas RZ, Mansoor MK, Alghamdi ES, Saeed M, Ayaz MM, Rahman M, Mahmood MS, Iqbal A, Manzoor M, Abbas A. An Insight into COVID-19: A 21st Century Disaster and Its Relation to Immunocompetence and Food Antioxidants. Frontiers in Veterinary Science. 2021;7:1168. DOI: 10.3389/fvets.2020.586637

[59] Quéro L, Girard V, Pawtowski A, Tréguer S, Weill A, Arend S, Cellière B, Polsinelli S, Monnin V, van Belkum A, Vasseur V. Development and application of MALDI-TOF MS for identification of food spoilage fungi. Food microbiology. 2019;81:76-88. DOI: 10.1016/j.fm.2018.05.001.

[60] Ahlberg SH, Joutsjoki V, Korhonen HJ. Potential of lactic acid bacteria in aflatoxin risk mitigation. International journal of food microbiology. 2015;207:87-102. DOI: 10.1016/j.ijfoodmicro.

[61] Chugh B, Kamal-Eldin A. Bioactive compounds produced by probiotics in food products. Current Opinion in Food Science. 2020;32:76-82. DOI: 10.1016/j.cofs.2020.02.003

[62] Ribeiro FC, Rossoni RD, de Barros PP, Santos JD, Fugisaki LR, Leão MP, Junqueira JC. Action mechanisms of probiotics on Candida spp. and candidiasis prevention: an update. Journal of applied microbiology. 2020;129(2):175-185. DOI: 10.1111/jam.14511.

Chapter 4

Probiotics as Potential Antimicrobials for the Treatment of Infections: Current Reality or Remote Future?

Diego Romario-Silva, Otavio Akira Souza Sakaguchi, Andrea Cristina Barbosa da Silva, Janaína Orlandi Sardi, Rafaela Parolina de Carvalho, Sindy Magri Roque, Lincoln Pires Silva Borges, Rodrigo Barros Esteves Lins, Letícia Targino Campos and Edja Maria Melo de Brito Costa

Abstract

Probiotics are microorganisms that live in symbiosis with the human body. The intake of probiotics in adequate amounts can improve biological functions bringing improvements in the health of the host. Many studies have demonstrated the indisputable antimicrobial activity of probiotics and their potential for an alternative treatment of infections. Nevertheless, the forms of encapsulation, as well as clinical trials on the clinical use of these microorganisms as a recognized and well-established protocol, are still incipient. In this chapter, we provide a general approach to the topic and point to future directions in the probiotics field for this purpose. Moreover, microbial resistance is a current public health problem and the search for new therapeutic alternatives is urgent. Probiotics and other natural therapies have been considered very promising. The approaches of future research should focus mainly on the isolation of new probiotic microorganisms, the definition of inoculum, forms of encapsulation for controlled delivery, and clinical trials for the definition of doses and mechanism of action in the fight against infections.

Keywords: probiotics, pharmacology, antimicrobial activity, microbiota, biomaterials

1. Introduction

The human body is inhabited by numerous microorganisms, including bacteria, fungi, viruses, and protozoa, which represent the human microbiota. Compared to the number of human cells, there is a much larger number of microorganisms [1], which affect the host's physiological functions in different ways [2]. After a long time of science focusing on pathogenic microorganisms that cause human diseases, the interest was also turned to those that provide benefits to the organism, such as probiotics.

The first time that probiotics were mentioned and defined was in 1965 and the concept was restricted to substances produced by bacteria that promote the growth of other bacteria [3]. In 2001, the Food and Agriculture Organization of the United Nations (FAO) updated the concept of probiotics for any living microorganisms that provide health benefits to the host when ingested in adequate quantities [4]. The most widely used and studied probiotics for human health benefits are generally gram-positive bacteria that function primarily as modulators and maintainers of gut health [5]. Examples of widely studied probiotics such as *Lactobacillus*, *Bifidobacterium*, *Escherichia*, *Enterococcus*, *Bacillus e Streptococcus* [6].

The commensal intestinal microbiota is related to important functions for maintaining the health of the organism, such as increased resistance against infections, differentiation of the immune system, and synthesis of nutrients [7]. Nevertheless, recent studies have shown that the benefits of probiotics for human health go beyond [8], including anti-inflammatory activities [9], anti-tumor activities [10], antioxidant [11], antimicrobial [12] and modulation of the microbiome [13]. Although, research on the antimicrobial activity of probiotic microorganisms remains incipient and its clinical applicability for the treatment of infections has not been fully explored [14].

Infections have been commonly treated with antibiotics. However, the unrestrained and irrational use of these drugs can range from individual harms, such as specific adverse effects of the drug for the patient, to serious public health problems, such as the selection of drug-resistant microorganisms [15]. Likewise, research on alternative therapies for the treatment of infectious diseases should be encouraged and the field of probiotic microorganisms is very promising. Therefore, in this chapter, we will discuss the current reality of treating infections using probiotic microorganisms and/or their by-products as well as the prospects for this therapy to become a reality in current medicine.

2. Probiotic microorganisms

In 1965, Lilly and Stillwell first used the term probiotic, describing substances that one organism secretes and can stimulate the growth of another [16]. Nonetheless, its use goes back to millennia, as the use of recipes with fermented milk by Greeks and Romans. There are also reports of the use of sour milk in the bible. Thus, it is observed that the benefits of the use of probiotics to human health have been discussed for millennia [17].

These microorganisms, when colonizing the gastrointestinal tract, interact directly with the cells of the immune system, playing an important role in the maintenance and balance of the immune system [18]. The mechanisms of action of probiotics are complex and, in most cases, likely, more than one mechanism occurs simultaneously. The main biological pathways of action include increased epithelial barrier, inhibition of microbial adhesion and competitive exclusion of pathogenic microorganisms in addition to the production of antimicrobial substances, modulation of the immune system, maintenance of normal levels of short-chain fatty acids, and regulation of intestinal absorption of electrolytes [19].

The word "probiotic" comes from Greek and means "for life" [20]. Probiotics are viable live microorganisms, bacteria, and yeasts, which confer benefits to the health of the host when ingested in adequate concentration. Probiotic microorganisms, in general, are part of the intestinal microflora, but can also be found in ecological environments. Many factors need to be considered before isolating a potential probiotic microorganism. Initially, it is necessary that the strain is not pathogenic and shows some type of behavior that reflects in biological activities

Genus	Specie	Main source	Reference
Lactobacillus	*L. casei*, *L. bulgaricus*, *L. acidophilus*, *L. rhamnosus*, *L. reuteri*, *L. pantarum* and *L. johnsonii*	Dairy and human gastrointestinal tract	[26, 27]
Bifidobacterium	*B. animalis*, *B. bifidum*, *B. breve*, *B. infantis*, *B. lactis*, *B. longum*	Human, Dog, Primate, Pig, Cow and Horse gastrointestinal tract	[28–30]
Streptococcus	*Streptococcus thermophilus*	Dairy	[31, 32]
Enterococcus	*Enterococcus faecalis*, *Enterococcus faecium*	Human, Cow and Pig gastrointestinal tract	[33–35]
Pediococcus	*Pediococcus pentosaceus*, *Pediococcus acidilactici*	Dry quark and rice wine	[36]

Table 1.
Main probiotic microorganisms that are cited in the literature for human health benefits.

for the benefit of the host [21]. Besides, it is important to consider that the probiotic action is not universal for all species and does not work the same in all tissues of the body [22].

Lactic acid bacteria (*Lactococcus*, *Lactobacillus*, *Streptococcus*, and *Enterococcus*) are among the most well-known microorganisms, used and studied by man for probiotic purposes. In addition to these, we can include, *Bifidobacterium* and *Saccharomyces* species, a non-pathogenic yeast [23–25]. **Table 1** summarizes the main probiotic microorganisms mentioned in the literature for the benefit of human health.

Microorganisms can produce lactic acid from different carbon sources, as well as release secondary metabolites, including bacteriocins, exopolysaccharides, and enzyme complexes with antimicrobial properties preventing the installation and growth of other microorganisms [21, 37]. The mechanisms involved in the action of these microbial products are well understood concerning the benefits generated to the human intestine. However, the use of probiotics for alternative antimicrobial therapy against infections, in general, is incipient, although promising. Subsequently, we will discuss how probiotics can affect a human microbiota, ways of encapsulation, and their main uses for treating infections.

3. Probiotics affect the microbiota

In recent years, several findings have revealed benefits in the administration of probiotics, ranging from direct inhibition of pathogenic microorganisms to improvements in host immune system functions [38–43].

Despite a large number of studies with probiotics, most efforts are focused on understanding the benefits for the intestinal health of the host. Probiotics can exert their antimicrobial activity through different mechanisms of action. Generally, it has been reported that these microorganisms control/kill the pathogenic microbiota through the production of inhibitory substances such as bacteriocins and hydrogen peroxide (capable of inhibiting Gram-negative and Gram-positive pathogenic bacteria); interference at adhesion sites; competition for nutrients in the microenvironment, among others [41, 42, 44, 45]. Besides, there is also the modulation of the immune system, which also plays a role in the control of infections, which can occur in several ways: increased non-specific phagocytic activity through the activation of macrophages [9, 45, 46].

Several probiotic species are widely used in research showing its benefits to the host [46, 47]. Among these benefits, antimutagenic properties [48], anticarcinogenic properties [49–51], antidiarrheal drugs [52–54], system stimulation [55], prevention of atopic dermatitis [56–58], reduced blood cholesterol [59, 60].

Therefore, the use of probiotics has been considered a promising strategy for the prevention and control of various infectious diseases [38–40, 42, 43, 48, 61–63].

Some studies have also demonstrated the importance of probiotics relating to multidrug-resistant bacteria [64]. Multidrug-resistant bacteria, such as vancomycin resistant enterococcus (VRE), carbapenemase-producing enterobacteria (CPE), and extended-spectrum beta-lactamase (ESBL)-carrying strains, represent a major public health issue because they are potential pathogens associated with a high mortality rate [64, 65]. Prevention strategies could be based on the use of probiotics to prevent the colonization of the colon microbiota. Transient colonization with multidrug-resistant bacteria could result in the transfer of antibiotic resistance genes in commensals or potential pathogens, resulting in the persistence of the resistance gene in the microbiota, which could be responsible for an increased risk of lethal infection due to the delay in introducing an effective antibiotic [64, 66]. Surprisingly, clinical cases demonstrated that fecal transplantation was able to cause decolonization of microbiota of naturally resistant Extended Spectrum β-lactamase (ESBL) bacterial strains [67–69]. Furthermore, there are reports that the composition of the microbiota of hospitalized patients is related to the susceptibility to colonization with multiresistant bacteria. The use of probiotic microorganisms such as *L. plantarum* or *L. fermentum* reduced the colonization of resistant pathogens such as *Acinetobacter baumannii*, *Pseudomonas aeruginosa* or *Candida albicans* [70, 71]. Nevertheless, an in vitro study showed that the culture supernatants of *Clostridium butyricum*, *C. difficile*, *Clostridium perfringens*, *Enterococcus faecium*, and *L. plantarum* were able to suppress the growth and transmission of gene resistance of bacteria carrying ESBL and Carbapenemase-Producing Enterobacteriaceae (CPE) [64]. It is undeniable that both colonization by probiotics and the use of their by-products have great potential in the treatment and prevention of infections, however these properties are still scarcely explored.

Vancomycin-resistant enterococci (VRE) seem less adapted to survival in the intestinal microbiota. Thus, these pathogens are more susceptible to decolonization when compared to other multiresistant bacteria. The intestinal microbiota in patients suffering from hematologic malignancies is less frequently colonized by VRE in the presence of *Barnesiella* [7]. In vivo evidence demonstrates that supplementing resident microbiota with *Barnesiella* or *Lactobacillus paracasei* CNCM I-3689 reduces VRE colonization in mice [72, 73]. In clinics, a case report showed VRE decolonization after fecal grafting for the treatment of *C. difficile colitis* [64].

The clinical use of probiotics in the treatment of infection is challenging the thinking of encapsulation for delivery. It is necessary to maintain the viability of these microorganisms long enough to compete with pathogenic microorganisms. Next, we'll discuss different potential encapsulation modalities for delivery.

4. Biomaterials for encapsulation of probiotics

The drug delivery systems through liposomes, micelles, carbon nanotubes, and dendrimers allowed the increase of therapeutic efficacy, reduction of toxicity, sustained and controlled release [74, 75]. The biotechnology industry has been aiming at the development of techniques for encapsulating probiotics, since their health benefits are indisputable. However, unlike inert substances, probiotics are live microorganisms, which in a way is a challenge in their manufacture, as they must be kept in a live/viable state during the processing, storage, and gastrointestinal transit steps to ensure its effectiveness on target sites [75].

The encapsulation technique consists of a set of physical–chemical or mechanical processes in which solid, liquid or gaseous materials are packaged, trapped in another material, usually hydrocolloidal materials, resulting in the formation of particles that vary in shape and size (from nanometer to millimeter) [76–78].

The encapsulated part is named core material, internal phase, active agent, or payload phase, and the encapsulating agent is called the carrier, shell, external phase, or matrix [78]. From these components, the encapsulation forms different structures: reservoir (where the core is surrounded by a shell), matrix (the internal phase is distributed on the surface), or coated matrix, in which matrix is surrounded by an additional coating layer [78].

The use of nanoencapsulation techniques (<1 μm) is not feasible because of the size of the bacteria (1 to 5 μm) [76]. On the other hand, it is possible to obtain microcapsules using other techniques [79, 80]. The first microencapsulation techniques applied were spray drying, freeze-drying or lyophilization, foam drying, and fluidized bed drying [78]. Other techniques used are extrusion, emulsion technologies, gel particles, coacervation, and electrospraying [76, 78, 81].

The encapsulation of probiotics can be made using natural polymers, such as polysaccharides, polypeptides, and polynucleotides, or synthetic polymers. Conventionally, three processes are involved in encapsulation. First, the cells must be incorporated into a matrix, which can be liquid (by dissolution or dispersion) or solid (by agglomeration or adsorption). Then the solution must be dispersed (liquids) or sprayed (solids) on the surface. The last process aims to stabilize the structure, through polymerization, gelling, solidification, evaporation, coacervation, or coalescence [79].

Before choosing the technique, it is necessary to consider some important criteria: the relationship between the composition of the material, type of bacteria, temperature and pH of the medium, as well as the host's immune response. The biocompatibility of the material used in the encapsulation is directly related to the viability of the probiotics, which must remain equal to or greater than 107 CFU/ml [82, 83]. Therefore, factors such as solubility, digestibility, and release capacity must also be carefully analyzed [84]. Consequently, it is expected that the biomaterial will be able to form an effective protective barrier to resist pH variations and ensure the survival of bacteria, without causing damage to the host organism. Next, some biomaterials commonly used for the encapsulation of probiotics will be discussed.

4.1 Alginate

It is a natural polysaccharide composed of alginic acid (β-D-manuronic acid and L-gunoronic acid), obtained through some types of seaweed (laminaria). It is considered the most used material for the encapsulation of probiotics. Calcium alginate is preferable because it associates the biocompatibility of the material with a simple and low-cost technique. However, some disadvantages are attributed, such as the high porosity of the particles, which can reduce the protection of cells in the matrix [85] and sensitization in an acid medium [86]. Nonetheless, the association of alginate with other polymeric components or the addition of additives to the surface of the particles can easily overcome these defects [87]. Alginate spheres reach the intestine satisfactorily, without undergoing significant degradation by stomach acids [88]. Besides, the structural configuration of the probiotic encapsulation to alginate is comparable to the beneficial biofilm formation by probiotics bacteria [89].

4.2 Chitosan

It is a biodegradable copolymer obtained from the deacetylation of chitin (polysaccharide) present in the crustacean exoskeleton. It consists of units of D-glucosamine, capable of forming polymeric networks through Cross-link due to the presence of free amino groups. It is commonly found associated with another polymer since studies have shown that its isolated use in the matrix does not contribute to the maintenance of cell viability [86]. When applied in multilayers together with calcium alginate, have shown promising results, where the particles are coated with chitosan forming polyelectrolyte complexes that reinforce the alginate structure [89, 90]. Although its use is relatively common, care should be taken when choosing this biomaterial to encapsulate some types of bacteria, such as those from lactic acid, since chitosan can cause their inhibition [91]. Additionally, its solubility is directly related to the pH of the medium, being insoluble at pH higher than 5.5 [92], which may result in null or insufficient release.

4.3 Carrageenan

These natural polymers are extracted from red algae (Rhodophyceae) and are commonly used as additives in the food industry. Three variables are found: (kappa) k-carryenink, (iota) i-carrageenan and (lambda) λ-carrageenan [93]. The use for encapsulation of probiotics is based on the sol–gel transition characteristics of the types k-carrageenan and i-carrageenan [93]. The dissolution of the polymer occurs after heating in a temperature range between 40 and 45°C, at which point the bacteria must be incorporated. Subsequently, the solution is stored at room temperature allowing gelation to occur, forming a three-dimensional gel [87]. Studies have shown that bacteria have been kept viable, demonstrating a promising effect of the use of carrageenan [94–96].

4.4 Gellan gum

This polysaccharide comes from the bacterium *Sphingomonas elodea*. It is composed of glucose (60%), rhamnose (20%), and gluconic acid (20%). These microbial polysaccharides are considered water-soluble polymers and are commonly used as solidifying, gelling, or stabilizing agents [97]. Other microbial polysaccharides, such as arabic gum, jamilam, and xanthan gum, when associated with gelam gum, become very promising for the encapsulation of probiotics [98].

4.5 Cellulose acetate phthalate (CAP)

They are polysaccharides derived from plants that have important characteristics, such as insolubility at pH below 5 and solubility at pH above 6. Thus, it can be used effectively to enable encapsulated probiotics to reach the intestine and be released gradually without being altered by stomach pH [99]. CAP does not form a gel, therefore, it is used as a coating agent for other biomaterials.

4.6 Starches

Another polysaccharide extracted from plants. Resistance to degradation by pancreatic enzymes present in the small intestine is an interesting characteristic that justifies its use as a probiotic delivery agent, guaranteeing the viability of bacteria when reaching the large intestine [86, 100]. It is commonly associated with alginate or carrageenan to form resistant capsules or gels [87, 101].

4.7 Synthetic polymers

The use of synthetic material for encapsulating probiotics requires that it must be a biodegradable material and provide bacterial viability. An example of these polymers is PVA - poly (vinyl alcohol), characterized by being soluble in water, chemically stable, and of low cost. Studies have shown that its use the use of this material alone [102] or associated with other biomaterials [103] is satisfactory while maintaining the viability of probiotic microorganisms. Poly(lactic acid) (PLA), poly(glycolic acid) (PGA), poly(lactic-co-glycolic acid) (PLGA), poly(ethylene glycol) (PEG), poly(ethylene oxide) (PEO), and poly(vinyl pyrrolidone) (PVP) are other synthetic polymers used for encapsulation of probiotics synthetic polymers used for encapsulation of probiotics [84]. The use of these polymers is linked to the technique of producing fibers through electrospinning.

All of these alternatives mentioned aim to encapsulate probiotics for intestinal delivery. Although they can be applied to other tissues of the body, the data in the literature are incipient and need to be better analyzed for application in the treatment of other infections, such as those discussed in the next topic.

5. Prevention and treatment of infection with probiotics

The resistance of pathogenic microorganisms to synthetic antimicrobials and, consequently, the ineffectiveness of conventional therapies and recurrence of infections reflects the need to seek alternative and/or supplementary methods in the treatment protocols [104]. Probiotics are one of the methods and are considered promising, as they provide satisfactory results when facing infections of a bacterial, fungal and viral nature, whether in the intestinal, urinary, respiratory, female genital tracts, and in the oral cavity. In addition, it is safe and does not promote adverse effects on the human body [105, 106]. **Figure 1** schematizes the delivery of microencapsulated probiotic microorganisms in an epithelium colonized by pathogenic microorganisms for the treatment of an infection.

One indication of probiotics refers to the treatment of *Helicobacter pylori* infection, which is one of the most common chronic bacterial infections in humans, with approximately 4.4 billion infected individuals worldwide in 2015 [107]. *H. pylori* infection is associated with the development of gastric cancer, which represents one of the main global causes of cancer-related deaths [108, 109]. The treatment of *H. pylori* infection is based on its eradication, with the use of antibiotics, such as amoxicillin, clarithromycin, and metronidazole. However, antibiotic therapy promotes an imbalance in the intestinal microbiota and increased levels of resistant bacteria [110], as well as species associated with persistent gastric inflammation and gastric carcinogenesis [111]. This situation justifies probiotic supplementation, aiming to reduce undesirable changes in the intestinal microbiota, promote the eradication of *H. pylori* [108, 112], produce significant improvements in gastrointestinal symptoms, and, consequently, in the quality of life of individuals [108, 109]. The combination of probiotics with antibiotic therapy for the eradication of *H. pylori* was suggested in the Thailand Consensus, held in 2015 [110].

Probiotics, in addition to reducing the density of *H. pylori*, promote immune responses with reduced inflammatory status [112–115], significantly reduce adverse events related to antibiotic treatment, and improve patient compliance [109, 116]. Despite this evidence, it was highlighted in the Thailand Consensus, that most studies that evaluated the effects of probiotics on the eradication of *H. pylori* are of poor quality, compromising general recommendations. It has been suggested that

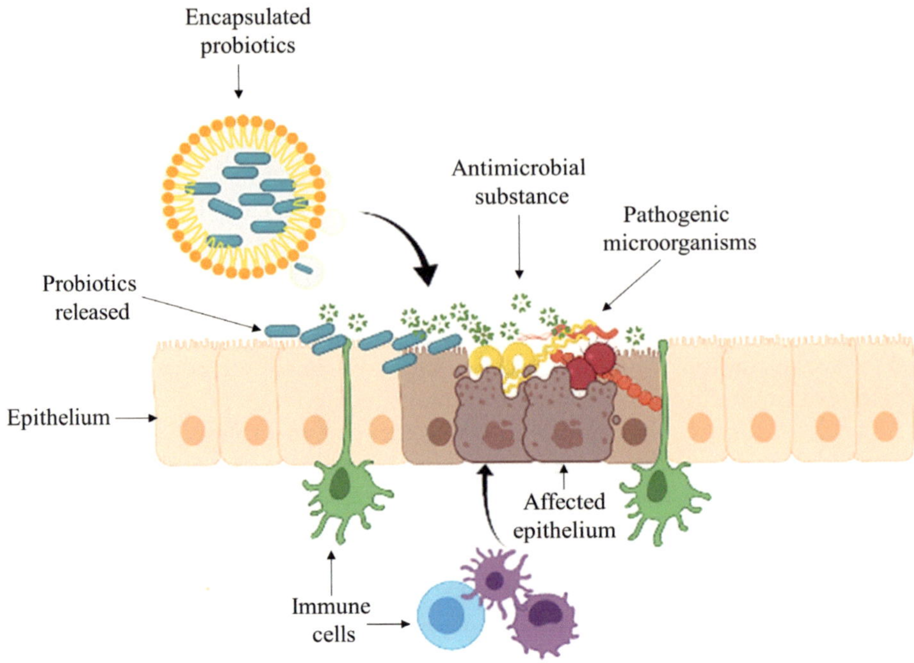

Figure 1.
Microencapsulated probiotics being delivered for the treatment of infection in epithelial tissue. Note that after the exit of the microorganisms from the micelle there is the colonization of the region and release of bacteriocins that in addition to acting as antimicrobials, stimulate the host's immune system.

further studies should be carried out to determine the best strain, the ideal dose, the duration of treatment, effectiveness, contraindications, and cost–benefit [110].

Probiotics are also indicated to reduce or prevent diarrhea associated with antibiotics and infections by *Clostridium difficile*, common in hospitalized patients [117, 118] and the elderly [119]. In children, its effectiveness in preventing antibiotic-associated diarrhea [120] and in treatment for acute gastroenteritis has not been confirmed, despite reducing the duration of hospitalization [121]. The use of probiotics in the treatment of infections by *Enterobacteriaceae* producing extended-spectrum β-lactamase has also been discussed. However, the results are incipient to indicate its use in eradication therapy in patients with prolonged intestinal transport of *Enterobacteriaceae* [122].

Some studies have suggested that supplementation with probiotics can improve the host's innate and acquired immune response, promoting a protective effect against respiratory infections [46, 123, 124]. The increase in the population of T cells, more precisely CD4 and CD8, is one of the most important mechanisms of the anti-infection effect of probiotics [125, 126]. Oral probiotics, when used in children, in addition to improving intestinal microecological balance can reduce the frequency of respiratory tract infections [89], mostly caused by viruses, such as the coronavirus [127], influenza [128], and bacteria, such as *Streptococcus pneumoniae*) [129]. Several studies have found that probiotics reduce episodes of acute respiratory tract infections in children, adults, the elderly, and athletes [89, 125, 126, 130, 131], proving its beneficial effect in these populations, with no reports of adverse effects in children [131].

The high recurrence of urinary tract infections in children [132] and the possibility of developing microbial resistance to drugs used against this disease have justified research with non-antibiotic alternatives, such as the use of probiotics for the prevention of recurrent urinary infections in this population

[133]. Probiotics appear to prevent recurrent urinary infections by contributing to the recovery and maintenance of microbiomes, by reducing the adherence, growth, and colonization of infectious pathogens in the urinary tract, in addition to improving host defenses, and attenuating or eliminating inflammation [105, 134–144]. Unlike the beneficial role of the use of probiotics in preventing urinary infections in children [132], it appears to have no protective effect in adults with severe spinal injuries, who have recurrent urinary infections [145], as well as in healthy young women [146].

Regarding the genital tract, the administration of probiotics, alone or as adjunctive therapy to the use of conventional antimicrobials, demonstrates success in the treatment of infections such as bacterial vaginosis and vulvovaginal candidiasis, common and recurrent infections in women of reproductive age. These infections that produce abnormal vaginal discharge, itching, vulvar odor, are associated with important health complications, such as the increased transmission of sexual infections, risk of premature birth, and pelvic inflammation, with negative impacts on quality of life [138, 147–149].

In infections that affect the mouth, candidiasis is also one of the most prevalent diseases, especially when local factors are predisposing the installation of the infection. Probiotics have been suggested for the treatment of oral candidiasis because they reduce the population of *Candida* ssp. [150], the course of treatment with conventional antifungal therapies [151], and the severity of clinical manifestations of the infection associated with prosthetic stomatitis [152, 153], including asymptomatic [62]. Besides, the immunological and antimicrobial potential of probiotics also can be used in the treatment of periodontal disease killing periodontopathogens, as Porphyromona gingivalis, and promoting the expression of some favorable immunoregulatory effects [154]. In summary, probiotics favor oral health, increasing fluids in the mucosa, reducing the accumulation of dental biofilm and gingival inflammation, improving the clinical signs characteristic of periodontal infection, such as redness and swelling [63, 155, 156].

Studies show beneficial effects of the combination of probiotics in the treatment regimen for different infections, with improvements in the clinical condition and patient adherence to treatment. Although, researchers warn of the need for further studies to define the best treatment protocol, including the determination of effects, contraindications, and cost–benefit [110].

6. Concluding remarks

Today's society is experiencing a public health problem related to an exponential increase in microbial resistance, compared to the slow evolution of new drug development. The human organism is attacked daily by countless pathogenic microorganisms, many of which cause lethal infections. The use of alternative therapies, alone or as an adjunct to antibiotics, is a reality. Concerning the use of probiotics, its effectiveness in modifying the microbial is unquestionable, either by the production of antimicrobial bacteriocins or by the modulation of the immune system. Nonetheless, there is no consensus or standardization for the clinical use of probiotics for the treatment of infectious diseases, except its use for the recomposition of the intestinal microbiota. Moreover, two important challenges need to be overcome: the standardization of carriers to deliver these microorganisms effectively to the treatment site and the definition of important factors, such as the mechanism of action, standardization of inoculum, and therapeutic protocols, based clinical trials. Thus, although promising, widespread antimicrobial therapy with probiotics is not yet a reality for clinical practice.

Conflict of interest

The authors declare no conflict of interest.

Author details

Diego Romario-Silva[1,2*], Otavio Akira Souza Sakaguchi[3], Andrea Cristina Barbosa da Silva[4], Janaína Orlandi Sardi[5], Rafaela Parolina de Carvalho[1], Sindy Magri Roque[1], Lincoln Pires Silva Borges[6], Rodrigo Barros Esteves Lins[7], Letícia Targino Campos[8] and Edja Maria Melo de Brito Costa[8]

1 Department of Physiological Sciences, Piracicaba Dental School, University of Campinas, Piracicaba, SP, Brazil

2 FAIPE-Institute of Research and Teaching Ltda, Cuiabá, MT, Brazil

3 Department of Dentistry, Northern College of Mato Grosso, Guarantã do Norte, MT, Brazil

4 Department of Pharmacy, Center of Biological and Health Sciences, State University of Paraiba, Campina Grande, PB, Brazil

5 Faculty of Pharmaceutical Sciences, Federal University of Mato Grosso do Sul, Pioneiros, MS, Brazil

6 Department of Dental Materials, Piracicaba Dental School, University of Campinas, Piracicaba, SP, Brazil

7 College of Dentistry, Science, Technology and Health Center, State University of Paraiba, Araruna, PB, Brazil

8 Department of Dentistry, State University of Paraiba, Campina Grande, PB, Brazil

*Address all correspondence to: diegoromarioo@gmail.com

References

[1] Sender R, Fuchs S, Milo R. Revised Estimates for the Number of Human and Bacteria Cells in the Body. PLoS biology. 2016;14(8):e1002533. DOI: 10.1371/journal.pbio.1002533

[2] Altveş S, Yildiz HK, Vural HC. Interaction of the microbiota with the human body in health and diseases. Bioscience of microbiota, food and health. 2020;39(2):23-32. DOI: 10.12938/bmfh.19-023

[3] Lilly DM, Stillwell RH. Probiotics: growth-promoting factors produced by microorganisms. Science. 1965;147:747-748. DOI: 10.1126/science.147.3659.747

[4] Food and Agriculture Organization and World Health Organization. FAO and WHO to hold first global forum of food safety regulators. [Internet]. 2001.1(101). Available from: https://fao.org/WAICENT/OIS/PRESS_NE/PRESSENG/2001/pren01101.htm [Accessed: 2021-05-22]

[5] Marco ML, Pavan S, Kleerebezem M. Towards understanding molecular modes of probiotic action. Curr Opin Biotechnol. 2006;17(2):204-10. DOI: 10.1016/j.copbio.2006.02.005

[6] Gupta V, Garg R. Probiotics. Indian J Med Microbiol. 2009;27(3):202-9. DOI: 10.4103/0255-0857.53201

[7] Ubeda C, Pamer EG. Antibiotics, microbiota, and immune defense. Trends Immunol. 2012;33(9):459-66. DOI: 10.1016/j.it.2012.05.003

[8] Tang C, Lu Z. Health promoting activities of probiotics. J Food Biochem. 2019;43(8):e12944. DOI: 10.1111/jfbc.12944

[9] Plaza-Díaz J, Ruiz-Ojeda FJ, Vilchez-Padial LM, Gil A. Evidence of the Anti-Inflammatory Effects of Probiotics and Synbiotics in Intestinal Chronic Diseases. Nutrients. 2017;9(6):555. DOI: 10.3390/nu9060555.

[10] Marinelli L, Tenore GC, Novellino E. Probiotic species in the modulation of the anticancer immune response. Semin Cancer Biol. 2017;46:182-190. DOI: 10.1016/j.semcancer.2017.08.007.

[11] Mishra V, Shah C, Mokashe N, Chavan R, Yadav H, Prajapati J. Probiotics as potential antioxidants: a systematic review. J Agric Food Chem. 2015;63(14):3615-26. DOI: 10.1021/jf506326t

[12] Baumgardner RM, Berreta A, Kopper JJ. Evaluation of commercial probiotics for antimicrobial resistance genes. Can Vet J. 2021;62(4):379-383.

[13] Quigley EMM. Prebiotics and Probiotics in Digestive Health. Clin Gastroenterol Hepatol. 2019;17(2):333-344. DOI: 10.1016/j.cgh.2018.09.028

[14] Silva DR, Sardi JCO, Pitangui NS, Roque SM, Silva ACB, Rosalen PL. Probiotics as an alternative antimicrobial therapy: Current reality and future directions. 2020:104080. DOI: 10.1016/j.jff.2020.104080

[15] Yang H, Sun Y, Cai R, Chen Y, Gu B. The impact of dietary fiber and probiotics in infectious diseases. Microbial Pathogenesis. 2019:103931.

[16] Lilly DM, Stillwell RH. Probiotics: Growth-promoting factors produced by microorganisms. Science. 1965;147(3659):747-8. DOI: 10.1126/science.147.3659.747.

[17] Hosono A. Fermented milk in the orient. In: Nakazawa Y, Hosono A. Functions of Fermented Milk: Challengers for the Health Sciences. Barking (UK): Elsevier Science Publishers Ltd; 1992. p. 61-78.

[18] Bezirtzoglou E, Stavropoulou E. Immunology and probiotic impact of the newborn and young children intestinal microflora. Anaerobe. 2011;17(6):369-74. DOI: 10.1016/j.anaerobe.2011.03.010.

[19] Bermudez-Brito M, Plaza-Díaz J, Muñoz-Quezada S, Gómez-Llorente C, Gil A. Probiotic mechanisms of action. Ann Nutr Metab. 2012;61(2):160-74. DOI: 10.1159/000342079.

[20] Reid G, Jass J, Sebulsky MT, McCormick JK. Potential uses of probiotics in clinical practice. Clin Microbiol Rev. 2003;16(4):658-72. DOI: 10.1128/cmr.16.4.658-672.2003.

[21] Melo Pereira GV, de Oliveira Coelho B, Magalhães Júnior AI, Thomaz-Soccol V, Soccol CR. How to select a probiotic? A review and update of methods and criteria. Biotechnol Adv. 2018;36:2060-2076.

[22] Stavropoulou E, Bezirtzoglou E. Probiotics in Medicine: A Long Debate. Frontiers in immunology. 2020;11:2192. DOI: 10.3389/fimmu.2020.02192

[23] Doron S, Snydman DR. Risk and safety of probiotics. Clin Infect Dis. 2015;60:S129–S134.

[24] Prado FC, Lindner JD, Inaba J, Thomaz-Soccol V, Brar SK, Soccol CR. Development and evaluation of a fermented coconut water beverage with potential health benefits. J Funct Foods. 2015;12:489-497.

[25] Soccol CR, Prado MRM, Garcia LMB, Rodrigues C, Medeiros ABP, Thomaz-Soccol V. Current developments in probiotics. J Microb Biochem Technol.118 2015;7:11-20.

[26] Karami S, Roayaei M, Hamzavi H, Bahmani M, Hassanzad-Azar H, Leila M, Rafieian-Kopaei M. Isolation and identification of probiotic Lactobacillus from local dairy and evaluating their antagonistic effect on pathogens. International journal of pharmaceutical investigation. 2017;7(3):137-141. DOI: 10.4103/jphi.JPHI_8_17

[27] Bazireh H, Shariati P, Azimzadeh Jamalkandi S, Ahmadi A, Boroumand MA. Isolation of Novel Probiotic Lactobacillus and Enterococcus Strains From Human Salivary and Fecal Sources. Front Microbiol. 2020;11:597946. DOI: 10.3389/fmicb.2020.597946.

[28] Jungersen M, Wind A, Johansen E, Christensen JE, Stuer-Lauridsen B, Eskesen D. The Science behind the Probiotic Strain Bifidobacterium animalis subsp. lactis BB-12(®). Microorganisms. 2014;2(2):92-110. doi: 10.3390/microorganisms2020092

[29] Reuter G. The Lactobacillus and Bifidobacterium microflora of the human intestine: composition and succession. Curr Issues Intest Microbiol. 2001;2(2):43-53.

[30] Milani C, Mangifesta M, Mancabelli L, Lugli GA, James K, Duranti S, Turroni F, Ferrario C, Ossiprandi MC, van Sinderen D, Ventura M. Unveiling bifidobacterial biogeography across the mammalian branch of the tree of life. ISME J. 2017;11(12):2834-2847. DOI: 10.1038/ismej.2017.138

[31] Yamamoto E, Watanabe R, Koizumi A, Ishida T, Kimura K. Isolation and characterization of Streptococcus thermophilus possessing prtS gene from raw milk in Japan. Biosci Microbiota Food Health. 2020;39(3):169-174. DOI: 10.12938/bmfh.2019-052

[32] Xiong ZQ, Kong LH, Lai PF, Xia YJ, Liu JC, Li QY, Ai LZ. Genomic and phenotypic analyses of exopolysaccharide biosynthesis in

Streptococcus thermophilus S-3. J Dairy Sci. 2019;102(6):4925-4934. DOI: 10.3168/jds.2018-15572

[33] Fisher K, Phillips C. The ecology, epidemiology and virulence of Enterococcus. Microbiology (Reading). 2009;155(Pt 6):1749-1757. DOI: 10.1099/mic.0.026385-0

[34] Reuben RC, Roy PC, Sarkar SL, Alam RU, Jahid IK. Isolation, characterization, and assessment of lactic acid bacteria toward their selection as poultry probiotics. BMC Microbiol. 2019;19(1):253. DOI: 10.1186/s12866-019-1626-0

[35] Madoshi BP, Mtambo MMA, Muhairwa AP, Lupindu AM, Olsen JE. Isolation of vancomycin-resistant Enterococcus from apparently healthy human animal attendants, cattle and cattle wastes in Tanzania. J Appl Microbiol. 2018;124(5):1303-1310. DOI: 10.1111/jam.13722

[36] Bhagat D, Raina N, Kumar A, Katoch M, Khajuria Y, Slathia PS, Sharma P. Probiotic properties of a phytase producing Pediococcus acidilactici strain SMVDUDB2 isolated from traditional fermented cheese product, Kalarei. Sci Rep. 2020;10(1):1926. DOI: 10.1038/s41598-020-58676-2

[37] Leroy F, De Vuyst L. Simulation of the effect of sausage ingredients and technology on the functionality of the bacteriocin-producing Lactobacillus sakei CTC 494 strain. Int J Food Microbiol. 2005;100(1-3):141-52. DOI: 10.1016/j.ijfoodmicro.2004.10.011

[38] Sajedinejad N, Paknejad M, Houshmand B, Sharafi H, Jelodar R, Shahbani Zahiri H, Noghabi KA. Lactobacillus salivarius NK02: a Potent Probiotic for Clinical Application in Mouthwash. Probiotics Antimicrob Proteins. 2018;10(3):485-495. DOI: 10.1007/s12602-017-9296-4

[39] Lopes EG, Moreira DA, Gullón P, Gullón B, Cardelle-Cobas A, Tavaria FK. Topical application of probiotics in skin: adhesion, antimicrobial and antibiofilm in vitro assays. J Appl Microbiol. 2017;122(2):450-461. DOI: 10.1111/jam.13349

[40] Rossoni RD, Fuchs BB, de Barros PP, Velloso MD, Jorge AO, Junqueira JC, Mylonakis E. Lactobacillus paracasei modulates the immune system of Galleria mellonella and protects against *Candida albicans* infection. PLoS One. 2017;12(3):e0173332. DOI: 10.1371/journal.pone.0173332

[41] Markowiak P, Śliżewska K. Effects of Probiotics, Prebiotics, and Synbiotics on Human Health. Nutrients. 2017;9(9):1021. DOI: 10.3390/nu9091021

[42] de Moraes GMD, de Abreu LR, do Egito AS, Salles HO, da Silva LMF, Nero LA, Todorov SD, Dos Santos KMO. Functional Properties of Lactobacillus mucosae Strains Isolated from Brazilian Goat Milk. Probiotics Antimicrob Proteins. 2017;9(3):235-245. DOI: 10.1007/s12602-016-9244-8

[43] Goderska K, Agudo Pena S, Alarcon T. Helicobacter pylori treatment: antibiotics or probiotics. Appl Microbiol Biotechnol. 2018;102(1):1-7. DOI: 10.1007/s00253-017-8535-7

[44] Neal-McKinney JM, Lu X, Duong T, Larson CL, Call DR, Shah DH, Konkel ME. Production of organic acids by probiotic lactobacilli can be used to reduce pathogen load in poultry. PLoS One. 2012;7(9):e43928. DOI: 10.1371/journal.pone.0043928

[45] Sikorska H, Smoragiewicz W. Role of probiotics in the prevention and treatment of meticillin-resistant *Staphylococcus aureus* infections. Int J Antimicrob Agents. 2013;42(6):475-81. DOI: 10.1016/j.ijantimicag.2013.08.003

[46] Dong H, Rowland I, Thomas LV, Yaqoob P. Immunomodulatory effects of a probiotic drink containing Lactobacillus casei Shirota in healthy older volunteers. Eur J Nutr. 2013;52(8):1853-1863.

[47] Ganguli K, Meng D, Rautava S, Lu L, Walker WA, Nanthakumar N. Probiotics prevent necrotizing enterocolitis by modulating enterocyte genes that regulate innate immune-mediated inflammation. Am J Physiol Gastrointest Liver Physiol. 2013;304(2):G132-41. DOI: 10.1152/ajpgi.00142.2012

[48] Matsubara VH, Wang Y, Bandara HMHN, Mayer MPA, Samaranayake LP. Probiotic lactobacilli inhibit early stages of *Candida albicans* biofilm development by reducing their growth, cell adhesion, and filamentation. Appl Microbiol Biotechnol. 2016;100(14):6415-6426. DOI: 10.1007/s00253-016-7527-3

[49] Yang HL, Xia HQ, Ye YD, Zou WC, Sun YZ. Probiotic *Bacillus pumilus* SE5 shapes the intestinal microbiota and mucosal immunity in grouper *Epinephelus coioides*. Dis Aquat Organ. 2014;111(2):119-27. DOI: 10.3354/dao02772

[50] Yu AQ, Li L. The Potential Role of Probiotics in Cancer Prevention and Treatment. Nutr Cancer. 2016;68(4):535-44. DOI: 10.1080/01635581.2016.1158300

[51] Wollowski I, Rechkemmer G, Pool-Zobel BL. Protective role of probiotics and prebiotics in colon cancer. Am J Clin Nutr. 2001;73(2):451S-455S. DOI: 10.1093/ajcn/73.2.451s

[52] Devaraj NK, Suppiah S, Veettil SK, Ching SM, Lee KW, Menon RK, Soo MJ, Deuraseh I, Hoo FK, Sivaratnam D. The Effects of Probiotic Supplementation on the Incidence of Diarrhea in Cancer Patients Receiving Radiation Therapy: A Systematic Review with Meta-Analysis and Trial Sequential Analysis of Randomized Controlled Trials. Nutrients. 2019;11(12):2886. DOI: 10.3390/nu11122886

[53] Clancy R. Immunobiotics and the probiotic evolution. FEMS Immunol Med Microbiol. 2003;38(1):9-12. DOI: 10.1016/S0928-8244(03)00147-0

[54] Liu MM, Li ST, Shu Y, Zhan HQ. Probiotics for prevention of radiation-induced diarrhea: A meta-analysis of randomized controlled trials. PLoS One. 2017;12(6):e0178870. DOI: 10.1371/journal.pone.0178870

[55] Casas-Solís J, Huizar-López M, Irecta-Nájera C, Pita-López M, Santerre A. Immunomodulatory Effect of Lactobacillus casei in a Murine Model of Colon Carcinogenesis. Probiotics and Antimicrobial Proteins. 2020;12. DOI: 10.1007/s12602-019-09611-z

[56] Rather IA, Bajpai VK, Kumar S, Lim J, Paek WK, Park YH. Probiotics and Atopic Dermatitis: An Overview. Front Microbiol. 2016;7:507. DOI: 10.3389/fmicb.2016.00507

[57] Huang R, Ning H, Shen M, Li J, Zhang J, Chen X. Probiotics for the Treatment of Atopic Dermatitis in Children: A Systematic Review and Meta-Analysis of Randomized Controlled Trials. Front Cell Infect Microbiol. 2017;7:392. DOI: 10.3389/fcimb.2017.00392

[58] Lise M, Mayer I, Silveira M. Use of probiotics in atopic dermatitis. Rev Assoc Med Bras (1992). 2018;64(11):997-1001. DOI: 10.1590/1806-9282.64.11.997

[59] Shimizu M, Hashiguchi M, Shiga T, Tamura HO, Mochizuki M. Meta-Analysis: Effects of Probiotic Supplementation on Lipid Profiles in Normal to Mildly Hypercholesterolemic

Individuals. PLoS One. 2015;10(10):e0139795. DOI: 10.1371/journal.pone.0139795

[60] Nath A, Molnár MA, Csighy A, Kőszegi K, Galambos I, Huszár KP, Koris A, Vatai G. Biological Activities of Lactose-Based Prebiotics and Symbiosis with Probiotics on Controlling Osteoporosis, Blood-Lipid and Glucose Levels. Medicina (Kaunas). 2018;54(6):98. DOI: 10.3390/medicina54060098

[61] Tahmourespour A, Kermanshahi RK. The effect of a probiotic strain (Lactobacillus acidophilus) on the plaque formation of oral Streptococci. Bosn J Basic Med Sci. 2011;11(1):37-40. DOI: 10.17305/bjbms.2011.2621

[62] Ishikawa KH, Mayer MP, Miyazima TY, Matsubara VH, Silva EG, Paula CR, Campos TT, Nakamae AE. A multispecies probiotic reduces oral Candida colonization in denture wearers. J Prosthodont. 2015;24(3):194-9. DOI: 10.1111/jopr.12198.

[63] Kuru BE, Laleman I, Yalnızoğlu T, Kuru L, Teughels W. The Influence of a Bifidobacterium animalis Probiotic on Gingival Health: A Randomized Controlled Clinical Trial. J Periodontol. 2017;88(11):1115-1123. DOI: 10.1902/jop.2017.170213.

[64] Wieërs G, Belkhir L, Enaud R, Leclercq S, Philippart de Foy JM, Dequenne I, de Timary P, Cani PD. How Probiotics Affect the Microbiota. Front Cell Infect Microbiol. 2020;9:454. DOI: 10.3389/fcimb.2019.00454

[65] Caballero S, Carter R, Ke X, Sušac B, Leiner IM, Kim GJ, Miller L, Ling L, Manova K, Pamer EG. Distinct but Spatially Overlapping Intestinal Niches for Vancomycin-Resistant Enterococcus faecium and Carbapenem-Resistant *Klebsiella pneumoniae*. PLoS Pathog. 2015;11(9):e1005132. doi: 10.1371/journal.ppat.1005132.

[66] Kaushik SB, Lebwohl MG. Psoriasis: Which therapy for which patient: Focus on special populations and chronic infections. J Am Acad Dermatol. 2019;80(1):43-53. DOI: 10.1016/j.jaad.2018.06.056

[67] Singh V, Kumar A, Raheja G, Anbazhagan AN, Priyamvada S, Saksena S, Jhandier MN, Gill RK, Alrefai WA, Borthakur A, Dudeja PK. Lactobacillus acidophilus attenuates downregulation of DRA function and expression in inflammatory models. Am J Physiol Gastrointest Liver Physiol. 2014;307(6):G623-31. DOI: 10.1152/ajpgi.00104.2014

[68] Crum-Cianflone NF, Sullivan E, Ballon-Landa G. Fecal microbiota transplantation and successful resolution of multidrug-resistant-organism colonization. J Clin Microbiol. 2015;53(6):1986-9. DOI: 10.1128/JCM.00820-15

[69] Millan B, Park H, Hotte N, Mathieu O, Burguiere P, Tompkins TA, Kao D, Madsen KL. Fecal Microbial Transplants Reduce Antibiotic-resistant Genes in Patients With Recurrent *Clostridium difficile* Infection. Clin Infect Dis. 2016;62(12):1479-1486. DOI: 10.1093/cid/ciw185

[70] Singhi SC, Kumar S. Probiotics in critically ill children. F1000Res. 2016;5:F1000 Faculty Rev-407. doi: 10.12688/f1000research.7630.1

[71] Soltan Dallal MM, Zamaniahari S, Davoodabadi A, Hosseini M, Rajabi Z. Identification and characterization of probiotic lactic acid bacteria isolated from traditional persian pickled vegetables. GMS Hyg Infect Control. 2017;12:Doc15. DOI: 10.3205/dgkh000300

[72] Tannock GW, Munro K, Harmsen HJ, Welling GW, Smart J, Gopal PK. Analysis of the fecal microflora of human subjects

consuming a probiotic product containing Lactobacillus rhamnosus DR20. Appl Environ Microbiol. 2000;66(6):2578-88. DOI: 10.1128/aem.66.6.2578-2588.2000

[73] Crouzet L, Derrien M, Cherbuy C, Plancade S, Foulon M, Chalin B, van Hylckama Vlieg JET, Grompone G, Rigottier-Gois L, Serror P. Lactobacillus paracasei CNCM I-3689 reduces vancomycin-resistant Enterococcus persistence and promotes Bacteroidetes resilience in the gut following antibiotic challenge. Sci Rep. 2018;8(1):5098. DOI: 10.1038/s41598-018-23437-9

[74] Singh MN, Hemant KS, Ram M, Shivakumar HG. Microencapsulation: A promising technique for controlled drug delivery. Res Pharm Sci. 2010;5(2):65-77.

[75] Sarao LK, Arora M. Probiotics, prebiotics, and microencapsulation: A review. Crit Rev Food Sci Nutr. 2017;57(2):344-371. DOI: 10.1080/10408398.2014.887055

[76] Champagne CP, Fustier P. Microencapsulation for the improved delivery of bioactive compounds into foods. Curr Opin Biotechnol. 2007;18(2):184-90.

[77] Chen MJ, Chen KN. Applications of Probiotic Encapsulation. In: Dairy Products. Encapsulation Control Release Technol Food Syst. 2007. p. 83-112. DOI: 10.1002/9780470277881.ch4

[78] Asgari S, Pourjavadi A, Licht TR, Boisen A, Ajalloueian F. Polymeric carriers for enhanced delivery of probiotics. Adv Drug Deliv Rev. 2020;161-162:1-21. DOI: 10.1016/j.addr.2020.07.014

[79] Burgain J, Gaiani C, Linder M, Scher J. Encapsulation of probiotic living cells: From laboratory scale to industrial applications. J Food Eng. Elsevier Ltd. 2011;104:467-83. DOI: 10.1016/j.jfoodeng.2010.12.031

[80] Sundus KSY, Sayantani N, Moses DJA. Targeted Delivery of Probiotics : Perspectives on Research and Commercialization. Probiotics Antimicrob. Proteins. Springer US. 2021. DOI: 10.1007/s12602-021-09791-7

[81] Rodrigues FJ, Cedran MF, Bicas JL, Sato HH. Encapsulated probiotic cells: Relevant techniques, natural sources as encapsulating materials and food applications – A narrative review. Food Res Int. 2020;137:109682. DOI: 10.1016/j.foodres.2020.109682

[82] Rossier-Miranda FJ, Schroën K, Boom R. Mechanical characterization and pH response of fibril-reinforced microcapsules prepared by layer-by-layer adsorption. Langmuir. 2010;26(24):19106-13. DOI: 10.1021/la1033542

[83] Serna L, Vallejo-Castillo, V. Probiotic encapsulation. African journal of microbiology research. 2013;7:4743. DOI: 10.5897/AJMR2013.5718.

[84] Yoha KS, Nida S, Dutta S, Moses JA, Anandharamakrishnan C. Targeted Delivery of Probiotics: Perspectives on Research and Commercialization. Probiotics Antimicrob Proteins. 2021;27:1-34. DOI: 10.1007/s12602-021-09791-7

[85] Gouin S. Microencapsulation: Industrial appraisal of existing technologies and trends. Trends Food Sci Technol. 2004;15:330-47.

[86] Mortazavian AM, Azizi A, Ehsani MR, Razavi SH, Mousavi SM, Sohrabvandi S, Reinheimer JA. Survival of encapsulated probiotic bacteria in Iranian yogurt drink (Doogh) after the product exposure to simulated gastrointestinal conditions. Milchwissenschaft. 2008;63(4):427-429.

[87] Krasaekoopt W, Bhandari B, Deeth H. Evaluation of encapsulation techniques of probiotics for yoghurt. Int Dairy J. 2003;13:3-13.

[88] Rayment P, Wright P, Hoad C, Ciampi E, Haydock D, Gowland P, et al. Investigation of alginate beads for gastro-intestinal functionality, Part 1: In vitro characterisation. Food Hydrocoll. Elsevier Ltd. 2009;23:816-22. DOI: 10.1016/j.foodhyd.2008.04.011

[89] Li KL, Wang BZ, Li ZP, Li YL, Liang JJ. Alterations of intestinal flora and the effects of probiotics in children with recurrent respiratory tract infection. World J Pediatr. 2019;15(3):255-261. DOI: 10.1007/s12519-019-00248-0.

[90] Lee JS, Cha DS, Park HJ. Survival of freeze-dried Lactobacillus bulgaricus KFRI 673 in chitosan-coated calcium alginate microparticles. J Agric Food Chem. 2004;52:7300-5.

[91] Groboillot AF, Champagne CP, Darling GD, Poncelet D, Neufeld RJ. Membrane formation by interfacial cross-linking of chitosan for microencapsulation of Lactococcus lactis. Biotechnol Bioeng. 1993;42(10):1157-63. DOI: 10.1002/bit.260421005

[92] Huguet ML, Neufeld RJ, Dellacherie E. Calcium-alginate beads coated with polycationic polymers: Comparison of chitosan and DEAE-dextran. Process Biochem. 1996;31:347-53.

[93] Yuguchi Y, Thu Thuy TT, Urakawa H, Kajiwara K. Structural characteristics of carrageenan gels: Temperature and concentration dependence. Food Hydrocoll. 2002;16:515-22.

[94] Dinakar P, Mistry VV. Growth and viability of Bifidobacterium bifidum in cheddar cheese. J Dairy Sci. 1994; 77(10):2854-64. DOI: 10.3168/jds.S0022-030(94)77225-8

[95] Dafe A, Etemadi H, Zarredar H, Mahdavinia GR. Development of novel carboxymethyl cellulose/k-carrageenan blends as an enteric delivery vehicle for probiotic bacteria. Int J Biol Macromol. Elsevier B.V. 2017;97:299-307. DOI: 10.1016/j.ijbiomac.2017.01.016

[96] Gutiérrez-Zamorano C, González-Ávila M, Díaz-Blas G, Smith CT, González-Correa C, García-Cancino A. Increased anti-Helicobacter pylori effect of the probiotic Lactobacillus fermentum UCO-979C strain encapsulated in carrageenan evaluated in gastric simulations under fasting conditions. Food Res Int. Elsevier. 2019;121:812-6. DOI: 10.1016/j.foodres.2018.12.064

[97] Bajaj IB, Survase SA, Saudagar PS, Singhal RS. Gellan gum: Fermentative production, downstream processing and applications. Food Technol Biotechnol. 2007;45:341-54.

[98] Jiménez-Pranteda ML, Poncelet D, Náder-Macías ME, Arcos A, Aguilera M, Monteoliva-Sánchez M, et al. Stability of lactobacilli encapsulated in various microbial polymers. J Biosci Bioeng [Internet]. The Society for Biotechnology, Japan. 2012;113:179-84. DOI: 10.1016/j.jbiosc.2011.10.010

[99] Fávaro-Trindade CS, Grosso CRF. Microencapsulation of L. acidophilus (La-05) and B. Lactis (Bb-12) and evaluation of their survival at the pH values of the stomach and in bile. Journal of Microencapsulation. 2002;19(4):485-494.

[100] Crittenden R, Laitila A, Forsell P, Matto J, Saarela M, Mattila-Sandholm T, Myllarinen P. Adhesion of bifidobacteria to granular starch and its implications in probiotic technologies. Applied and Environmental Microbiology. 2001;67(8):3469-3475.

[101] Martin MJ, Lara-Villoslada F, Ruiz MA, Morales ME. Effect of unmodified starch on viability of alginate-encapsulated Lactobacillus

fermentum CECT5716. LWT - Food Sci Technol. Elsevier Ltd. 2013;53:480-6. DOI: 10.1016/j.lwt.2013.03.019

[102] López-Rubio A, Sanchez E, Sanz Y, Lagaron JM. Encapsulation of living bifidobacteria in ultrathin PVOH electrospun fibers. Biomacromolecules. 2009;10:2823-9.

[103] Çanga EM, Dudak FC. Improved digestive stability of probiotics encapsulated within poly(vinyl alcohol)/cellulose acetate hybrid fibers. Carbohydr Polym. Elsevier Ltd. 2021;264.

[104] Klarin B, Adolfsson A, Torstensson A, Larsson A. Can probiotics be an alternative to chlorhexidine for oral care in the mechanically ventilated patient? A multicentre, prospective, randomised controlled open trial. Crit Care. 2018;22(1):272. DOI: 10.1186/s13054-018-2209-4.

[105] Rostok M, Hütt P, Rööp T, Smidt I, Štšepetova J, Salumets A, Mändar R. Potential vaginal probiotics: safety, tolerability and preliminary effectiveness. Benef Microbes. 2019;10(4):385-393. DOI: 10.3920/BM2016.0123.

[106] De Gregorio PR, Maldonado NC, Pingitore EV, Terraf MCL, Tomás MSJ, de Ruiz CS, Santos V, Wiese B, Bru E, Paiz MC, Reina MF, Schujman DE, Nader-Macías MEF. Intravaginal administration of gelatine capsules containing freeze-dried autochthonous lactobacilli: a double-blind, randomised clinical trial of safety. Benef Microbes. 2020;11(1):5-17. DOI: 10.3920/BM2019.0081.

[107] Hooi JKY, Lai WY, Ng WK, Suen MMY, Underwood FE, Tanyingoh D, Malfertheiner P, Graham DY, Wong VWS, Wu JCY, Chan FKL, Sung JJY, Kaplan GG, Ng SC. Global Prevalence of Helicobacter pylori Infection: Systematic Review and Meta-Analysis. Gastroenterology. 2017;153(2):420-429. DOI: 10.1053/j.gastro.2017.04.022

[108] Oh B, Kim BS, Kim JW, Kim JS, Koh SJ, Kim BG, Lee KL, Chun J. The Effect of Probiotics on Gut Microbiota during the Helicobacter pylori Eradication: Randomized Controlled Trial. Helicobacter. 2016;21(3):165-74. DOI: 10.1111/hel.12270.

[109] Poonyam P, Chotivitayatarakorn P, Vilaichone RK. High Effective of 14-Day High-Dose PPI-Bismuth-Containing Quadruple Therapy with Probiotics Supplement for Helicobacter Pylori Eradication: A Double Blinded-Randomized Placebo-Controlled Study. Asian Pac J Cancer Prev. 2019;20(9):2859-2864. DOI: 10.31557/APJCP.2019.20.9.2859

[110] Mahachai V, Vilaichone RK, Pittayanon R, Rojborwonwitaya J, Leelakusolvong S, Kositchaiwat C, Mairiang P, Praisontarangkul OA, Ovartlarnporn B, Sottisuporn J, Pisespongsa P, Maneerattanaporn M, Sony R, Sirinthornpunya S, Chaiyamahapurk O, Wiwattanachang O, Sansak I, Harnsomboon P, Chitapanarux T, Chuenrattanakul S. Thailand Consensus on Helicobacter pylori Treatment 2015. Asian Pac J Cancer Prev. 2016;17(5):2351-2360. DOI: 10.7314/APJCP.2016.17.5.2351

[111] Sung JJY, Coker OO, Chu E, Szeto CH, Luk STY, Lau HCH, Yu J. Gastric microbes associated with gastric inflammation, atrophy and intestinal metaplasia 1 year after Helicobacter pylori eradication. Gut. 2020;69:1572-1581. DOI: 10.1136/gutjnl-2019-319826

[112] Yoon JY, Cha JM, Hong SS, Kim HK, Kwak MS, Jeon JW, Shin HP. Fermented milk containing Lactobacillus paracasei and *Glycyrrhiza glabra* has a beneficial effect in patients with Helicobacter pylori infection. A

randomized, double-blind, placebo-controlled study. Medicine. 2019;98:35. DOI: 10.1097/MD.0000000000016601

[113] Çekin AH, Şahintürk Y, Harmandar FA, Uyar S, Yolcular BO, Çekin Y. Use of probiotics as an adjuvant to sequential *H. pylori* eradication therapy: impact on eradication rates, treatment resistance, treatment-related side effects, and patient compliance. Turk J Gastroenterol. 2017;28(1):3-11. DOI: 10.5152/tjg.2016.0278.

[114] Chen L, Xu W, Lee A, He J, Huang B, Zheng W, Su T, Lai S, Long Y, Chu H, Chen Y, Wang L, Wang K, Si J, Chen S. The impact of Helicobacter pylori infection, eradication therapy and probiotic supplementation on gut microenvironment homeostasis: An open-label, randomized clinical trial. EBioMedicine. 2018;35: 87-96. DOI: 10.1016/j.ebiom.2018.08.028

[115] Underwood MA. Probiotics and the prevention of necrotizing enterocolitis. Journal of Pediatric Surgery. 2019;54(3):405-412. DOI: 10.1016/j.jpedsurg.2018.08.055

[116] Seddik H, Boutallaka H, Elkoti I, Nejjari F, Berraida R, Berrag S, Loubaris K, Sentissi S, Benkirane A. Saccharomyces boulardii CNCM I-745 plus sequential therapy for Helicobacter pylori infections: a randomized, open-label trial. Eur J Clin Pharmacol. 2019;75(5):639-645. DOI: 10.1007/s00228-019-02625-0

[117] Barker AK, Duster M, Valentine S, Hess T, Archbald-Pannone L, Guerrant R, Safdar N. A randomized controlled trial of probiotics for *Clostridium difficile* infection in adults (PICO). J Antimicrob Chemother. 2017;72:3177-3180. DOI: 10.1093/jac/dkx254

[118] Alberda C, Marcushamer S, Hewer T, Journault N, Kutsogiannis D. Feasibility of a Lactobacillus casei Drink in the Intensive Care Unit for Prevention of Antibiotic Associated Diarrhea and *Clostridium difficile*. Nutrients. 2018;10:539. DOI: 10.3390/nu10050539

[119] van Wietmarschen HA, Busch M, van Oostveen A, Pot G, Jong MC. Probiotics use for antibiotic-associated diarrhea: a pragmatic participatory evaluation in nursing homes. BMC Gastroenterology. 2020;20:151. DOI: 10.1186/s12876-020-01297-w

[120] Kołodziej M, Szajewska H. Lactobacillus reuteri DSM 17938 in the prevention of antibiotic-associated diarrhoea in children: a randomized clinical trial. Clinical Microbiology and Infection. 2019;25:699-704. DOI: 10.1016/j.cmi.2018.08.017 1198-743

[121] Szymański H, Szajewska H. Lack of Efficacy of Lactobacillus reuteri DSM 17938 for the Treatment of Acute Gastroenteritis: A Randomized Controlled Trial. Pediatr Infect Dis J. 2019;38(10):e237-e242. DOI: 10.1097/INF.0000000000002355

[122] Ljungquist O, Kampmann C, Resman F, Riesbeck K, Tham J. Probiotics for intestinal decolonization of ESBL-producing Enterobacteriaceae: a randomized, placebo-controlled clinical trial. Clinical Microbiology and Infection. 2020;26:456-462. DOI: 10.1016/j.cmi.2019.08.019 1198-743X

[123] Nova E, Wärnberg J, Gómez-Martínez S, Díaz LE, Romeo J, Marcos A. Immunomodulatory effects of probiotics in different stages of life. Br J Nutr. 2007;98(1):90-95.

[124] Kawase M, He F, Kubota A, Yoda K, Miyazawa K, Hiramatsu M. Heatkilled Lactobacillus gasseri TMC0356 protects mice against influenza virus infection by stimulating gut and respiratory immune responses. FEMS Immunol Med Microbiol. 2012;64(2):280-288.

[125] Pu F, Guo Y, Li M, Zhu H, Wang S, Shen X, He M, Huang C, He F. Yogurt

supplemented with probiotics can protect the healthy elderly from respiratory infections: A randomized controlled open-label trial. Clin Interv Aging. 2017;12:1223-1231. DOI: 10.2147/CIA.S141518.

[126] Michalickova D, Minic R, Dikic N, Andjelkovic M, Kostic-Vucicevic M, Stojmenovic T, Nikolic I, Djordjevic B. Lactobacillus helveticus Lafti L10 supplementation reduces respiratory infection duration in a cohort of elite athletes: a randomized, double-blind, placebo-controlled trial. Appl Physiol Nutr Metab. 2016;41(7):782-9. DOI: 10.1139/apnm-2015-0541.

[127] Peiris JS. Severe acute respiratory syndrome (SARS). J Clin Virol. 2003;28:245-7.

[128] Peiris JS, Tu WW, Yen HL. A novel H1N1 virus causes the first pandemic of the 21st century. Eur J Immunol. 2009;39:2946-54.

[129] Marsland BJ, Gollwitzer ES. Host– microorganism interactions in lung diseases. Nat Rev Immunol. 2014;14:827– 835. DOI: 10. 1038/nri3769

[130] Wang B, Hylwka T, Smieja M, Surrette M, Bowdish DME, Loeb M. Probiotics to Prevent Respiratory Infections in Nursing Homes: A Pilot Randomized Controlled Trial. J Am Geriatr Soc. 2018;66(7):1346-1352. DOI: 10.1111/jgs.15396

[131] Campanella V, Syed J, Santacroce L, Saini R, Ballini A, Inchingolo F. Oral probiotics influence oral and respiratory tract infections in pediatric population: a randomized double-blinded placebo-controlled pilot study. Eur Rev Med Pharmacol Sci. 2018;22(22):8034-8041. DOI: 10.26355/eurrev_201811_16433.

[132] Sadeghi-Bojd S, Naghshizadian R, Mazaheri M, Ghane Sharbaf F, Assadi F. Efficacy of Probiotic Prophylaxis After The First Febrile Urinary Tract Infection in Children With Normal Urinary Tracts. J Pediatric Infect Dis Soc. 2020;9(3):305-310. DOI: 10.1093/jpids/piz025.

[133] Nelson CP, Hoberman A, Shaikh N, et al. Antibiotic resistance and urinary tract infection recurrence. Pediatrics. 2016;137:pii:e20152490. DOI: 10.1542/peds.2015-2490.

[134] Libertucci J, Young VB. The role of the microbiota in infectious diseases. Nat Microbiol. 2019;4:35-45.

[135] Matsuzaki T, Chin J. Modulating immune responses with probiotic bacteria. Immunol Cell Biol. 2000;78:67-73.

[136] Cadieux PA, Burton J, Devillard E, Reid G. Lactobacillus by-products inhibit the growth and virulence of uropathogenic *Escherichia coli*. J Physiol Pharmacol. 2009;60(6):13-8.

[137] Kovachev SM, Vatcheva-Dobrevska RS. Local Probiotic Therapy for Vaginal *Candida albicans* Infections. Probiotics Antimicrob Proteins. 2015;7(1):38-44. DOI: 10.1007/s12602-014-9176-0.

[138] Pendharkar S, Brandsborg E, Hammarström L, Marcotte H, Larsson PG. Vaginal colonisation by probiotic lactobacilli and clinical outcome in women conventionally treated for bacterial vaginosis and yeast infection. BMC Infect Dis. 2015;15:255. DOI: 10.1186/s12879-015-0971-3.

[139] Barthow C, Wickens K, Stanley T, Mitchell EA, Maude R, Abels P, Purdie G, Murphy R, Stone P, Kang J, Hood F, Rowden J, Barnes P, Fitzharris P, Craig J, Slykerman RF, Crane J. The Probiotics in Pregnancy Study (PiP Study): rationale and design of a double-blind randomised controlled trial to improve maternal health during pregnancy and prevent infant eczema and allergy. BMC Pregnancy Childbirth.

2016;16(1):133. DOI: 10.1186/s12884-016-0923-y.

[140] Davar R, Nokhostin F, Eftekhar M, Sekhavat L, Bashiri Zadeh M, Shamsi F. Comparing the Recurrence of Vulvovaginal Candidiasis in Patients Undergoing Prophylactic Treatment with Probiotic and Placebo During the 6 Months. Probiotics Antimicrob Proteins. 2016;8(3):130-3. DOI: 10.1007/s12602-016-9218-x.

[141] Russo R, Superti F, Karadja E, De Seta F. Randomised clinical trial in women with Recurrent Vulvovaginal Candidiasis: Efficacy of probiotics and lactoferrin as maintenance treatment. Mycoses. 2019;62(4):328-335. DOI: 10.1111/myc.12883.

[142] Vladareanu R, Mihu D, Mitran M, Mehedintu C, Boiangiu A, Manolache M, Vladareanu S. New evidence on oral *L. plantarum* P17630 product in women with history of recurrent vulvovaginal candidiasis (RVVC): a randomized double-blind placebo-controlled study. Eur Rev Med Pharmacol Sci. 2018;22(1):262-267. DOI: 10.26355/eurrev_201801_14128.

[143] Reznichenko H, Henyk N, Maliuk V, Khyzhnyak T, Tynna Y, Filipiuk I, Veresniuk N, Zubrytska L, Quintens J, Richir K, Gerasymov S. Oral Intake of Lactobacilli Can Be Helpful in Symptomatic Bacterial Vaginosis: A Randomized Clinical Study. J Low Genit Tract Dis. 2020;24(3):284-289. DOI: 10.1097/LGT.0000000000000518.

[144] Sgibnev A, Kremleva E. Probiotics in addition to metronidazole for treatment Trichomonas vaginalis in the presence of BV: a randomized, placebo-controlled, double-blind study. Eur J Clin Microbiol Infect Dis. 2020;39(2):345-351. DOI: 10.1007/s10096-019-03731-8.

[145] Toh SL, Lee BB, Ryan S, Simpson JM, Clezy K, Bossa L, Rice SA, Marial O, Weber GH, Kaur J, Boswell-Ruys CL, Goodall S, Middleton JW, Tuderhope M, Kotsiou G. Probiotics [LGG-BB12 or RC14-GR1] versus placebo as prophylaxis for urinary tract infection in persons with spinal cord injury [ProSCIUTTU]: a randomised controlled trial. Spinal Cord. 2019;57(7):550-561. DOI: 10.1038/s41393-019-0251-y.

[146] de Wolff MG, Johansen M, Ersbøll AS, Rosthøj S, Brunsgaard A, Midtgaard J, Tabor A, Hegaard HK. Efficacy of a midwife-coordinated, individualized, and specialized maternity care intervention (ChroPreg) in addition to standard care in pregnant women with chronic disease: protocol for a parallel randomized controlled trial. Trials. 2019;20(1):291. DOI: 10.1186/s13063-019-3405-5

[147] Gallo MF, Macaluso M, Warner L, Fleenor ME, Hook EW 3rd, Brill I, Weaver MA. Bacterial vaginosis, gonorrhea, and chlamydial infection among women attending a sexually transmitted disease clinic: a longitudinal analysis of possible causal links. Ann Epidemiol. 2012;22(3):213-20. DOI: 10.1016/j.annepidem.2011.11.005.

[148] Macklaim JM, Clemente JC, Knight R, Gloor GB, Reid G. Changes in vaginal microbiota following antimicrobial and probiotic therapy. Microb Ecol Health Dis. 2015;26:27799. DOI: 10.3402/mehd.v26.27799.

[149] Russo R, Karadja E, De Seta F. Evidence-based mixture containing Lactobacillus strains and lactoferrin to prevent recurrent bacterial vaginosis: a double blind, placebo controlled, randomised clinical trial. Benef Microbes. 2019;10(1):19-26. DOI: 10.3920/BM2018.0075.

[150] Doppalapudi R, Vundavalli S, Prabhat MP. Effect of probiotic bacteria on oral Candida in head- and neck-radiotherapy patients: A randomized

clinical trial. J Cancer Res Ther. 2020;16(3):470-477. DOI: 10.4103/jcrt.JCRT_334_18.

[151] Hu L, Mao Q, Zhou P, Lv X, Hua H, Yan Z. Effects of Streptococcus salivarius K12 with nystatin on oral candidiasis-RCT. Oral Dis. 2019;25(6):1573-1580. DOI: 10.1111/odi.13142.

[152] Lee X, Vergara C, Lozano CP. Severity of Candida-associated denture stomatitis is improved in institutionalized elders who consume Lactobacillus rhamnosus SP1. Aust Dent J. 2019;64(3):229-236. DOI: 10.1111/adj.12692.

[153] Miyazima TY, Ishikawa KH, Mayer M, Saad S, Nakamae A. Cheese supplemented with probiotics reduced the Candida levels in denture wearers-RCT. Oral Dis. 2017;23(7):919-925. DOI: 10.1111/odi.12669.

[154] Invernici MM, Furlaneto FAC, Salvador SL, Ouwehand AC, Salminen S, Mantziari A, Vinderola G, Ervolino E, Santana SI, Silva PHF, Messora MR. Bifidobacterium animalis subsp lactis HN019 presents antimicrobial potential against periodontopathogens and modulates the immunological response of oral mucosa in periodontitis patients. PLoS One. 2020;15(9):e0238425. DOI: 10.1371/journal.pone.0238425.

[155] Sabatini S, Lauritano D, Candotto V, Silvestre FJ, Nardi GM. Oral probiotics in the management of gingivitis in diabetic patients: a double blinded randomized controlled study. J Biol Regul Homeost Agents. 2017;31(2 Suppl 1):197-202.

[156] Tobita K, Watanabe I, Tomokiyo M, Saito M. Effects of heat-treated Lactobacillus crispatus KT-11 strain consumption on improvement of oral cavity environment: a randomised double-blind clinical trial. Benef Microbes. 2018;9(4):585-592. DOI: 10.3920/BM2017.0137.

Chapter 5

Probiotics and Postbiotics from Food to Health: Antimicrobial Experimental Confirmation

Janet Cheruiyot Kosgey, Mercy W. Mwaniki and Fengmin Zhang

Abstract

The field of probiotics is up-and-coming, especially in management of microbial pathogens. Probiotics confer nutritional benefits, reduce inflammation and infection. Probiotics have also shown to be helpful in the management of microbial pathogens, which include bacteria, fungi, and viruses. To ernes this potential maximumly, there is a need for an elaborate screening system for new isolates. This entails; rigorous screening methods and thorough confirmatory systems. There is need also to come up with standard methods used to evaluate the probiotics mechanism of action both in vivo and in vitro. In summary, there is a need for a standard screening process for probiotic microorganisms that is reproducible. The aim is to ensure that, the candidate microbial cultures are not written off without proper investigations. This will also fasten the screening process and save time and resources wasted in pre-screening experiments.

Keywords: probiotics, screening methods, confirmatory methods, postbiotics, animal model, coculture

1. Introduction

Fermentation is one of the oldest technologies used for food preservation. It involves converting carbohydrates to alcohol, carbon dioxide, and organic acids using microorganisms under anaerobic conditions. The fermentation process improves food by developing diverse flavors, aromas, and textures in food substrates. Also, it enriches food substrates with protein, essential amino acids, essential fatty acids, and vitamins. The primary mechanism of the preservation of foods is the production of acid, which lowers the pH to a level at which most of the spoilage-causing microorganisms cannot grow, hence prolonging the shelf life of such foods [1]. At present, various fermented foods are produced worldwide at household and industrial levels, in both small-scale and large commercial enterprises. Associated with fermentation are beneficial microorganisms known as probiotics. The vast majority of the probiotics are lactic acid microorganisms [2] to produce fermented dairy products.

Among the beneficial effects of probiotics include improved intestinal health, enhancement of the immune response, reduction of serum cholesterol, and cancer prevention [3–5]. There is also substantial evidence to support probiotic use in treating acute diarrhoeal diseases, prevention of antibiotic-associated diarrhea, and improvement of lactose metabolism [6]. The range of food products containing probiotic strains is vast and still growing. And so is the list of beneficial effects. More so, with an increasing desire for quality life, preference for minimal use of chemicals, and the rising cost of healthcare. Natural products like probiotics is a promising alternative. Related to probiotics are prebiotics. Biogenics involves the use of beneficial bioactive substances produced by probiotic bacteria whose activities are independent of the viability of probiotic bacteria.

This book chapter focuses on the use of probiotics in the management of microbial pathogens, emphasizing the need to have a reproducible standard screening process both *in vivo* and *in vitro*. This will highlight areas in the used technologies that need harmonization, technologies for investigation and confirmation of the antimicrobial activities of probiotics, and finally, the future prospects of probiotics and antimicrobial agents.

1.1 Mechanism of action of probiotics

WHO/FAO defines probiotics as "live microorganisms that, when administered in adequate amounts, confer a health benefit on the host" [7, 8]. Prebiotics refer to the substrates that are selectively utilized by host microorganisms that result in conferring a health benefit to the host [8–11]. Furthermore, postbiotics entails the use of beneficial bioactive compounds produced by probiotic bacteria. The activity of postbiotics is independent of probiotic bacteria's viability [11]. The term synbiotics is where both prebiotics and probiotics are utilized simultaneously [11, 12].

The probiotics have myriad of mechanisms in which it protects against infection. These include; (1) they lower pH, (2) pathogen antagonism by producing antimicrobial compounds for example, bacteriocins and or other metabolic products, (3) competitive exclusion with the pathogen for binding sites and receptors sites, (4) competition for substrates that is, nutrients and growth factors, therefore, limiting resources, (5) stimulate immunomodulatory cells, (6) production of enzymes example, enzymes that neutralize toxins produced by pathogens (7) improve the barrier function of the intestinal mucosa, (8) modulate inflammatory responses, (9) aggregate with pathogens, (10) produce hydrogen peroxide (H_2O_2) a strong oxidizing agent that damage nucleic acids and proteins, (11) produce organic acids like lactic acid, acetic acid among others (12) produce CO_2 thus creating anaerobic microenvironment (**Figure 1**) [3, 4, 13–16].

The probiotics are generally regarded as safe [17]. The few results obtained when probiotics are administered together with conventional drugs clinically are promising and include synergy with the drug, half dose of conventional drug needed, and faster healing [18–21]. Further research is needed in this area.

1.2 Probiotics as antimicrobial agents

Besides the health-improving benefits, the antimicrobial activity of probiotics has been well documented, with promising results against microbial pathogens. Probiotics have been deemed as the following most crucial immune defense systems according to WHO [7]. This is due to increasing antibiotic resistance to commonly prescribed antibiotics [22, 23]. There is a need, therefore, to come up with reproducible screening protocols for *in vitro*, *in vivo*, and clinical studies. Therefore, this book chapter will highlight protocols used in screening probiotics and postbiotics, cite their strengths and drawbacks, and point areas that need harmonization.

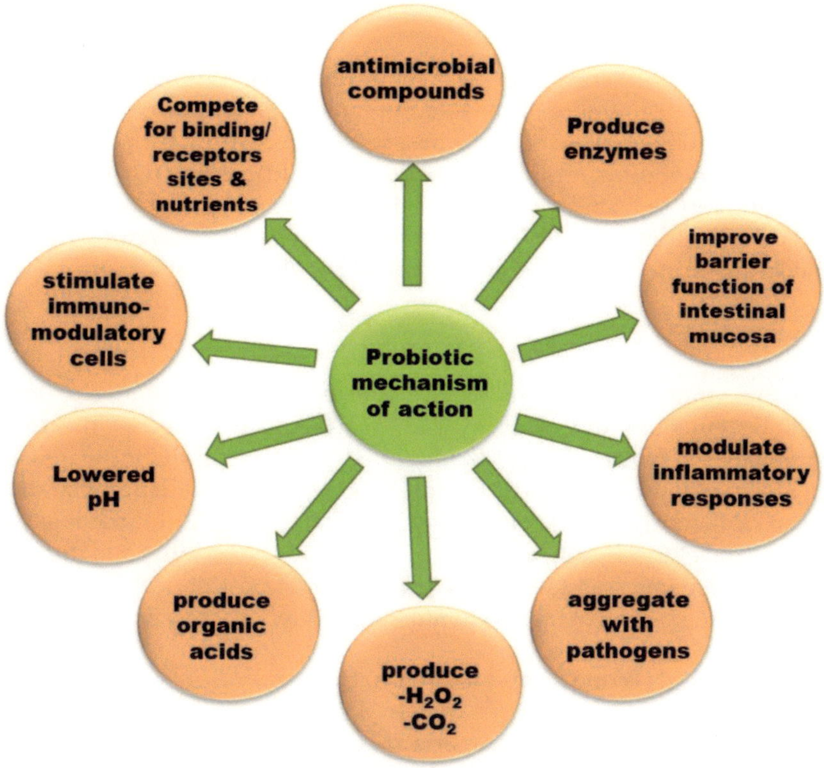

Figure 1.
Mechanisms in which probiotics protect against infection.

2. Areas in the used technology that need harmonization

To obtain reproducible and conclusive results of probiotic antimicrobial activity, standardization of protocols is essential. This section reviews the essential areas that will inform on the choice of indicator pathogen, probiotic microorganism, inoculum size, incubation time and conditions, and technique of production of postbiotics (also referred to as cell-free supernatant (CFS)/ Biogenic/spent media) used in previous research and the need for harmonization.

2.1 The selection of experimental indicator pathogen

The choice has relied on the target disease that the probiotic is thought to treat. Thus, for vulvovaginal candidiasis *C. albicans,* the predominant pathogen has been chosen [24, 25], even though *Candida glabrata* has also been screened [26, 27]. Enterotoxigenic *E. coli* and *Salmonella typhimurium* is the choice for studying gastrointestinal infection [28]. However, while screening new probiotic microorganisms for general antimicrobial activity, major classes of pathogens of medical importance should be representatively tested [29]. For example, studies on fungal pathogens should include at least a dermatophyte, non-dermatophyte, and yeast. Antibacterial should consist of a Gram-positive and a Gram-negative bacterial pathogen. Furthermore, clinical, typed microorganism and drug-resistant strains should be included due to emerging resistance [10].

2.2 The choice of probiotic microorganism and postbiotics

The WHO/FAO has listed the criteria for evaluation of probiotic microorganism, which include; the ability of the microorganism to adhere to epithelial cells, bile salts, resist stomach acid and enzymes, persistence within the system, produce antimicrobial compounds, antibiotic resistance profile inability to confer resistance or genome stability and ability to stabilize the normal microbiota among others [7, 15, 30]. Probiotic antimicrobial activity is strain-specific; therefore, the species level and strain of the selected probiotic should be identified.

2.3 Inoculum size

The actual number of viable indicator pathogens in the inoculum size directly influences the outcome. Too little may lead to false-positive results, while too heavy inoculum may give a false negative result [29, 31]. A foundation for the inoculum size can be suggested by CLSI [32]. Researchers have used different inoculum size, incubation temperature, and time for both probiotic and indicator pathogen in *in vitro*, *in vivo* and clinical studies [9]. We propose that the viability and dose of probiotic microorganisms used (also in the production of postbiotics) be established by dose-dependent experiments. This should be indicated in experimental reports.

2.4 The experimental conditions and incubation time

Lactic acid bacteria and Bifidobacteria are fastidious; subsequently, the media chosen should have a specific nutrient requirement, for example, growth factors. MRS, which is an appropriate media for the growth of probiotic microorganisms, is widely used. MRS is both a selective and an enriched media for the growth and isolation of only lactic acid bacteria and other bacteria. Therefore, if this medium cannot support the indicator pathogen, for example, dermatophytes (J. [33]), probiotic growth factors can be incorporated in any media of choice such as potato dextrose agar (PDA), sabouraud dextrose agar (SDA) and nutrient agar (NA) to favor the growth of both the indicator pathogen and the probiotic microorganism. Proper choice of media and specific modifications is key to a successful experiment [33, 34]. Therefore, media supplemented with growth factors should be screened for the ability to grow both probiotic microorganisms and indicator pathogen. We propose that the specific incubation conditions such as time and oxygen requirements for both probiotic microorganisms and indicator pathogen be optimized before the experiment and confirmed by the growth curve of individual microorganisms (**Figure 2**). Furthermore, fresh media should always be prepared and used for reproductive results, especially in the case of disc diffusion results.

2.5 The technique of production of postbiotics

The postbiotics is also referred to as cell-free supernatant (CFS) or biogenics or spent media. The preparation of postbiotics is varied and attests to the need to harmonize the methods. The process entails the following steps; the probiotic microorganism is inoculated in broth media and incubated in an incushaker [35]. Cells are then removed by centrifuging to obtain the CFS ([36]; J. [33, 35, 37]). The supernatant obtained can then be screened for antimicrobial activity [35], or the supernatant is further filter-sterilized [35, 36]. The CFS is then used to screen for the microbial activity or concentrated to obtain concentrated CFS (cCFS) [36, 38] or freeze-dried [36].

The advantage of using postbiotics is that the properties of the active component can be deduced. To ascertain if the active ingredient is proteinaceous, heat treatment and enzymes are used. If the activity is reduced or is lost compared to non-treated postbiotic, it infers that the antimicrobial agent is proteinaceous [33, 38]. To ascertain if the antimicrobial activity is pH-related, the postbiotic is neutralized and buffered [30].

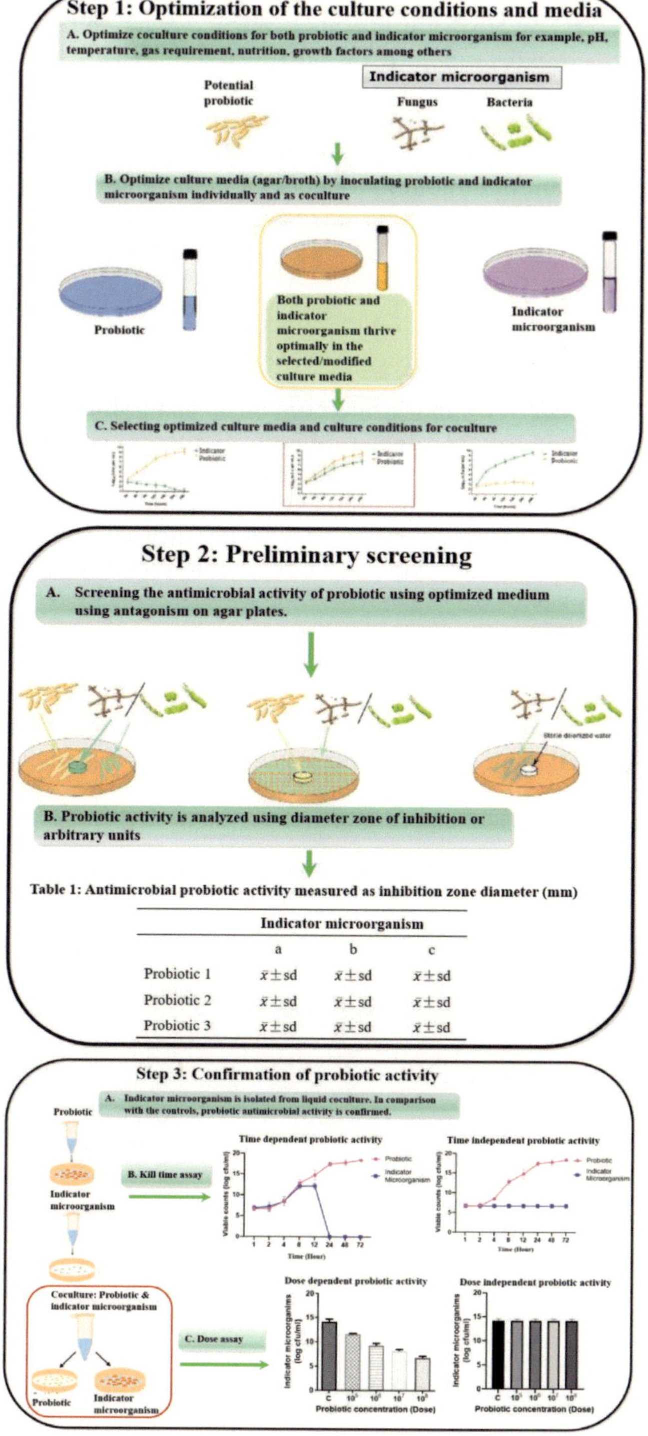

Figure 2.
Detailed proposed method for conclusively screening probiotic antimicrobial activity. Step 1 entails choice of optimal media and growth conditions, step 2 is the preliminary screening on agar and step 3 is the confirmation of probiotic antimicrobial activity in liquid cocultures.

3. Technology for investigation and confirmation of the antimicrobial activity of probiotics

3.1 Experiments for investigation of antimicrobial potential of probiotics *In vitro*

Included in this section are the *In vitro* antagonism methods on agar plates and liquid coculture for checking probiotic antimicrobial activity with their strengths and drawbacks. In antagonism on agar plate's methods, probiotic and indicator microorganism is introduced in the same plate. The difference is the sequence and manner of the inoculation of either indicator pathogen or probiotic microorganisms. After incubation, the diameter zone of inhibition which is the clear zones around the inoculated area, is then read in millimeters or reported or arbitrary units (AU) (**Figures 2** and **3**).

3.1.1 Antagonism on agar plate methods

3.1.1.1 Simple spot-on lawn assay

To screen postbiotics or probiotic microorganism using this method, the indicator pathogen is first inoculated, then probiotic microorganisms are spotted at specific points on solid media [37]. **Modification** to the method entails spotting probiotic microorganisms as parallel lines [33]. Its strength includes (a) media can be modified [33, 34], (b) it has an option of different incubation conditions, i.e., probiotic microorganism incubation conditions are first optimized, followed by optimizations for indicator pathogen.

3.1.1.2 Spot on agar assay

Probiotic microorganisms are first spotted on agar media and then incubated [39]. An indicator pathogen is added, and soft agar at around 45–50°C is poured to

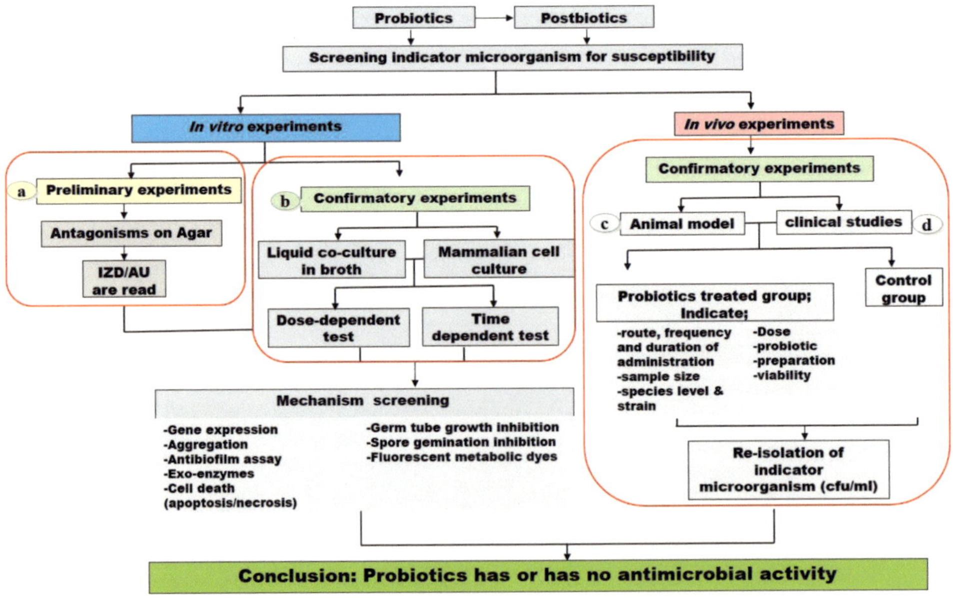

Figure 3.
Abridgement of methods involved in screening probiotic microorganisms both In vitro *and* In vivo.
(a) In vitro *preliminary screening experiments on agar. (b)* In vitro *confirmatory experiments. (c)* In vivo *animal confirmatory experiment. (d)* In vivo *clinical confirmatory experiment.*

the previously prepared plate spotted with a probiotic microorganism [25, 35]. The advantage of the Agar spot test is that two different media can be used, one for spotting and the other as overlaid soft agar. Indicator and probiotic microorganisms can be grown at different times, meaning incubation conditions can be adjusted for each microorganism. The disadvantage is the high temperature of soft agar, i.e., between 45°C and 50°C, killing heat-labile indicator microorganisms. The strict aerobes may not grow well due to the pour plate method.

3.1.1.3 Spot on lawn assay with wells also referred to as Agar well diffusion assay or as conventional whole plate method

The wells are dug and indicator pathogen inoculated. Then postbiotic/Probiotic is dispensed [37, 40]. Unlike the simple spot-on lawn assay method, the probiotic microorganism can be allowed to grow first before introducing the indicator microorganisms or vice versa.

3.1.1.4 Paper disc assay

The postbiotic/probiotic is dispensed on the paper discs and placed on the inoculated media. The inoculation of both indicator pathogen and probiotic microorganism is simultaneous. The disadvantage of this method is that the results are not reproducible [41]. This is mainly attributed to the production of non-diffusible antimicrobials.

3.1.1.5 Cross streak on agar assay

Entails streaking the probiotic microorganism as parallel lines on media. A perpendicular line of indicator pathogen is then streaked. Growth inhibition is determined at the interception point [40].

3.1.1.6 The radial streak on agar assay

The probiotic microorganism is inoculated as a circle in the middle of the agar plate. The indicator pathogen is then streaked as radial lines from the edge of the petri dish to the center, and growth inhibition is examined [42]. Another method closely related to this method is cutting the media with the probiotic microorganisms and placing it on top of the indicator pathogen inoculated plate.

3.1.2 Liquid coculture method

The probiotic and indicator pathogens are both introduced to optimized broth culture media, then incubated. Samples are intermittently collected, and viability (cfu/ml) of indicator pathogen is established. It is used to determine if the probiotic effect is static or cidal [13, 24]. It may also be used to reveal the mechanism by which the probiotic bacteria exert their antimicrobial activity [35]. Microtitre assay is used to screen minimum inhibitory concentration (MIC) of postbiotics using microdilution method, macro serial dilution, or conventional kill time assay [35, 43]. Liquid coculture assay is recommended as a confirmatory test (**Figures 2** and **3**).

3.1.3 Summary of antagonism assay

Antagonism assay on agar plates has the advantage of being fast and straightforward. The disadvantage is that it does not directly interact with the probiotic microorganism or postbiotics and indicator pathogen. Consequently, the probiotic microorganism should produce sufficient antimicrobial agent that should have the potential to diffuse through solid media in terms of size and spatial centrifugation [44]. Accordingly, it is not prudent to use these methods solely to ascertain antimicrobial activity of probiotic microorganisms. Hence, it is recommended to combine antagonism on agar plates and liquid coculture to establish the antimicrobial activity of probiotic microorganisms and postbiotics (**Figures 2** and **3**).

3.1.4 Cell culture and tissues

To closely mimic human infection, human cell cultures are infected with indicator pathogen, then treated with probiotic cultures or postbiotics [41].

3.2 Experiments for the discovery of antimicrobial mechanisms of probiotics

The methods used to ascertain probiotic microorganism mechanisms of antimicrobial activity include; the ability to inhibit virulence factors and cell death.

3.2.1 Ability to inhibit virulence factors

The virulence factors of pathogenic microorganisms vary from one microorganism to the other. For example, the virulence factor in bacteria includes adhesion, immunoevasion and immunosuppression, exo-enzymes, and exotoxin, among others [45]. The virulent factors in *Candida* include secretion of hydrolases, yeast to hypha transition, contact sensing, thigmotropism, biofilm formation, phenotypic switching, and range of fitness attributes [27, 37]. The following methods can be used to examine the ability of the probiotic microorganism to inhibit the virulence factors;

3.2.1.1 Gene expression levels

The expression levels of specific genes controlling one or more of these virulence factors can be ascertained when checking for probiotic activity [14, 25, 35, 36, 46–48]. The methods used include microarray analysis, RT-PCR techniques, and western blot [49].

3.2.1.2 Aggregation and coaggregation assay

Aggregation assay using spectrophotometric autoaggregation and coaggregation is used to ascertain the antimicrobial activity of probiotics [26, 38, 50]. The morphological transition of *C. albicans* that is, germ tube formation contributes to adherence and invasion to the host tissue and increases virulence [51, 52]. Lactobacilli build aggregates and co-aggregates with Candida cells, and this process neutralizes germ tube growth [53]. In addition, the coaggregation protects access of pathogens to a cell receptor and, as a result, inhibit pathogen adhesion which is a prerequisite step for colonization and the subsequent development of disease [26, 44, 50, 54].

3.2.1.3 Antibiofilm Assay

Biofilm produced by pathogens serves as a physical barrier and increases virulence. Antibiofilm assay includes (a) **static systems** like microtiter plate, Molony biofilm, Calgary biofilm device, biofilm ring test (b) **open systems** such as Kadouri system, flow cell, perfused (membrane) biofilm fermenter, microfermentors, Modified Robbins Device, sorbarod devices (SBF), drip flow reactor, constant depth film fermenter, microfluidic biochips, rotating disc reactor, BioFlux device, annular reactors, CDC biofilm reactors (c) **microcosm** example airway epithelial cell model, reconstituted human epithelia (RHE), endothelial cells under flow model, Zürich oral biofilm-model, microfluidic coculture model, Zürich burn biofilm-model, multiple Sorbarod devices (MSD) (d) **ex-vivo which include;** candidiasis in the vaginal mucosa, RWV bioreactor, cardiac valve *ex vivo* model, root canal biofilms [55]. Viable colonies can also be used. While fluorescent labeling of biofilm coupled with mathematical labeling is used [41].

3.2.1.4 Exo-enzymes

The indicator microorganisms are treated with probiotics or CFS. The indicator microorganism is then examined for the ability to produce exo-enzymes on agar plate assays. The agar plate contains a suitable substrate specific to each enzyme activity [56].

3.2.1.5 Electron microscopy

Scanning electron microscopy and Transmission electron microscope are used to examine cell integrity which includes morphological adherence, distortion, biofilm, or apoptosis [27, 50, 57].

3.2.1.6 Germ tube and hyphal growth inhibition

The pelleted spores of dermatophytes and dimorphic pathogenic fungus are allowed to develop germ tubes and hyphae. Probiotic or CFS is then added and incubated. Growth is determined by examining germ tubes and hyphae [36, 58].

3.2.1.7 Spore germination inhibition assay

The pelleted mycelia and probiotic or CFS are added to media and incubated. Samples are withdrawn and microscopically examined. Percentage spore germination is calculated by the following formula [33, 36, 58]:

% spore germination = [Numbers of germinated spores /Numbers of total spores] × 100

3.2.1.8 Fluorescent metabolic dyes and Confocal laser scanning microscopy

The indicator microorganisms are treated with probiotic cultures or CFS then stained with fluorescent dyes according to the manufacturer's instructions. The live or dead cells are counted, and their metabolic activity is ascertained [26, 27]. Live/dead cells can also be confirmed by viable counts (cfu/ml).

3.2.2 Ability to induce cell death

A sequence of unique morphological changes outlines apoptosis. These include; visible cell shrinkage, extensive plasma membrane blebbing, chromatin condensation, nuclear fragmentation, formation of apoptotic bodies, which later undergoes decomposition within the phagosome and finally terminates with complete recycling of the components [59, 60]. Accumulation of reactive oxygen species (ROS) decreased membrane potential, biochemical and cytological responses well known in programmed cell death (PCD), for instance, apoptosis [60]. Very high ROS concentrations induce necrosis [61]. These changes can be used to determine cell integrity. Of the biochemical and cytological methods used to check pathogen cell integrity after treatment with probiotics include but are not limited to; nuclear fragmentation using DAPI/Tunnel [62–67]; *in situ* ligation assay [65]; DNA laddering [65, 66]; externalization of Annexin V/PI by cell membrane [62, 64, 67–70]; mitochondrial and cytosolic calcium [66, 67, 69, 71]; depolarization of the mitochondria using mitochondria membrane potential detection kits for instance, JC fluorescent probes [62, 63, 66–71]; reactive oxygen species (ROS) accumulation [66, 67, 69–71]; detecting cytochrome c in cytoplasm using western blotting or color metric kits [63, 66–69, 71, 72]; cytosol / mitochondria intracellular glutathione [67, 69]lipid peroxidation [67, 69]; potassium release [67] and metacaspace activation detection using kits like CaspACE FITC-VAD-FMK *in situ* Marker [63, 67–69]. The antimicrobial activity of a probiotic microorganism can be assessed using a combination of a number of these methods, which can corroborate the integrity of the indicator pathogen. Careful choice of positive (example, antimicrobial drug) and negative (untreated) controls are important for interpreting the results.

3.3 Experiments that confirm the antimicrobial activity of probiotics *in vivo*

The *in vitro* studies offer required information about antimicrobial agents on susceptibility responses [73], exposure times, and optimal concentrations [74]. However, these studies have their limitations, for instance, the bulk of antimicrobial agents that are active *in vitro* lack significant antimicrobial activity *in vivo,* and vice versa sometimes occurs [73]. The strength of animal models in determining antimicrobial efficacy is that the study can be ascertained at specific body sites, for example, skin, thigh, lung, peritoneum, meninges, and endocardia [74]. Furthermore, antimicrobial agents are altered by host factors such as metabolism and the immune system in an animal model [74]. Consequently, animal models bridge the gap between in vitro and clinical trials [73] and are indispensable for authentication of probiotic antimicrobial activity. In brief, *in vivo* animal models and clinical studies are an absolute requirement to provide proof of beneficial activities of probiotic antimicrobial activity. To achieve this, appropriate infectious models for the two groups are critical. One infected with indicator pathogen and treated with probiotic cultures, and the other group infected with indicator pathogen only (negative control).

3.3.1 In vivo experiments on animal models

The infection route of dermatophytes is strictly dependent on the goal of the study, indicator fungus, and animal disease model of interest. Examples, to study geophilic and anthrophilic dermatophytes; *Microsporum gypseum* and *Trichophyton rubrum* that is difficult to establish infections in laboratory animals', zoophilic dermatophytes especially *Trichophyton metangrophytes* var. *mentagrophtes*, var. *quinckeanum* and var. *granulae*, *Trichophyton verrucosum,* and *Microsporum canis* are used instead. The most recommended animal model for dermatophytoses is hairless guinea pigs as the infection resembles infections in humans, and topical treatment is applicable. Mouse, rat, hamster, and dog are disadvantaged for dermatophytoses animal model since they defecate, lick, and bite itching or irritating lesions intensively [75].

C. albicans and *Candida tropicalis* have high virulence in systemically induced mice model [76–79]. Pregnant mice [75], zebrafish [80] and *Caenorhabditis elegans* [46] have also been utilized in disseminated systemic infection models. *Candida metapsilosis* is virulent in the vaginal mouse model [81]. Furthermore, oophectomised rats are used for chronic vaginitis [47, 75]. However, *C. parapsilosis, C. glabrata,* and *C. krusei* do not induce mice mortality [77]. Further, *C. albicans* [82], *Ctropicalis, C. parapsilosis* complex (*C. parapsilosis, C. orthopsilosis,* and *C. metapsilosis*), are virulent in the invertebrate *Galleria monella* model [77]. Induced immunosuppressed mice in murine oral candidiasis model of choice. To cause the immunosuppressed condition, administration of prednisolone 100 mg per kg [83] or ketamine: xylazine 90-100 mg/kg and 10 mg/kg respectively [84] of body weight administered by injected subcutaneously 24 h before inoculation with Candida orally is given. Additionally, avian and rats species can be used as oral candidiasis models [75, 84]; a summary of these *in vivo* models is given in **Table 1**.

Disease	Animal	Route of infection	Target organ	Reference
Dermatomycosis				
Dermatomycosis	Guinea pig	Skin abrasion	Skin localized infection	[75]
Dermatomycosis	Guinea pig	Intravenous	cutaneous disseminated infection	[75]
Candidosis				
Bacterial and fungal systemic infection	*Caenorhabditis elegans* (Round worm)	Skin	media	[46]
Bacterial and fungal systemic infection	Pregnant mice	Intravascular	placenta	[75]
Bacterial and fungal systemic infection	*Galleria mellonella* (Wax moth caterpillar)	Injection	systemic	[20, 85]
Bacterial and fungal systemic infection	Zebra fish (*Danio rerio)*	Microinjection	disseminated infection	[80]
Chronic vaginitis	Rats; oophectomised and kept permanently in pseudoestrous-weekly injection of estrogen	Intravaginal with blastospores	Vaginal swabs	[47, 75]
Localized oral candidosis (thrush)	Rats and several avian species	Peroral challenge with blastospores; favored by carbohydrate rich diet, antibiotic treatment and use of germ free or specific pathogen free animals	Mouth swabs	[75, 84]

Table 1.
Précis of in vivo *animal models for dermatomycosis, candidiasis and bacterial infections.*

3.3.2 Clinical trials

Clinical trials are conducted after promising *in vitro* and *in vivo* animal model experiments. The randomized placebo-controlled clinical trial is the most recommended method [10]. The number of clinical researches conducted on probiotics is about 1000, with *Lactobacillus rhamnosus* GG and *B. animalis* sp. *Lactis* being the most studied [41, 86]. The majority of these studies are on gastrointestinal diseases and the digestive system [86]. However, currently, there is a shift to metabolic disorders, communicable and infection [86]. The primary concerns in these clinical studies that need to be addressed for harmonization of probiotic clinical research include:

1. The probiotic dosage administered; only 42% of the clinical studies reported dosage correctly. It is recommended that the probiotic dosage is reported in colony-forming unit (CFU). Some clinical studies reported the number of drops, grams, or not indicated at all [86].

2. The amount of probiotic administered should be adequate [7, 87]; however, the amount used varied from 10^7 to 9×10^{11} per day [86].

3. The description of how the probiotic was prepared was incomplete in many studies [86].

4. Viability, which is the overall health of cells. It is crucial to check the viability of probiotics before administration and after a given duration since storage, transportation, and handling condition could kill some microorganisms.

5. It is essential to describe probiotic microorganisms not only to the species level but also to strain. This is because the diversity of probiotic microorganisms is enormous. Further, the probiotic activity is species and strain-specific [88–90]. This is incomplete in the majority of the clinical studies done. Only 49% of the studies conducted complete strain identification.

6. Route, frequency, and duration [91] of probiotic administration should always be reported. Many studies omit this vital aspect.

7. Sample size affects the power of the study to draw a conclusion and the precision of estimates. Therefore, the sample size should be big enough to reduce bias, especially when some patients discontinue the study.

It is important to note that, these details including probiotic dosage used in clinical studies, should be extrapolated from *in vitro* and *in vivo* models. Therefore, this emphasizes the importance of prior quality research.

Few clinical trials on confirmation of the antimicrobial effect of probiotics have been reported so far, yet they have been considered the final confirmative experiment. Probiotics are regarded as safe [13, 17]; thus, many researchers skip this critical step. This is the case in which many commercially marketed probiotics have pending clinical studies [92]. Probiotics clinical studies on the management of oral pathogens [9, 21, 93–95], urogenital infections [20, 96–99] and gastrointestinal systems [100] had promising results thus, supporting some probiotics as potential antimicrobial agents [10].

In conclusion, clinical studies are essential. Successful clinical studies require thorough *in vitro* and *in vivo* experiments, especially estimating the dosage, duration, and frequency of probiotic administration. Areas that need urgent reporting and harmonization in clinical studies include probiotic viability, probiotic species and strain, dosage (CFU), duration, frequency of administration, and route of probiotics administration.

4. Summary and future prospects of probiotics as antimicrobial agents

The probiotics are offering a ray of hope to solve dwindling antibiotic efficacy. Further, the number of immunocompromised persons, number of microbial infections and drug resistance, and probiotics could come in handy to solve these problems. Therefore, there is a need for detailed conclusive research on *in vitro, in vivo,* and clinical trials of probiotic microorganisms, prebiotics, and postbiotics administration including, the benefits and side effects. The choice of probiotics, methods, and experimental designs need to be emphasized. Research has demonstrated that probiotics of a particular strain may have antimicrobial activity against one pathogen and not another [9, 10, 14]. This has been attributed to the great diversity of virulence factors expressed by these pathogens. Some pathogens can produce exoenzymes, encode resistance genes, form biofilms, and induce inflammatory responses, among others [37, 101, 102]. The probiotic dosage, duration, frequency, formulation, viability, species-level, and strain, among others, should always be reported for conclusive studies. Otherwise, it would be pretty challenging to compare these experiments and draw a definite conclusion. Some particular probiotics do not show any antimicrobial activity *in vitro* but present significant activity *in vivo* and vice versa. Hence, there is a need for meticulous screening of probiotic microorganisms before the antimicrobial activity is or is not confirmed.

Author details

Janet Cheruiyot Kosgey[1,2,3*], Mercy W. Mwaniki[1] and Fengmin Zhang[2,3]

1 School of Biological and Life Sciences, Technical University of Kenya, Kenya

2 Department of Microbiology, Harbin Medical University, Harbin, China

3 WU Lien-Teh Institute, Harbin Medical University, Harbin, China

*Address all correspondence to: jantomeli@yahoo.com; janet.kosgey@tukenya.ac.ke

References

[1] Kalui, C. M., Mathara, J. M., & Kutima, P. M. J. A.J.o.B. (2010). Probiotic potential of spontaneously fermented cereal based foods–A review. 9(17), 2490-2498.

[2] FAO/WHO. (2006). Guidelines for the evaluation of probiotics in food. Report of a Joint FAO/WHOWorking Group on Drafting Guidelines for the Evaluation of Probiotics in Food, Ontario, Canada, April 30 and May 1, 2002 (pp. 1-11).

[3] Amara, A., & Shibl, A. J. S. p. j. (2015a). Role of probiotics in health improvement, infection control and disease treatment and management 23(2), 107-114.

[4] Amara, A. A., & Shibl, A. (2015b). Role of Probiotics in health improvement, infection control and disease treatment and management. Saudi Pharm J, 23(2), 107-114. doi:10.1016/j.jsps.2013.07.001

[5] Kechagia, M., Basoulis, D., Konstantopoulou, S., Dimitriadi, D., Gyftopoulou, K., Skarmoutsou, N., & Fakiri, E. M. J. I. S. R. N. (2013). Health benefits of probiotics: a review 2013.

[6] Kosgey, J. C., Jia, L., Fang, Y., Yang, J., Gao, L., Wang, J., Wekesa, V. J. J.o.m.m.. (2019). Probiotics as antifungal agents: Experimental confirmation and future prospects. 162, 28-37.

[7] Additives, J. F. W. E. C. o. F., Meeting, J. F. W. E. C. o. F. A., & Organization, W. H (2002). Evaluation of Certain Food Additives and Contaminants: Fifty-seventh Report of the Joint FAO/WHO Expert Committee on Food Additives (Vol. 57): World Health Organization.

[8] Gibson, G. R., Hutkins, R., Sanders, M. E., Prescott, S. L., Reimer, R. A., Salminen, S. J., Cani, P. D. (2017). The International Scientific Association for Probiotics and Prebiotics (ISAPP) consensus statement on the definition and scope of prebiotics. Nat Rev Gastroenterol Hepatol, 14(8), 491-502.

[9] Matsubara, V. H., Bandara, H. M., Ishikawa, K. H., Mayer, M. P., & Samaranayake, L. P. (2016a). The role of probiotic bacteria in managing periodontal disease: a systematic review. Expert Rev Anti Infect Ther, 14(7), 643-655. doi:10.1080/14787210.20 16.1194198

[10] Matsubara, V. H., Bandara, H. M., Mayer, M. P., & Samaranayake, L. P. (2016b). Probiotics as Antifungals in Mucosal Candidiasis. Clin Infect Dis, 62(9), 1143-1153. doi:10.1093/ cid/ciw038

[11] Ohshima, T., Kojima, Y., Seneviratne, C. J., & Maeda, N. (2016). Therapeutic Application of Synbiotics, a Fusion of Probiotics and Prebiotics, and Biogenics as a New Concept for Oral Candida Infections: A Mini Review. Frontiers in Microbiology, 7(10). doi:10.3389/fmicb.2016.00010

[12] Kojima, Y., Ohshima, T., Seneviratne, C. J., & Maeda, N. (2016). Combining prebiotics and probiotics to develop novel synbiotics that suppress oral pathogens. Journal of Oral Biosciences, 58(1), 27-32.

[13] Deidda, F., Amoruso, A., Allesina, S., Pane, M., Graziano, T., Del Piano, M., & Mogna, L. (2016). In Vitro Activity of Lactobacillus fermentum LF5 Against Different Candida Species and Gardnerella vaginalis: A New Perspective to Approach Mixed Vaginal Infections?, J Clin Gastroenterol, 50 Suppl 2, Proceedings from the 8th Probiotics, Prebiotics & New Foods for Microbiota and Human Health meeting held in Rome Italy on September 13-15,

2015, S168-S170. doi:10.1097/MCG.0000000000000692

[14] Guo, Wei, Liu, C., Li, D., Sun, J., Huang, H., & Zhou, H. (2015). Inhibitory effects of oral Actinomyces on the proliferation, virulence and biofilm formation of Candida albicans. 60, 1368-1374. doi:10.1016/j.archoralbio.2015.06.015

[15] Matsubara, V. H., Wang, Y., Bandara, H. M., Mayer, M. P., & Samaranayake, L. P. (2016c). Probiotic lactobacilli inhibit early stages of Candida albicans biofilm development by reducing their growth, cell adhesion, and filamentation. Appl Microbiol Biotechnol, 100(14), 6415-6426. doi:10.1007/s00253-016-7527-3

[16] Shehata, M. G., El Sohaimy, S. A., El-Sahn, M. A., & Youssef, M. M. (2016). Screening of isolated potential probiotic lactic acid bacteria for cholesterol lowering property and bile salt hydrolase activity. Annals of Agricultural Sciences, 61(1), 65-75. doi: 10.1016/j.aoas.2016.03.001

[17] Sulik-Tyszka, B., Snarski, E., Niedzwiedzka, M., Augustyniak, M., Myhre, T. N., Kacprzyk, A., Wroblewska, M. (2018). Experience with Saccharomyces boulardii Probiotic in Oncohaematological Patients. Probiotics Antimicrob Proteins, 10(2), 350-355. doi:10.1007/s12602-017-9332-4

[18] Lau, C. S. M., Ward, A., & Chamberlain, R. S. (2016). Probiotics improve the efficacy of standard triple therapy in the eradication of Helicobacter pylori: a meta-analysis. Infection and Drug Resistance, 9, 275-289. doi:10.2147/IDR.S117886

[19] Rishi, P., Preet, S., & Kaur, P. (2011). Effect of L. plantarum cell-free extract and co-trimoxazole against Salmonella Typhimurium: a possible adjunct therapy. Annals of Clinical Microbiology and Antimicrobials, 10, 9-9. doi:10.1186/1476-0711-10-9

[20] Russo, R., Superti, F., Karadja, E., & De Seta, F. (2018). Randomized clinical trial in women with Recurrent Vulvovaginal Candidiasis: efficacy of probiotics and lactoferrin as maintenance treatment. Mycoses, doi:10.1111/myc.12883

[21] Shah, M. P., Gujjari, S. K., & Chandrasekhar, V. S. (2013). Evaluation of the Effect of Probiotic (Inersan®) Alone, Combination of Probiotic with Doxycycline and Doxycycline Alone on Aggressive Periodontitis – A Clinical and Microbiological Study. Journal of Clinical and Diagnostic Research : JCDR, 7(3), 595-600. doi:10.7860/JCDR/2013/5225.2834

[22] Kailasapathy, K., Chin, J. J. I., & biology, c. (2000). Survival and therapeutic potential of probiotic organisms with reference to Lactobacillus acidophilus and Bifidobacterium spp. 78(1), 80-88.

[23] Levy, S. J. J. (2002). Active efflux, a common mechanism for biocide and antibiotic resistance. 92, 65S-71S.

[24] Denkova, R. V., Yanakieva, Z., Denkova, V., & Radeva N. V. (2013). In vitro inhibitory activity of Bifidobacterium and Lactobacillus strains against Candida albicans. Bulgarian Journal of Veterinary Medicine, 16((No. 3)), 186–197.

[25] Kohler, G. A., Assefa, S., & Reid, G. (2012). Probiotic interference of Lactobacillus rhamnosus GR-1 and Lactobacillus reuteri RC-14 with the opportunistic fungal pathogen Candida albicans. Infect Dis Obstet Gynecol, 2012, 636474. doi:10.1155/2012/636474

[26] Chew, S. Y., Cheah, Y. K., Seow, H. F., Sandai, D., & Than, L. T. (2015a). Probiotic Lactobacillus rhamnosus GR-1 and Lactobacillus reuteri RC-14 exhibit strong antifungal effects against vulvovaginal candidiasis-causing Candida glabrata isolates. J Appl

Microbiol, 118(5), 1180-1190. doi:10.1111/jam.12772

[27] Tan, Y., Leonhard, M., Moser, D., Ma, S., & Schneider-Stickler, B. (2018). Inhibitory effect of probiotic lactobacilli supernatants on single and mixed non-albicans Candida species biofilm. Arch Oral Biol, 85, 40-45. doi:10.1016/j.archoralbio.2017.10.002

[28] Munoz-Quezada, S., Bermudez-Brito, M., Chenoll, E., Genovés, S., Gomez-Llorente, C., Plaza-Diaz, J. Ramón, D. J. B.. (2013). Competitive inhibition of three novel bacteria isolated from faeces of breast milk-fed infants against selected enteropathogens. 109(S2), S63-S69.

[29] Panda, S. K. (2012). Screening methods in the study of antimicrobial properties of medicinal plants. International Journal of Biotechnology and Research (IJBTR), Vol. 2(Issue 1), 1-35.

[30] Aarti, C., Khusro, A., Varghese, R., Arasu, M. V., Agastian, P., Al-Dhabi, N. A., Choi, K. C. (2018). In vitro investigation on probiotic, anti-Candida, and antibiofilm properties of Lactobacillus pentosus strain LAP1. Arch Oral Biol, 89, 99-106. doi:10.1016/j.archoralbio.2018.02.014

[31] CLSI. (2008). M38-A2 Reference Method for Broth Dilution Antifungal Susceptibility Testing of Filamentous Fungi; Approved Standard—Second Edition. Available at: http://shop.clsi.org/site/Sample_pdf/M38A2_sample.pdf

[32] Fridkin, S. K., & Jarvis, W. R. (1996). Epidemiology of nosocomial fungal infections. Clin Microbiol Rev, 9(4), 499-511.

[33] Guo, J., Mauch, A., Galle, S., Murphy, P., Arendt, E. K., & Coffey, A. (2011). Inhibition of growth of Trichophyton tonsurans by Lactobacillus reuteri. J Appl Microbiol, 111(2), 474-483. doi:10.1111/j.1365-2672.2011.05032.x

[34] Martinez, R. C., Seney, S. L., Summers, K. L., Nomizo, A., De Martinis, E. C., & Reid, G. (2009). Effect of Lactobacillus rhamnosus GR-1 and Lactobacillus reuteri RC-14 on the ability of Candida albicans to infect cells and induce inflammation. Microbiol Immunol, 53(9), 487-495. doi:10.1111/j.1348-0421.2009.00154.x

[35] Tao, X. B., Qian, L. H., Li, Y., Wu, Q., Ruan, J. J., Cai, D. Z., & Peng, H. (2014). Hospital-acquired infection rate in a tertiary care teaching hospital in China: a cross-sectional survey involving 2434 inpatients. Int J Infect Dis, 27, 7-9. doi:10.1016/j.ijid.2014.05.011

[36] Crowley, S., Mahony, J., Morrissey, J. P., & van Sinderen, D. (2013). Transcriptomic and morphological profiling of Aspergillus fumigatus Af293 in response to antifungal activity produced by Lactobacillus plantarum 16. Microbiology, 159(Pt 10), 2014-2024. doi:10.1099/mic.0.068742-0

[37] Mehdi-Alamdarloo, S., Ameri, A., Moghimipour, E., Gholipour, S., & Saadatzadeh, A. (2016). Formulation Development of a Topical Probiotic Gel for Antidermatophytosis Effect. Jundishapur J Nat Pharm Prod, 11(3), e35893. doi:10.17795/jjnpp-35893

[38] Lara-Hidalgo, C. E., Dorantes-Alvarez, L., Hernandez-Sanchez, H., Santoyo-Tepole, F., Martinez-Torres, A., Villa-Tanaca, L., & Hernandez-Rodriguez, C. (2018). Isolation of Yeasts from Guajillo Pepper (Capsicum annuum L.) Fermentation and Study of Some Probiotic Characteristics. Probiotics Antimicrob Proteins. doi:10.1007/s12602-018-9415-x

[39] Pfaller, M. A., Pappas, P. G., & Wingard, J. R. (2006). Invasive Fungal

Pathogens: Current Epidemiological Trends. Clinical Infectious Diseases 43(Supplement 1), S3-S14. doi:10.1086/504490

[40] Fijan, S. (2016). Chapter 10: Antimicrobial Effect of Probiotics against Common Pathogens. In V. Rao & L. G. Rao (Eds.), Probiotics and Prebiotics in Human Nutrition and Health Rijeka: IntechOpen.

[41] Silva, D. R., Sardi, J. D. C. O., de Souza Pitangui, N., Roque, S. M., da Silva, A. C. B., & Rosalen, P. L. J. J. O. F. F. (2020). Probiotics as an alternative antimicrobial therapy: Current reality and future directions 73, 104080.

[42] Coman, M. M., Verdenelli, M. C., Cecchini, C., Silvi, S., Orpianesi, C., Boyko, N., & Cresci, A. (2014). In vitro evaluation of antimicrobial activity of Lactobacillus rhamnosus IMC 501((R)), Lactobacillus paracasei IMC 502((R)) and SYNBIO((R)) against pathogens. J Appl Microbiol, 117(2), 518-527. doi:10.1111/jam.12544

[43] Kheradmand, E., Rafii, F., Yazdi, M. H., Sepahi, A. A., Shahverdi, A. R., & Oveisi, M. R. (2014). The antimicrobial effects of selenium nanoparticle-enriched probiotics and their fermented broth against Candida albicans. DARU Journal of Pharmaceutical Sciences, 22(1), 48. doi:10.1186/2008-2231-22-48

[44] Santos, C. M. A., Pires, M. C. V., Leão, T. L., Hernández, Z. P., Rodriguez, M. L., Martins, A. K. S., Nicoli, J. R. (2016). Selection of Lactobacillus strains as potential probiotics for vaginitis treatment. Microbiology, 162(7), 1195-1207. 10.1099/mic.0.000302

[45] Gospodarek, E., Bogiel, T., & Zalas-Wiecek, P. J. P. J.M. (2009). Communication between microorganisms as a basis for production of virulence factors. 58(3), 191-198.

[46] de Barros, P. P., Scorzoni, L., Ribeiro, F. C., Fugisaki, L. R. O., Fuchs, B. B., Mylonakis, E., Rossoni, R. D. (2018). Lactobacillus paracasei 28.4 reduces in vitro hyphae formation of Candida albicans and prevents the filamentation in an experimental model of Caenorhabditis elegans. Microb Pathog, 117, 80-87. doi:10.1016/j.micpath.2018.02.019

[47] Gabrielli, E., Pericolini, E., Ballet, N., Roselletti, E., Sabbatini, S., Mosci, P., Vecchiarelli, A. (2018). Saccharomyces cerevisiae-based probiotic as novel anti-fungal and anti-inflammatory agent for therapy of vaginal candidiasis. Benef Microbes, 9(2), 219-230. doi:10.3920/bm2017.0099

[48] Oliveira, V. M. C. S., Silva, C.R.G.; Jorge, A. O. C., Leão, M. V. P. (2016). Lactobacillus is able to alter the virulence and the sensitivity profile of Candida albicans. Journal of applied microbiology, 121(6), 1737-1744.

[49] Pan, W., Lin, J., & Le, C. T. J. G. b. (2002). How many replicates of arrays are required to detect gene expression changes in microarray experiments? A mixture model approach. 3(5), 1-10.

[50] Chew, S. Y., Cheah, Y. K., Seow, H. F., Sandai, D., & Than, L. T. L. (2015b). In vitro modulation of probiotic bacteria on the biofilm of Candida glabrata. Anaerobe, 34, 132-138.

[51] Henriques, M., Azeredo, J., & Oliveira, R. (2006). Candida albicans and Candida dubliniensis: comparison of biofilm formation in terms of biomass and activity. British journal of biomedical science, 63(1), 5-11.

[52] Lu, Y., Su, C., Unoje, O., & Liu, H. (2014). Quorum sensing controls hyphal initiation in Candida albicans through Ubr1-mediated protein degradation. Proceedings of the National Academy of Sciences, 111(5), 1975-1980.

[53] Mason, K. L., Downward, J. R. E., Mason, K. D., Falkowski, N. R., Eaton, K. A., Kao, J. Y., Huffnagle, G. B. (2012). Candida albicans and bacterial microbiota interactions in the cecum during recolonization following broad-spectrum antibiotic therapy. Infection and immunity, 80(10), 3371-3380.

[54] Martín, R., Sánchez, B., Suárez, J. E., & Urdaci, M. C. (2012). Characterization of the adherence properties of human Lactobacilli strains to be used as vaginal probiotics. FEMS microbiology letters, 328(2), 166-173.

[55] Lebeaux, D., Chauhan, A., Rendueles, O., & Beloin, C. J. P. (2013). From in vitro to in vivo models of bacterial biofilm-related infections.2(2), 288-356.

[56] Hossain, T. J., Chowdhury, S. I., Mozumder, H. A., Chowdhury, M. N., Ali, F., Rahman, N., & Dey, S. J. F. i. m. (2020). Hydrolytic Exoenzymes Produced by Bacteria Isolated and Identified From the Gastrointestinal Tract of Bombay Duck. 11, 2097.

[57] Zhao, C., Lv, X., Fu, J., He, C., Hua, H., & Yan, Z. (2016). In vitro inhibitory activity of probiotic products against oral Candida species. Journal of Applied Microbiology, 121(1), 254-262. doi:10.1111/jam.13138

[58] Guo, J., Brosnan, B., Furey, A., Arendt, E., Murphy, P., & Coffey, A. (2012). Antifungal activity of Lactobacillus against Microsporum canis, Microsporum gypseum and Epidermophyton floccosum. Bioeng Bugs, 3(2), 104-113. doi:10.4161/bbug.19624

[59] Eisenberg-Lerner, A., Bialik, S., Simon, H.-U., & Kimchi, A. (2009). Life and death partners: apoptosis, autophagy and the cross-talk between them. Cell death and differentiation, 16(7), 966.

[60] Elmore, S. (2007). Apoptosis: a review of programmed cell death. Toxicologic pathology, 35(4), 495-516.

[61] Avery, S. V. (2011). Molecular targets of oxidative stress. Biochemical Journal, 434(2), 201-210.

[62] Hao, B., Cheng, S., Clancy, C. J., & Nguyen, M. H. (2013). Caspofungin kills Candida albicans by causing both cellular apoptosis and necrosis. Antimicrob Agents Chemother, 57(1), 326-332. doi:10.1128/aac.01366-12

[63] Hwang, J., Choi, H., Kim, A., Yun, J., Yu, R., Woo, E. R., & Lee, D. (2014). Hibicuslide C-induced cell death in C andida albicans involves apoptosis mechanism. Journal of applied microbiology, 117(5), 1400-1411.

[64] Khan, A., Ahmad, A., Khan, L. A., & Manzoor, N. (2014). Ocimum sanctum (L.) essential oil and its lead molecules induce apoptosis in Candida albicans. Research in microbiology, 165(6), 411-419.

[65] Ribeiro, G. F., Côrte-Real, M., & Johansson, B. (2006). Characterization of DNA damage in yeast apoptosis induced by hydrogen peroxide, acetic acid, and hyperosmotic shock. Molecular biology of the cell, 17(10), 4584-4591.

[66] Seong, M., & Lee, D. G. (2018). Reactive oxygen species-independent apoptotic pathway by gold nanoparticles in Candida albicans. Microbiological research, 207, 33-40.

[67] Yun, J., Hwang, J.-S., & Lee, D. G. (2017). The antifungal activity of the peptide, periplanetasin-2, derived from American cockroach Periplaneta americana. Biochemical Journal, 474(17), 3027-3043.

[68] Hwang, I. s., Lee, J., Hwang, J. H., Kim, K. J., & Lee, D. G. (2012). Silver

nanoparticles induce apoptotic cell death in Candida albicans through the increase of hydroxyl radicals. The FEBS journal, 279(7), 1327-1338.

[69] Lee, H., Hwang, J.-S., & Lee, D. G. (2016). Scolopendin 2 leads to cellular stress response in Candida albicans. Apoptosis, 21(7), 856-865.

[70] Ma, F., Zhang, Y., Wang, Y., Wan, Y., Miao, Y., Ma, T., Li, M. (2016). Role of Aif1 in regulation of cell death under environmental stress in Candida albicans. Yeast, 33(9), 493-506.

[71] Lee, J., & Lee, D. G. (2015). Novel antifungal mechanism of resveratrol: apoptosis inducer in Candida albicans. Current microbiology, 70(3), 383-389.

[72] Yun, D. G., & Lee, D. G. (2016). Silibinin triggers yeast apoptosis related to mitochondrial Ca2+ influx in Candida albicans. The international journal of biochemistry & cell biology, 80, 1-9.

[73] Zak, O., & O'Reilly, T. (1991). Animal models in the evaluation of antimicrobial agents. Antimicrobial agents and chemotherapy, 35(8), 1527.

[74] Craig, W. A. (2014). In vitro and animal PK/PD models. In Fundamentals of Antimicrobial Pharmacokinetics and Pharmacodynamics (pp. 23-44): Springer.

[75] Hau, J., & Schapiro, S. J. (2010). Handbook of Laboratory Animal Science, Volume I: Essential Principles and Practices: CRC press.

[76] Hebecker, B., Vlaic, S., Conrad, T., Bauer, M., Brunke, S., Kapitan, M., Jacobsen, I. D. (2016). Dual-species transcriptional profiling during systemic candidiasis reveals organ-specific host-pathogen interactions. Scientific reports, 6, 36055.

[77] Jacobsen, I. D. (2014). Galleria mellonella as a model host to study virulence of Candida. Virulence, 5(2), 237-239.

[78] Jacobsen, I. D., Lüttich, A., Kurzai, O., Hube, B., & Brock, M. (2014). In vivo imaging of disseminated murine Candida albicans infection reveals unexpected host sites of fungal persistence during antifungal therapy. Journal of Antimicrobial Chemotherapy, 69(10), 2785-2796.

[79] Pierce, C. G., Chaturvedi, A. K., Lazzell, A. L., Powell, A. T., Saville, S. P., McHardy, S. F., & Lopez-Ribot, J. L. (2015). A novel small molecule inhibitor of Candida albicans biofilm formation, filamentation and virulence with low potential for the development of resistance. NPJ Biofilms and Microbiomes, 1, 15012.

[80] Bergeron, A. C., Seman, B. G., Hammond, J. H., Archambault, L. S., Hogan, D. A., & Wheeler, R. T. (2017). Interact To Enhance Virulence of Mucosal Infection in Transparent Zebrafish. Infection and Immunity, 85(11), e00475-e00417. doi:10.1128/IAI.00475-17

[81] Németh, T., Tóth, A., Szenzenstein, J., Horváth, P., Nosanchuk, J. D., Grózer, Z., Vágvölgyi, C. (2013). Characterization of virulence properties in the C. parapsilosis sensu lato species. PloS one. 8(7), e68704.

[82] Hamamoto, H., Kurokawa, K., Kaito, C., Kamura, K., Razanajatovo, I. M., Kusuhara, H., Sekimizu, K. (2004). Quantitative evaluation of the therapeutic effects of antibiotics using silkworms infected with human pathogenic microorganisms. Antimicrobial agents and chemotherapy, 48(3), 774-779.

[83] Ishijima, S. A., Hayama, K., Burton, J. P., Reid, G., Okada, M., Matsushita, Y., & Abe, S. (2012). Effect of

Streptococcus salivarius K12 on the in vitro growth of Candida albicans and its protective effect in an oral candidiasis model. Appl Environ Microbiol, 78(7), 2190-2199. doi:10.1128/aem.07055-11

[84] Leao, M. V. P., Tavares, T. A. A., Goncalves, E. S. C. R., Dos Santos, S. S. F., Junqueira, J. C., de Oliveira, L. D., & Jorge, A. O. C. (2018). Lactobacillus rhamnosus intake can prevent the development of Candidiasis. Clin Oral Investig, 22(7), 2511-2518. doi:10.1007/s00784-018-2347-8

[85] Vilela, S. F. G., Barbosa, J. O., Rossoni, R. D., Santos, J. D., Prata, M. C. A., Anbinder, A. L., Junqueira, J. C. (2015). Lactobacillus acidophilus ATCC 4356 inhibits biofilm formation by C. albicans and attenuates the experimental candidiasis in Galleria mellonella. Virulence, 6(1), 29-39. doi:10.4161/21505594.2014.981486

[86] Dronkers, T. M., Ouwehand, A. C., & Rijkers, G. T. J. H. (2020). Global analysis of clinical trials with probiotics. 6(7), e04467.

[87] Hill, C., Guarner, F., Reid, G., Gibson, G. R., Merenstein, D. J., Pot, B., Hepatology. (2014). The International Scientific Association for Probiotics and Prebiotics consensus statement on the scope and appropriate use of the term probiotic 11(8), 506-514.

[88] Manzoni, P., Mostert, M., Leonessa, M. L., Priolo, C., Farina, D., Monetti, C., Gomirato, G. (2006). Oral Supplementation with Lactobacillus casei Subspecies rhamnosus Prevents Enteric Colonization by Candida Species in Preterm Neonates: A Randomized Study. Clinical Infectious Diseases, 42(12), 1735-1742. doi:https://doi.org/10.1086/504324

[89] Sutula, J., Coulthwaite, L., Thomas, L., & Verran, J. (2012). The effect of a commercial probiotic drink on oral microbiota in healthy complete denture wearers. Microb Ecol Health Dis, 23.

[90] Sutula, J., Coulthwaite, L. A., Thomas, L. V., & Verran, J. (2013). The effect of a commercial probiotic drink containing Lactobacillus casei strain Shirota on oral health in healthy dentate people. Microb Ecol Health Dis, 24.

[91] Pirotta, M., Gunn, J., Chondros, P., Grover, S., O'Malley, P., Hurley, S., & Garland, S. (2004). Effect of lactobacillus in preventing post-antibiotic vulvovaginal candidiasis: a randomised controlled trial. BMJ, 329(7465), 548-548. doi:10.1136/bmj.38210.494977.DE

[92] Degnan, F. H. (2012). Clinical studies involving probiotics: When FDA's investigational new drug rubric applies—and when it may not. Gut Microbes, 3(6), 485-489. doi:10.4161/gmic.22158

[93] Keller, M. K., & Kragelund, C. (2018). Randomized pilot study on probiotic effects on recurrent candidiasis in oral lichen planus patients. Oral Dis, 24(6), 1107-1114. doi:10.1111/odi.12858

[94] Mishra, R., Tandon, S., Rathore, M., & Banerjee, M. (2016). Antimicrobial efficacy of probiotic and herbal oral rinses against Candida albicans in children: a randomized clinical trial. International journal of clinical pediatric dentistry, 9(1), 25.

[95] Santos, A. L. D.; Jorge, A. O. C.; Santos, S. S. F. D.; & Leão, M. V. P. (2009). Influence of probiotics on Candida presence and IgA anti-Candida in the oral cavity. Brazilian Journal of Microbiology, 40(4), 960-964.

[96] Davar, R., Nokhostin, F., Eftekhar, M., Sekhavat, L., Zadeh, M. B., & Shamsi, F. (2016). Comparing the recurrence of vulvovaginal candidiasis in patients undergoing prophylactic treatment with probiotic and placebo during the 6 months. Probiotics and antimicrobial proteins, 8(3), 130-133.

[97] Fu, J., Ding, Y., Wei, B., Wang, L., Xu, S., Qin, P., Jiang, L. (2017). Epidemiology of Candida albicans and non-C.albicans of neonatal candidemia at a tertiary care hospital in western China. BMC Infectious Diseases, 17(1), 329. doi:10.1186/s12879-017-2423-8

[98] Mezzasalma, V., Manfrini, E., Ferri, E., Boccarusso, M., Di Gennaro, P., Schiano, I., Labra, M. (2017). Orally administered multispecies probiotic formulations to prevent uro-genital infections: a randomized placebo-controlled pilot study. Archives of gynecology and obstetrics, 295(1), 163-172.

[99] Reid, G. (2016). The development of probiotics for women's health. Canadian journal of microbiology, 63(4), 269-277.

[100] Zuo, T., & Ng, S. C. (2018). The Gut Microbiota in the Pathogenesis and Therapeutics of Inflammatory Bowel Disease. Frontiers in microbiology, 9, 2247-2247. doi:10.3389/fmicb.2018.02247

[101] Benjamin, D. K., Stoll, B. J., Fanaroff, A. A., & McDonald, S. A. (2006). National Institute of Child Health and Human Development neonatal research network. Neonatal candidiasis among extremely low birth weight infants: risk factors, mortality rates, and neurodevelopmental outcomes at 18 to 22 months. Pediatrics, 117. doi:10.1542/peds.2004-2292

[102] Shetty, S. S., Harrison, L. H., Hajjeh, R. A., & Taylor, T. (2005). Determining risk factors for candidemia among newborn infants from population-based surveillance: Baltimore, Maryland, 1998-2000. Pediatr Infect Dis J, 24. doi:10.1097/01.inf.0000168751.11375.d6

Chapter 6

Single Strain Probiotic Bifidobacteria Approach in Health and Non-Health Fields

Hüseyin Sancar Bozkurt and Havva Bozkurt

Abstract

Single strain probiotic bifidobacteria approach is promising for the future in health and non-health fields. Recent studies show that intestinal lumen microbial content and tissue microbial content are different, so the personalized microbiome approach with the 16S rRNA analysis comes to the fore with the single strain probiotic bifidobacteria (BB-12,Infantis) approach. In addition to their immune modulation effect, they have beneficial effects such as preventing pathogens from binding to the intestinal mucosa via the biofilm layer they produce, and also their electrophysical properties in various atmospheric conditions, They have the ability to be used in non-health areas such as microplastic biodegradition, nanostructures, food and agriculture fields. The availability of single strain probiotic bifidobacteria in health, ecological and food systems are signs that progress in the single strain probiotic bacteria approach will be more accurate.

Keywords: probiotic, bifidobacteria, health, ecology

1. Introduction

Probiotic bifidobacteria are living microorganisms that have beneficial immunomodulatory effects on human health and have fermentation properties. They can play a role in the management of dysbiosis-related intestinal disorders such as colon cancer, IBD, Celiac, IBS, as well as virological disorders such as SARS-Cov-2 and neurologic disorders. Although there are many scientific studies on the effects of single strain of probiotic bifidobacteria on human health, there are very few publications on their behavior and interactions in various atmospheric conditions other than the human body. In this section, we present the effects of single strain of probiotic bifidobacteria approach in the field of health, as well as the electrophysiological behaviors and interactions in various atmospheric conditions with different materials.

1.1 Single strain of probiotic Bifidobacteria approach in the field of health

1.1.1 Single strain of probiotic Bifidobacteria in gastrointestinal disorders

As we discussed in detail in our previous work [1], the human intestinal microbiota includes commensal, symbiotic, and pathogenic bacteria species [2, 3]. It was demonstrated that intestinal microbiota have anti-inflammatory features and contribute to the immune, neuroendocrine, and metabolic homeostasis of the host [4, 5]. The genus Bifidobacterium in gut microbiota is Gram-positive, non-motile, often branched anaerobic bacteria and it belongs to the phylum Actinobacteria [1]. Bifidobacteria are one of the dominant species in the human gut microbiota and are frequently used as probiotics [6]. *B. animalis* subsp. *lactis* exerts the highest level of intracellular hydrogen peroxide resistance among Bifidobacteria and provide protection against reactive cellular oxygen species [7]. Reduced bifidobacteria levels are associated with inflammatory bowel disease (IBD) [8, 9]. *B. infantis* 35624 has been shown that reduced plasma pro-inflammatory biomarkers in IBD and extra-intestinal inflammatory disorders [10].

Also, the administration of *B. infantis* 35624 was associated with a significant reduction in plasma pro-inflammatory biomarkers in patients with psoriatic disorder and oral administration of *B. infantis* 35624 modulates the cytokine across both gastrointestinal and non-gastrointestinal inflammatory disorders and healthy subjects. In our previous study [11], endoscopic single *Bifidobacterium animalis* subsp. *lactis* and xyloglucan administration was found effective in the mucosal healing and resolution of colonic symptoms in ulcerative colitis patients (**Figures 1** and 2) [11].

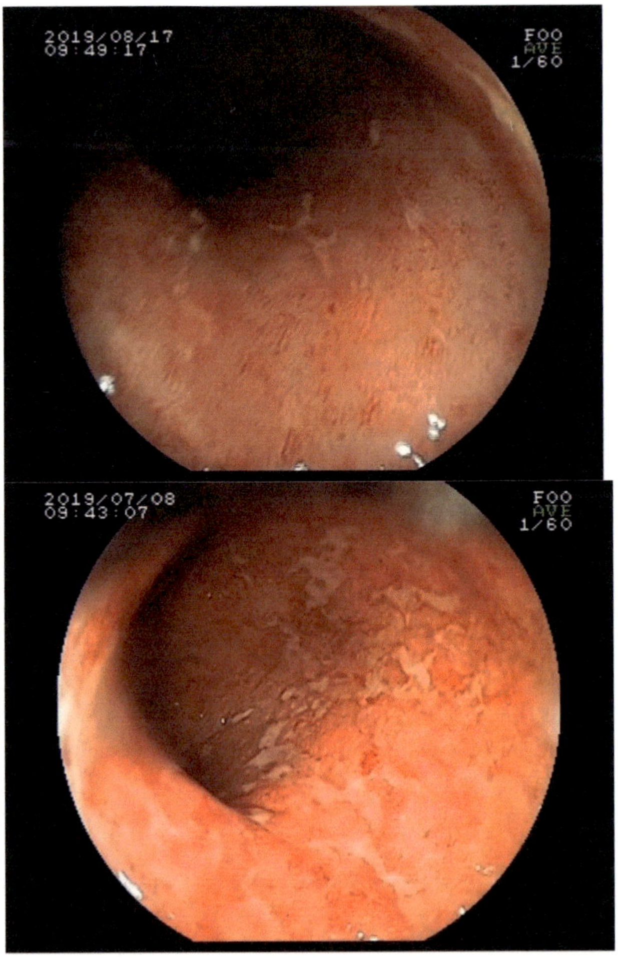

Figure 1.
Mucosal healing (upper) within one month after a single intracolonic application of 200 billion colony forming units (CFUs) of Bifidobacterium animalis *sp.* Lactis *and 4 gr Xyloglucan combination in unresponsive ulcerative colitis (below) [11].*

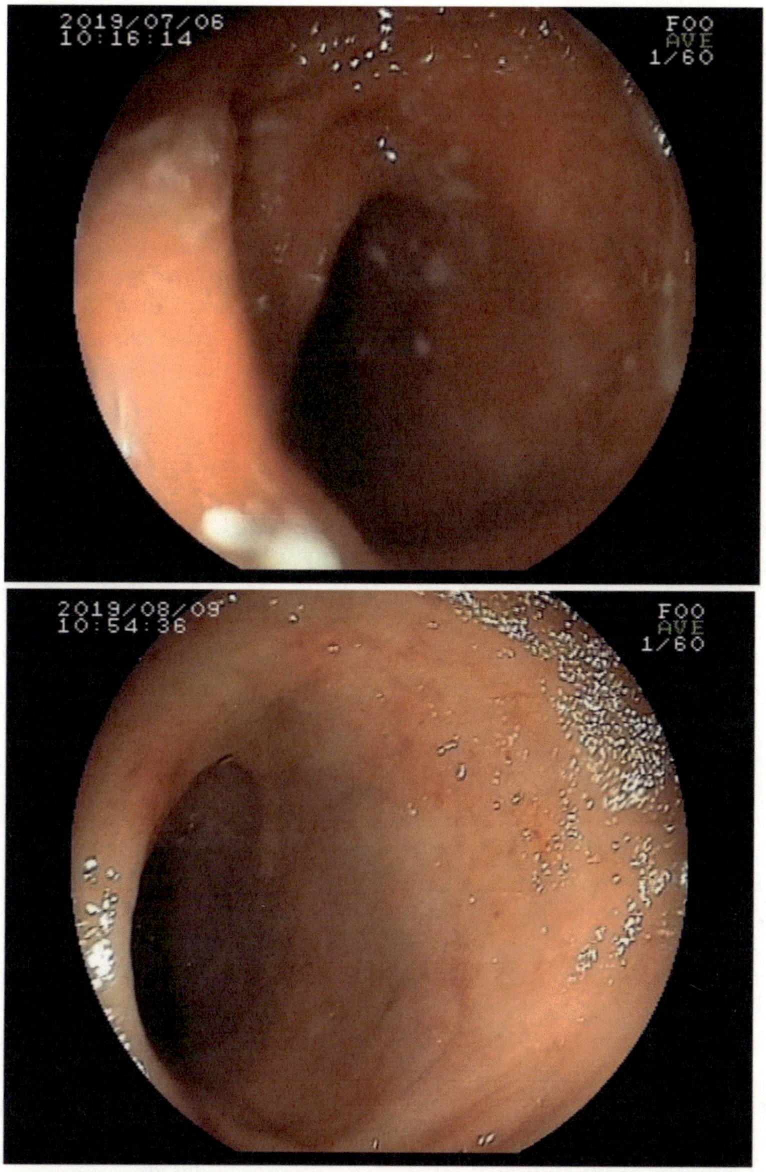

Figure 2.
Mucosal healing (below) within one month after a single intracolonic application of 200 billion colony forming units (CFUs) of Bifidobacterium animalis *sp.* Lactis *and 4 gr Xyloglucan combination in unresponsive ulcerative proctosigmoid colitis (upper) [11].*

The use of single strain probiotic bifidobacteria such as BB-12 and Infantis in effective and appropriate doses can be considered an effective treatment method for intestinal and extraintestinal disorders.

Another aspect of the single strain probiotic bifidobacteria is that they are suitable candidates for the next generation probiotic. As we discussed in detail our previous study [1], With the Open Reading Frame (ORF) method, these species can be guided by genetic coding for postbiotic production [12]. Mycosporin amino acids are a viable target for this situation. Mycosporin-like amino acids (MAAs) are low molecular weight amino acids. MAAs act as absorbers of ultraviolet (UV) light and as photo protectants which are unique components of red seaweeds [13]. Seaweed products are used as nutritional supplements in the management of bowel diseases.

MAAs also play a key role in protecting against sunlight damage by acting as antioxidant molecules scavenging toxic oxygen radicals. MAAs have been described to affect the intestinal mucosa, enhancing villus structure, as well as the intestinal microbiota, increasing the abundance of Bifidobacterium and, importantly, reducing the prevalence of Clostridium species in animal models [14]. Also, modulation of NF-κB and tryptophan metabolism via MAAs has a beneficial effect on the gut immune system. Besides these features, MAAs also inhibit thiobarbituric acid reactive oxygen species which are increased in colon cancer.

In this context, MAA-producing single strain *Bifidobacteria* species via ORF could result in a bacterium that is more potent in the prevention of dysbiosis associated disorders such as IBD, CRC, Chronic inflammation. Also, MAAs produced via ORF might be used not only as a probiotic but also as a pharmacological agent in intestinal disorders.

1.1.2 Single strain probiotic Bifidobacteria in Sars-Cov-2 management

As we reported in our previous study [15], Sars-Cov-2 is a pandemic virus that manifests itself with respiratory distress as well as leading to symptoms and signs associated with the gastrointestinal tract. Sars-Cov-2 is especially manifested by the disturbed adaptive immune status in lung and intestinal tissues which is called 'cytokine storm'. During their cellular replication, viral pathogens such as Sars-Cov-2 increase endoplasmic reticulum stress and exert their autophagy inducing effects through the adaptive TH17 / IL17 system and this leads to an uncontrolled immune response [15]. The cytokine storm can be modulated through immune effects of strain specific probiotic bifidobacteria. In our previous study, *Bifidobacterium animalis* sp. Lactis-BB12 led to rapid mucosal healing in ulcerative colitis patients [11] and this effect was related to the IL-17 inhibitory effect of the BB-12 strain. IL-6 promotes the generation of Th17 cells and that IL-6 and IL-17 synergistically promote viral replication and *B. infantis* 35624 could reduce the systemic inflammatory biomarkers such as IL-6,CRP, TNF alpha [15]. Also, *Bifidobacterium infantis* reduced the duration of acute respiratory infections illness in children and adults [16]. The administration of booster of an appropriate strain of bifidobacterium (such as BB-12, or infantis) especially in patients with gastrointestinal symptoms (diarrhea, abdominal pain, vomiting), may be postulated to have a role in the management of coronavirus infected patients (**Figure 3**).

1.1.3 Single strain probiotic Bifidobacteria in vaccine development

Gut dysbiosis might play a role in the failure to respond to vaccines. In this regard, gut microbiota could affect intestinal immune responses by acting as

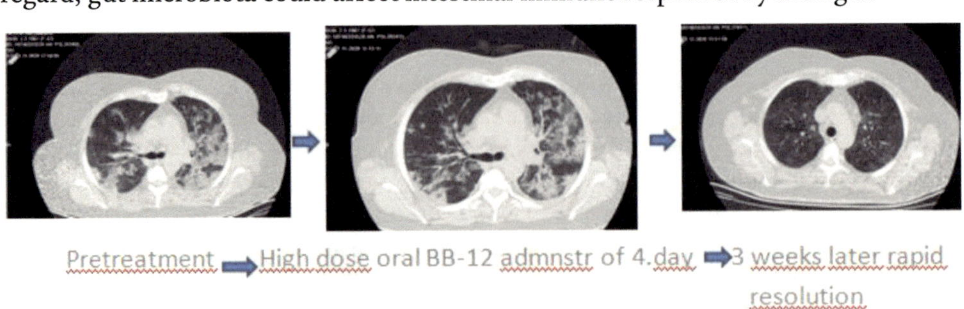

Figure 3.
Rapid radiologic enhancement of high dose oral Bifidobacterium *BB-12 administration in severe Sars-Cov-2 [15].*

immune modulators as well as natural vaccine adjuvants [17]. The administration of the probiotic strain *Bifidobacterium* BB-12 significantly increased antigen-specific immune responses in healthy individuals receiving influenza vaccination [18]. Also, Exopolysaccharide produced by *B. longum* 35624 played an essential role in the anti-inflammatory effects of this bacterium and removal of exopolysaccharide (EPS) resulted, not only in loss of these anti-inflammatory effects, but to a transformation to become an inducer of local TH17 responses [19]. In some experiments, EPS- protein conjugate vaccines could enhance immunogenity [20]. Our studies revealed that the maintenance of the unique electrophysiological properties of BB-12,Infantis in an aerobic environment for up to 6 months could be attributed to the integrity of their unique EPS structure [21]. Hence, the single strain probiotic bifidbacterial polysaccharide cell structure can be considered as a lipopeptide based vaccines.

Since the relationship between viral replication and gastrointestinal immunity is very close, an appropriate approach over probiotic bifid bacteria can play an important role in reducing viral replication. New approaches to the single strain probiotic bacteria can be promising, both in terms of vaccination and treatment models.

2. Single strain probiotic Bifidobacteria in non-health fields

2.1 Electrophysiological properties of Bifidobacterium BB12 and infantis

2.1.1 Bifidobacterium BB-12

As we cited in our previous study [1], BB-12 is technologically well suited, expressing fermentation activity, high aerotolerance, good stability and a high acid and bile tolerance. Because of high redox potential in the colon microbiota ecosystem, BB-12 is highly resistant bacteria in distress condition. The BB-12 cell envelope is an electrical and physical barrier that that consist of redox proteins. Bacterial cellular electron transfer systems (CET) are defined microbial bioelectrochemical processes in which electrons are transferred from the cytosol to the membrane of the cell [22, 23]. Charge transport behavior and the effect of the Relative Humidity (RH) level on it in the BB-12 film have been investigated by means of I-V measurements. Within aqua moisture environment, electrical conductivity of the BB-12 increased more than six decades while under N environment conductivity returns to the initial current value (**Figure 4**).

This behavior in conductivity modulation was reversible at least in the three cycle [21].

As we stated in our study [21], this experimental findings showed us that there was no structural transformation under relative humidity. On the other side, increase in the conductivity was interpreted by the increase in the population of charge carries, supplied by the interaction BB-12 with the water moisture, monitored by amine and carboxyl group through FTIR and Zeta potential measurements. The type of surface charge of *Bifidobacterium animalis* subsp. *lactis* BB-12 was found to be negative by zeta potential measurements, claiming that electrons were the charge carriers. Overall, obtained result in this study indicated that *Bifidobacterium* BB-12 has a great potential for humidity sensing device at room temperature.

2.1.2 Bifidobacterium Infantis

B. infantis 35624 is probiotic commensal bacteria that dominates the intestinal microbiota of breastfed babies and by accelerating and balancing the maturation of

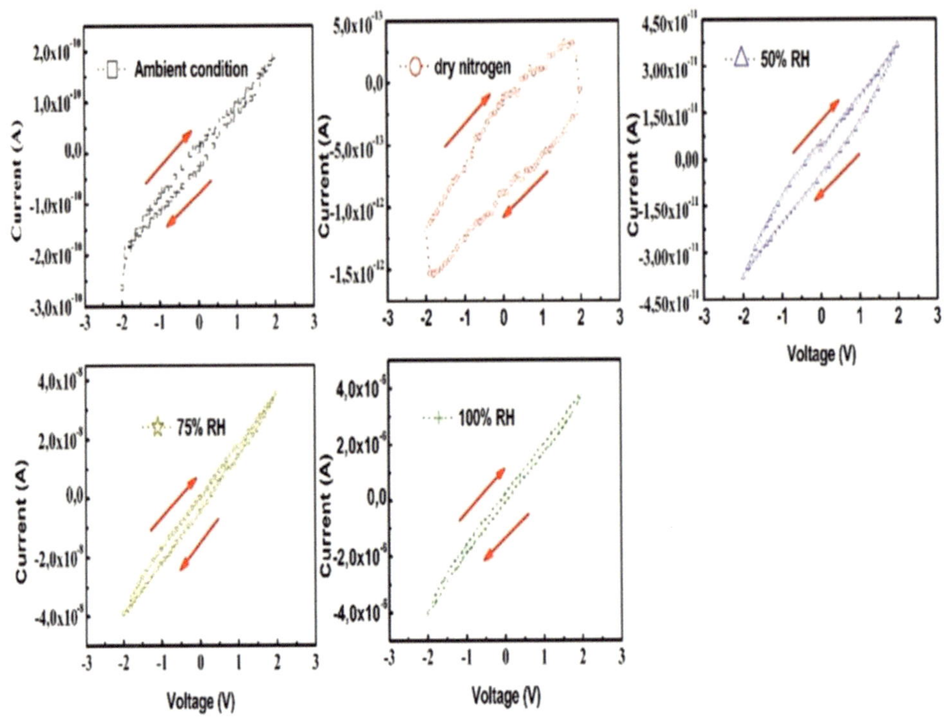

Figure 4.
I–V characteristics of the film of Bifidobacterium animalis subsp. lactis BB-12 at various RH levels.

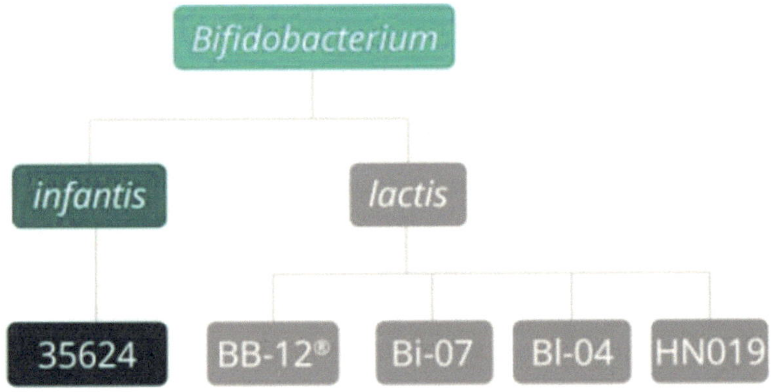

Figure 5.
Bifidobacterium Infantis.

the system and that improves intestinal barrier function and also benefits the host by increasing acetate production (**Figure 5**).

Interaction of aqua molecules with the surface of the *Bifidobacterium infantis* film leads to an increase. Increase in sensor current to a nearly constant value within a few minutes. Increase in sensor current, with aqua molecules, the interaction between bifidobacteria and aqua is highly dependent on the molecular structure of the assays.

Sensor sensitivity increases with the increase in relative humidity, aqua on the film surface reveals that adsorption of molecules is a multilayer process. Room linear increase in sensitivity with relative humidity, sensors 0–90% relative humidity indicates that it can be used for practical applications in the sensing range (**Figure 6**).

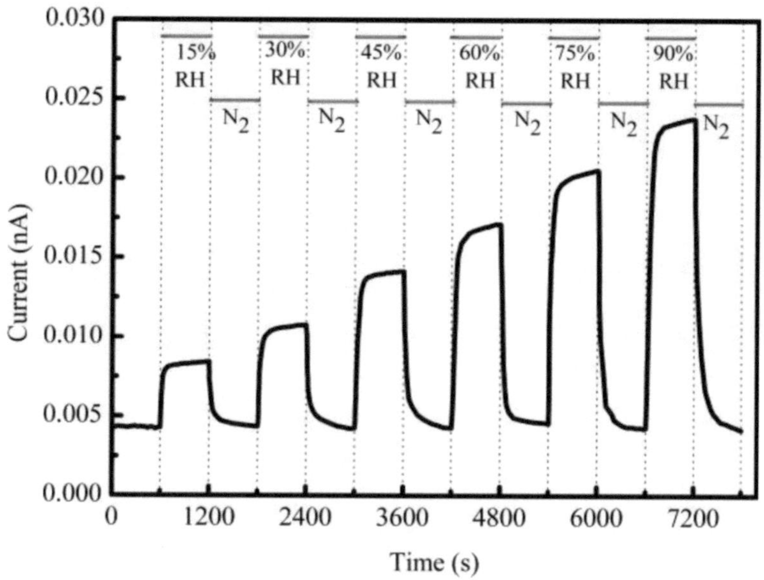

Figure 6.
Response-recovery behavior of Bifidobacterium infantis*-based sensor for various RH levels.*

3. Future approaches with single strain probiotic Bifidobacteria

Infection of medical equipment is one of the most common problems in the healthcare field, medical equipment infection can be prevented by probiotic bifidobacterial adhesion (**Figure 7**). Also, depending on the electrophysiological properties of these single strain probiotic bifidobacteria species, which have antimicrobial,

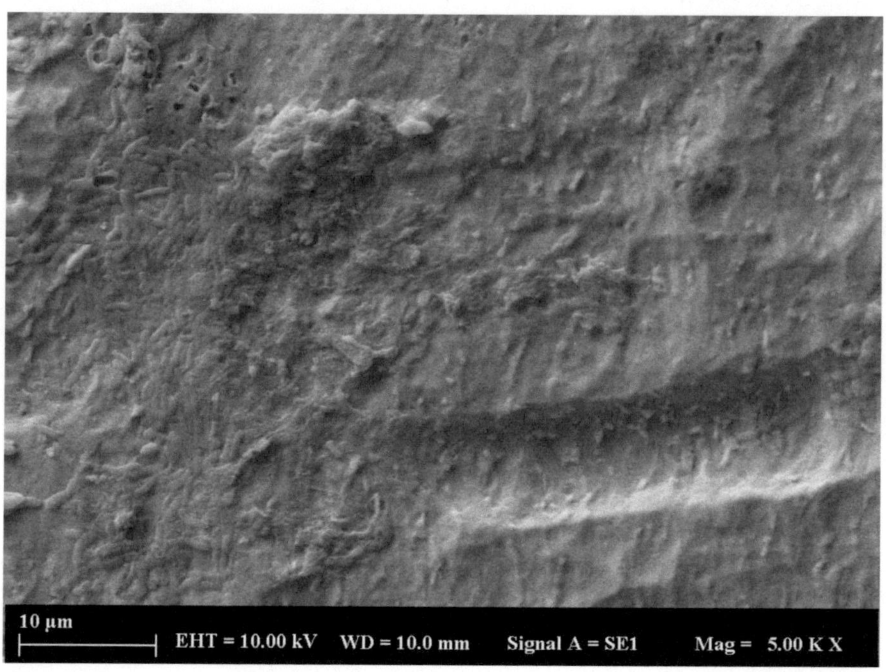

Figure 7.
Single strain probiotic bifidobacteria adhesion on medical orthopedic implant on scanning electron microscope (SEM) appearance.

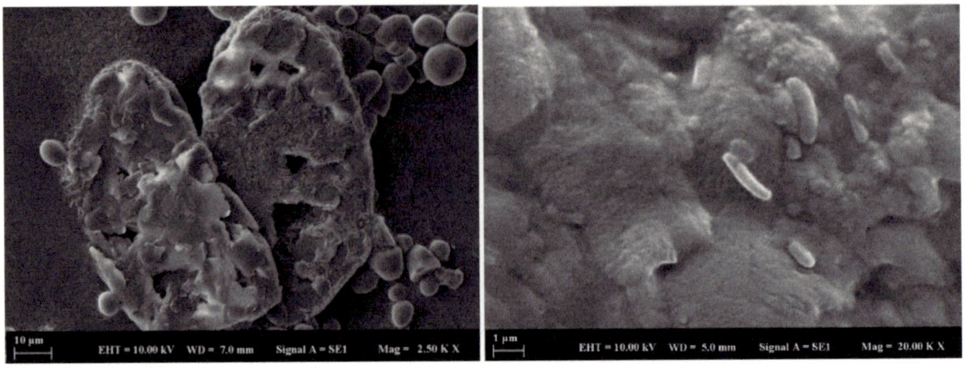

Figure 8.
Single strain probiotic bifidobacteria adhesion (left appearance of SEM) and biodegradation (right appearance of SEM EDS) on polypropylene microplastic.

immunomodulatory and beneficial effects on human health, they have paved the way for a new era in many areas such as agriculture, food, biodegradation of microplastics (**Figure 8**) and a healthy ecological system.

4. Conclusion

Single strain probiotic bifidbacteria approach is a promising approach in cases such as inflammatory bowel diseases, bowel disorders, virological disorders and colon cancer. Beside these, single strain probiotic bifidobacteria approach is promising for a healthy ecosystem depending on its behavior in atmospheric conditions.

Conflict of interest

The authors declare no conflict of interest.

Author details

Hüseyin Sancar Bozkurt[1*] and Havva Bozkurt[2]

1 Clinic of Gastroenterology, Internal Medicine, Medicine Faculty, Maltepe University, Istanbul, Turkey

2 Medicine Laboratuary, İstanbul, Turkey

*Address all correspondence to: sancarb79@gmail.com

References

[1] Bozkurt, H.S.; Quigley, E.M.; Kara, B. Bifidobacterium animalis subspecies lactis engineered to produce mycosporin-like amino acids in colorectal cancer prevention. SAGE Open Med. 2019, 7.

[2] The NIH HMP Working Group; Peterson, J.; Garges, S.; Giovanni, M.; McInnes, P.; Wang, L.; Schloss, J.A.; Bonazzi, V.; McEwen, J.E.; Wetterstrand, K.A.; et al. The NIH Human Microbiome Project. Genome Res. 2009, 19, 2317-2323.

[3] Sherwood, L.; Willey, J.; Woolverton, C.J. Prescott's Microbiology, 9th ed.; McGraw-Hill Education: New York, NY, USA, 2013; pp. 713-721

[4] 4.Cahenzli, J.; Balmer, M.L.; McCoy, K.D. Microbial-immune cross-talk and regulation of the immune system. Immunology 2012, 138, 12-22.

[5] Sunkara, T.; Rawla, P.; Ofosu, A.; Gaduputi, V. Fecal microbiota transplant—A new frontier in inflammatory bowel disease. J. Inflamm. Res. 2018, 11, 321-328.

[6] Bozkurt, H.S.; Quigley, E.M.M. Bifidobacteria and Mucosal-Associated Invariant T (MAIT) Cells: A New Approach to Colorectal Cancer Prevention? Gastrointest. Disord. 2019, 1, 266-272.

[7] Oberg, T.S.; Steele, J.L.; Ingham, S.C.; Smeianov, V.V. Intrinsic and inducible resistance to hydrogen peroxide in Bifidobacterium species. J. Ind. Microbiol. Biotechnol. 2011, 38, 1947-1953.

[8] 8.Hughes, K.R.; Harnisch, L.C.; Alcon-Giner, C.; Mitra, S.; Wright, C.J.; Ketskemety, J.; van Sinderen, D.; Watson, A.J.; Hall, L.J. Bifidobacterium breve reduces apoptotic epithelial cell shedding in an exopolysaccharide and MyD88-dependent manner. Open Biol. 2017, 7, 1.

[9] Duranti, S.; Gaiani, F.; Mancabelli, L.; Milani, C.; Grandi, A.; Bolchi, A.; Santoni, A.; Lugli, G.A.; Ferrario, C.; Mangifesta, M.; et al. Elucidating the gut microbiome of ulcerative colitis: Bifidobacteria as novel microbial biomarkers. FEMS Microbiol. Ecol. 2016, 92.

[10] David Groeger, Liam O'Mahony, Eileen F. Murphy, John F. Bourke, Timothy G. Dinan, Barry Kiely, Fergus Shanahan & Eamonn M.M. Quigley (2013) Bifidobacteriuminfantis 35624 modulates host inflammatory processes beyond the gut, Gut Microbes, 4: 4, 325-339.

[11] 11.Bozkurt HS, Kara B. A new treatment for ulcerative colitis: Intracolonic Bifidobacterium and xyloglucan application. European Journal of Inflammation. January 2020. doi:10.1177/2058739220942626.

[12] Bozkurt HS, Quigley EM, Kara B. *Bifidobacterium animalis* subspecies lactis engineered to produce mycosporin-like amino acids in colorectal cancer prevention. SAGE Open Med. 2019;7:2050312119825784. Published 2019 Jan 22. doi:10.1177/2050312119825784.

[13] Llewellyn CA, Airs RL. Distribution and abundance of MAAs in 33 species of microalgae across 13 classes. Mar Drugs 2010; 8(4): 1273-1291.

[14] Cian RE, Drago SR, de Medina FS, et al. Proteins and carbohydrates from red seaweeds: evidence for beneficial effects on gut function and microbiota. Mar Drugs 2015; 13(8): 5358-5383

[15] Bozkurt HS, Quigley EM. The probiotic Bifidobacterium in the management of Coronavirus: A

theoretical basis. International Journal of Immunopathology and Pharmacology. January 2020. doi:10.1177/2058738420961304.

[16] King, S, Glanville, J, Sanders, ME, et al. (2014) Effectiveness of probiotics on the duration of illness in healthy children and adults who develop common acute respiratory infectious conditions: A systematic review and meta-analysis. British Journal of Nutrition 112(1): 41-54.

[17] Ciabattini A, Olivieri R, Lazzeri E, et al. (2019) Role of the microbiota in the modulation of vaccine immune responses. Frontiers in Microbiology 10: 1305.

[18] Rizzardini G, Eskesen D, Calder PC, et al. (2012) Evaluation of the immune benefits of two probiotic strains *Bifidobacterium animalis* ssp. lactis, BB-12 and *Lactobacillus paracasei* ssp. paracasei,*L. casei* 431w in an influenza vaccination model: A randomised, double-blind,placebo-controlled study. British Journal of Nutrition 107(6): 876-884.

[19] Schiavi E, Gleinser M, Molloy E, et al. (2016) The surface-associated exopolysaccharide of Bifidobacterium longum 35624 plays an essential role in dampening host proinflammatory responses and repressing local TH17 responses. Applied and Environmental Microbiology 82(24): 7185-7196.

[20] Lee CJ, Lee LH, Lu CS, et al. (2001) Bacterial polysaccharides as vaccines—immunity and chemical characterization. Advances in Experimental Medicine and Biology 491: 453-471.

[21] Bozkurt K, Denktas C, Ozdemir O, et al. (2019) Charge Transport in Bifidobacterium animalis subsp. lactis BB-12 under various Atmospheres. Open Journal of Applied Sciences 9(6): 506-514.

[22] Shi, L., Dong, H., Reguera, G., Beyenal, H., Lu, A., Liu, J., Yu, H.Q. and Fredrickson, J.K. (2016) Extracellular Electron Transfer Mechanisms between Microorganisms and Minerals. Nature Reviews Microbiology, 14, 651-662.

[23] Light, S.H., Su, L., Rivera-Lugo, R., Cornejo, J.A. and Louie, A. (2018) A Flavin-Based Extracellular Electron Transfer Mechanism in Diverse Gram-Positive Bacteria. Nature, 562, 140-144.

Chapter 7

Propionibacterium freudenreichii: General Characteristics and Probiotic Traits

Vinícius de Rezende Rodovalho, Diego Lucas Neres Rodrigues, Gwénaël Jan, Yves Le Loir, Vasco Ariston de Carvalho Azevedo and Eric Guédon

Abstract

Propionibacterium freudenreichii is a Gram-positive dairy probiotic bacterial species that has been used as a ripening starter in the production of Swiss-type cheese for a long time. It has been exploited for the optimization of cheese production, including ripening capacities and aroma compounds production, but also for the production of vitamin B12 and organic acids. Furthermore, it has emerged in the probiotics landscape owing to several beneficial traits, including tolerance to stress in the gastrointestinal tract, adhesion to host cells, anti-pathogenic activity, anticancer potential and immunomodulatory properties. These beneficial properties have been confirmed with *in vitro* and *in vivo* investigations, using several omics approaches that allowed the identification of important molecular actors, such as surface proteins, short-chain fatty acids and bifidogenic factors. The diversity within the species was shown to be an important aspect to take into consideration, since many of these properties were strain-dependent. New studies should dive further into the molecular mechanisms related to the beneficial properties of this species and of its products, while considering the complexities of strain diversity and the interactions with the host and its microbiota. This chapter reviews current knowledge on the possible impact of *P. freudenreichii* on human health.

Keywords: *Propionibacterium freudenreichii*, propionibacteria, probiotics, immunomodulation, food microbiology

1. Introduction

The denomination "probiotics" comprises living microorganisms, including bacteria and yeasts, with health-promoting properties and suitable for safe consumption, as confirmed by their dietary uses for thousands of years of human history [1–3]. Lactic acid bacteria and bifidobacteria comprise traditional probiotic bacteria species, widely documented and commercialized [3, 4]. However, different species have emerged in the probiotics landscape, such as the dairy species *Propionibacterium freudenreichii* [4, 5], which is phylogenetically related to bifidobacteria (**Figure 1**) [4].

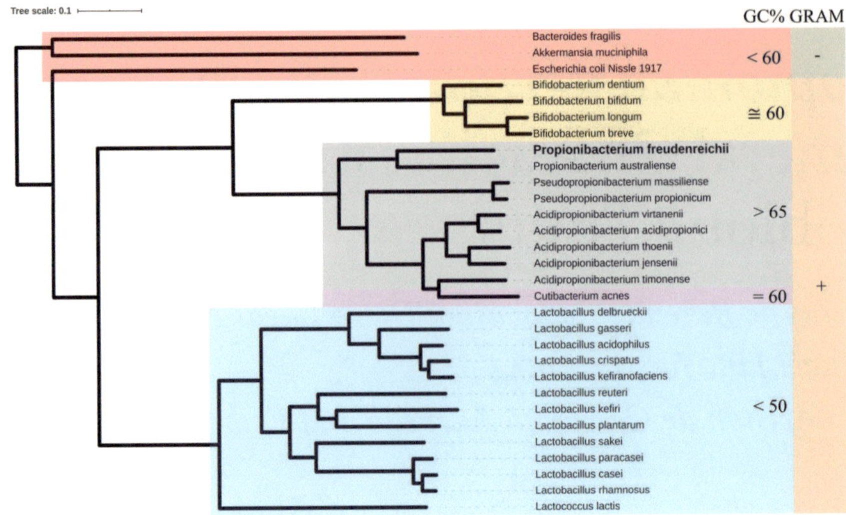

Figure 1.
Phylogenetic tree showing genomic similarity between health-promoting P. freudenreichii *species, other probiotic or closely-related species.*

The former *Propionibacterium* genus encompassed a group of microorganisms with importance in industry and health, due to the production of valuable metabolites, food, cosmetic and pharmacological products [6]. Previously, this genus included classic dairy propionibacteria species and skin-associated pathogenic propionibacteria [7]. However, a genome-based taxonomy reevaluation suggested the reclassification of cutaneous bacteria into the *Cutibacterium* genus, together with the inclusion of two other new genera for formerly classic propionibacteria, *Acidipropionibacterium* and *Pseudopropionibacterium* [7]. *P. freudenreichii*, which is one of the most notable dairy propionibacteria species, kept its former taxonomic classification [4, 7].

P. freudenreichii is a Gram-positive, high GC-content, mesophilic, aerotolerant, non-motile, non-spore forming bacterium, that shows low nutritional requirements and survives in harsh environments [5, 8, 9]. Regarding morphology, it is a pleomorphic rod microorganism, with aggregation tendency, forming clusters that resemble Chinese characters [5] (**Figure 2**). This bacterium, isolated from samples of Emmental cheese, was first described by Orla Jensen and von Freudenreich in 1906 [10]. Recently, *P. freudenreichii* strains have been identified in fecal samples from a discrete cohort of human preterm breast-fed infants, suggesting that it could be a component of the healthy human gut microbiota [11].

P. freudenreichii is able to use several carbon sources (e.g., glycerol, erythriol, L-arabinose, adonitol, galactose, D-glucose, D-fructose, D-manose, inositol, arbutine, esculine, lactose, lactate and gluconate) in the fermentation process to produce propionate, together with acetate, succinate and carbon dioxide (CO_2) [9, 12, 13]. Unlike other species, *P. freudenreichii* is able to reduce pyruvate into propionate via the transcarboxylase cycle (also referred to as Wood–Werkman cycle), which is a cyclic process coupled to oxidative phosphorylation, that allows a higher ATP yield than in other propionate-producing bacteria [9]. In its turn, pyruvate is a metabolic node molecule, which may be used either for the NADH-generating synthesis of acetate, or for the NADH-consuming synthesis of propionate [14]. In a strain-dependent manner, the bacterium modulates the proportions of pyruvate that are reduced into propionate or oxidized into acetate and CO_2, thus maintaining the

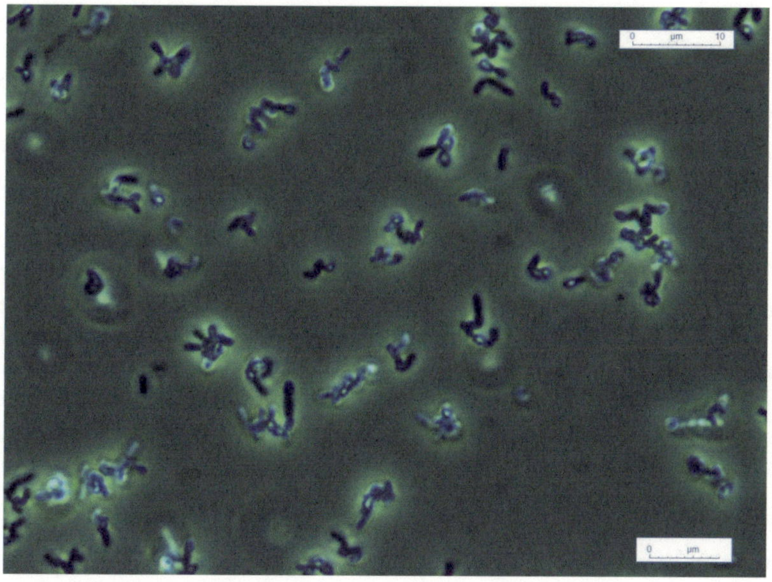

Figure 2.
Optical microscopy image showing the morphological aspect of a P. freudenreichii *CIRM-BIA129 culture, with typical aggregates resembling Chinese characters.*

redox equilibrium [9]. Therefore, this species encompasses biochemically versatile strains, that find different applications in several contexts [5].

2. Technological importance

P. freudenreichii is widely used for the production of Swiss-type cheeses, such as Emmental [5, 15] (**Figure 3**). In such dairy matrices, the CO_2 gas that is produced during fermentation forms bubbles that diffuse slowly, creating characteristic holes, or "eyes", in cheese architecture [9, 12]. Cheese flavor is related to propionate and acetate, as well as the products of amino acids catabolism and fat hydrolysis by propionibacteria [16, 17]. Importantly, these dairy products containing *P. freudenreichii* displayed anti-inflammatory properties *in vivo* [18–20], increasing the recognition of this bacterium and of its products as health-promoting. Therefore, dairy propionibacteria are considered 2-in-1 bacteria, with both fermentative and probiotic properties, which makes them ideal for the development of health-promoting fermented food [5, 18].

This bacterium is also well recognized to encompass a pathway for vitamin B12 (cobalamin) synthesis [8, 9]. Vitamin B12 is a water-soluble vitamin, which plays a key role in the functioning of the brain, of the nervous system and in the

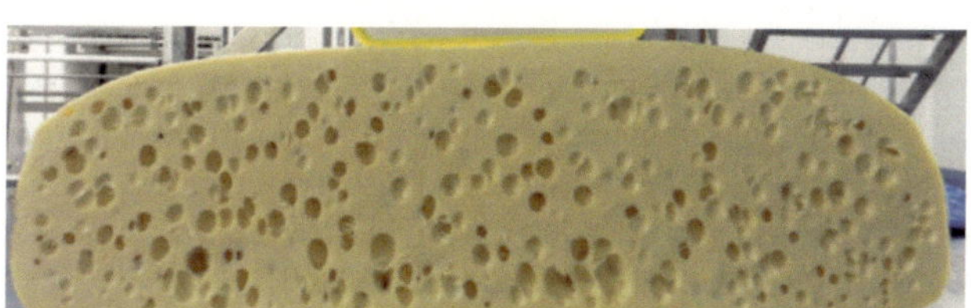

Figure 3.
Emmental cheese produced using P. freudenreichii *CIRM-BIA129, in conjunction with* Streptococcus thermophilus *and* Lactobacillus delbrueckii.

production of blood [21]. It is also a co-factor of methylmalonyl-CoA mutase, which catalyzes a crucial step in the fermentative route to produce propionate [22]. Therefore, the growth conditions of *P. freudenreichii* have been optimized for the production of vitamin B12, using substrates such as cereal matrices [23, 24], waste frying sunflower oil [25], tofu wastewater [26] and soybean agroindustry residue [27]. Moreover, *P. freudenreichii* has been genetically engineered to enhance vitamin B12 and propionate production [6, 28].

The production of vitamin B12, organic acids, trehalose and other metabolites, together with the safe use as cheese ripening starter and probiotic characteristics, make this bacterium attractive for several biotechnological and industrial applications [5, 6, 29, 30]. A wide range of genetic and environmental optimizations have been conducted to improve these properties [6, 29]. Moreover, some optimizations of the growth and processing conditions allowed the improvement of resistance towards storage and towards several industrial processes, such as freeze-drying and spray-drying [30–33].

3. Strain variability

The interesting properties of this bacterium, such as health-promoting features, and participation to industrial vitamin B12 and cheese production, were shown to be strain-dependent, suggesting the need for analysis that account for that variability [9]. As an example, some strains presented differences in nitrogen and sugar degradation, which had a genetic origin, probably resulting from horizontal transfers, duplications, transpositions and other mutations [13]. This strain diversity was confirmed at the genomic level by another study and attributed to transposable elements, in such a way that genome plasticity enabled bacterial adaptation to several environments [34].

In view of this strain-related variability, there have been efforts to specify criteria for the selection of probiotic strains. These criteria include tolerance to stresses encountered within the gastrointestinal tract, adhesion to host cells, antipathogenic activity, anticancer potential, immunomodulatory properties, industrial requirements and molecular characterization using omics methodologies [3]. Mounting evidence shows that *P. freudenreichii* fulfills these criteria [5].

4. Stress tolerance

Regarding stress tolerance and adaptation to the gastrointestinal tract (GIT), some *P. freudenreichii* strains presented adaptations, including morphological and proteomic modifications [35–37]. For example, those modifications were verified during the acid tolerance response in the strain *P. freudenreichii* SI41, which was investigated using a kinetic study of stress proteins production during acid adaptation [35]. As a result, biotin carboxyl carrier and proteins involved in DNA synthesis and repair were associated to early acid stress response, whereas chaperonins GroEL and GroES were associated to late acid stress response [35]. Analysis with the same strain showed that bile salts (a mixture of cholate and deoxycholate) triggered drastic morphological changes and induced proteins related to signal sensing and transduction, general stress and an alternative sigma factor [36]. The same strain was used in a follow-up comprehensive study that included heat, acid, and bile salts conditions to study *P. freudenreichii* tolerance. As a result, each form of stress induced specific proteins, but six of them were common to all stresses, including chaperones and proteins involved in energetic metabolism and oxidative stress remediation [37]. An *in vitro* study that involved 13 strains of *P. freudenreichii* showed that most of them had high capacity of tolerance to simulated gastric juices with varying pH and small intestine conditions [38].

Moreover, this resistance was also evidenced *in vivo*. The mRNA of *P. freudenreichii* methylmalonyl-transcarboxylase was detected in human fecal samples using real time reverse transcriptase polymerase chain reaction (RT-PCR) [39]. Methylmalonyl-transcarboxylase is a key enzyme of the transcarboxylase cycle, only expressed when propionic fermentation is active, therefore its detection in fecal samples indicated that the bacterium survived and remained metabolically active, transcribing genes within the human digestive tract [39]. A multi-strain study using human microbiota-associated rats monitored intestinal microbiota composition and short-chain fatty acids production, confirming that *P. freudenreichii* stress tolerance in the GIT is also strain-dependent [40]. *P. freudenreichii* CIRM-BIA1 was shown to adapt metabolically and physiologically to the colon environment of pigs, with changes in carbohydrate metabolism, down-regulation of stress genes and up-regulation of cell division genes [41]. Furthermore, the use of food vehicles for *P. freudenreichii* delivery, such as cheese and fermented milk, improved its resistance towards the GIT stressing environment [15, 18, 19, 42, 43].

Other aspects of *P. freudenreichii* resistance to stress conditions have also been studied, such as long-term nutritional shortage [44, 45]. A screening was performed with eight *P. freudenreichii* strains, which were incubated for several days after the beginning of the stationary phase, without further supplementation of nutrients. They displayed high survival rates and no lysis, indicating that these strains adapt to long-term nutritional shortage, using a viable, yet nonculturable state [45]. The strain *P. freudenreichii* CIRM-BIA138 was further studied in these conditions of incubation, and it was shown that a high population was maintained, even after exhaustion of lactate, the preferred carbon source. RNA-seq analysis showed that several metabolic and information processing pathways were down-regulated [44].

Another important feature of *P. freudenreichii* during stress response is the accumulation of trehalose. A study that investigated this bacterium during adaptation to osmotic, oxidative and acid stress, showed that the trehalose-6-phosphate synthase/phosphatase (OtsA–OtsB) pathway, related to trehalose synthesis, was enhanced in these conditions [46]. Another study focused in stress response to low temperature (4°C), a condition that mimicked cheese ripening conditions. As a result, seven *P. freudenreichii* strains displayed a slowed-down cell machinery, cold stress response and the accumulation of trehalose and glycogen [47]. *P. freudenreichii* also accumulated glycine betaine, glycogen, trehalose and polyphosphates when cultured in hyperconcentrated media [48]. The accumulation of trehalose, together with glycine betaine, was further verified in a technological context, when bacterial viability was increased during spray drying and storage, through the optimization of the growth medium composition and thermal adaptation [31]. The ratio of the concentrations of these intracellular osmoprotectants, trehalose and glycine betaine, was further shown to modulate the stress tolerance during the technological processes of freeze-drying and of spray-drying [32].

5. Adhesion properties

Adhesion to host cells is another important feature of probiotics, which favors their local beneficial action. Early studies revealed the ability of several probiotic bacteria, including *P. freudenreichii*, to adhere to glycoproteins and mucus from human intestinal tract [49, 50]. In the case of *P. freudenreichii*, the adhesion of some strains to pig ileum cells (IPEC-J2) was between 25 and 35%, and that proportion was higher with the addition of $CaCl_2$ [51]. In the case of human host, several bacterial strains were tested for adhesion to HT-29 colon cells *in vitro*; the most adhesive strain was *P. freudenreichii* CIRM-BIA129 and surface layer protein B (slpB) key role in adhesion was demonstrated by using gene inactivation [52, 53]. Another study demonstrated that bacterial adhesion to immobilized mucus could be synergistically improved by administration of strains combinations, such as *P. freudenreichii* ssp. *shermanii* JS in combination with *Bifidobacterium breve* or *Lactobacillus rhamnosus* strains [54].

6. Anti-pathogenic activity

There are also several evidences of an anti-pathogenic activity in this species. *P. freudenreichii* JS reduced by 39% the adhesion of *S. aureus* to human intestinal mucus and by 27% its viability, probably due to the production of organic acids [55]. *P. freudenreichii* PTCC 1674 was reported to secrete a lipopeptide biosurfactant with antimicrobial activity mainly against *Rhodococcus erythropolis*, and anti-adhesive activity mainly against *Pseudomonas aeruginosa* [56]. Moreover, *P. freudenreichii* DSM 20270 significantly inhibited *E. coli* O157:H7 growth *in vitro* [51].

P. freudenreichii also showed anti-pathogenic properties in animals. *P. freudenreichii* B-3523 and B-4327 impacted *Salmonella* strains multiplication, motility and adhesion to avian epithelial cells *in vitro* [57]. The follow up study indicated that the cell-free culture supernatants of the same probiotic strains were bactericidal against multidrug-resistant *Salmonella enterica* serovar Heidelberg [58]. *In vivo* assays further showed that the probiotic strains reduced the pathogen cecal colonization and dissemination to the liver in turkey poults [58]. *P. freudenreichii* consumption was furthermore shown to limit and to delay colonization of the mice intestinal tract by the pathogen *Citrobacter rodentium* [59].

In line with the synergies observed in terms of adhesion, probiotic combinations were proposed to improve anti-pathogenic activity, such as a combination of *P. freudenreichii* JS, *L. rhamnosus* GG and LC705, and *B. breve* 99, which promoted the inhibition, displacement and competition with several pathogenic species, such as *S. enterica*, *Listeria monocytogenes* and *Clostridium difficile* [60]. In another study, *P. freudenreichii* JS decreased the adhesion of *Helicobacter pylori* to Caco-2 intestinal cells when used individually, but also inhibited membrane leakage, improved epithelial barrier function and modulated inflammatory cytokines when used in combination with *L. rhamnosus* and *B. breve* strains [61].

7. Anticancer potential

Promising results, in the context of intestinal carcinogenesis, were also reported in this species. A pioneer study showed that *P. freudenreichii* ITGP18 and *P. freudenreichii* SI41 could induce apoptosis of cultured human colorectal carcinoma cell lines *in vitro* and this effect was mediated by short-chain fatty acids (SCFAs), such as propionate and acetate, acting on cancer cells mitochondria [62]. Following up, it was further clarified that the effect of SCFAs was modulated by extracellular pH shifts; and in acidic pH, cell death mode changed from apoptosis to necrosis in human colon HT-29 cells [63]. These effects were confirmed *in vivo*, with *P. freudenreichii* TL133 inducing the apoptosis of colon cells in human microbiota-associated rats treated with 1,2-dimethylhydrazine, yet not in healthy rats [64].

Another strain, *P. freudenreichii* ITG P9, was also employed for the development of a fermented milk with anti-oncogenic potential, since it induced apoptosis in cultured HGT-1 human gastric cancer cells *in vitro* [43]. Next, this fermented milk was proposed as an adjuvant in colorectal cancer therapy based on TNF-related apoptosis-inducing ligand (TRAIL), due to possible synergistic effect between the bacterium and TRAIL, which was confirmed with the enhancement of cytotoxic activity in HT-29 cells [65]. Another study investigated the crosstalk between bacterium and cancer cells: the latters produce lactate as a result of the metabolic shift referred as "aerobic" glycolysis or "Warburg effect"; lactate may then be used by this bacterium as a carbon source, stimulating its production of SCFAs [66].

8. Modulation of microbiota composition

Regarding the modulation of microbiota composition, consumption of dairy propionibacteria was shown to enhance intestinal populations of bifidobacteria in humans [67, 68]. In line with this, the stimulation of bifidogenic growth was observed in cell-free filtrate and cellular methanol extract derived from *P. freudenreichii* 7025 cultures [69]. Following analysis with the same strain allowed the purification of a bifidogenic growth stimulator component, the identification of its chemical structure (2-amino-3-carboxy-1,4-naphthoquinone, ACNQ) and the demonstration of its bifidogenic activity in the concentration of 0.1 ng/mL [70]. Another strain, *P. freudenreichii* ET-3 was reported to produce 1,4-dihydroxy-2-naphthoic acid (DHNA) in concentrations of 10 μg/mL, which also stimulated the growth of bifidobacteria [71]. The beneficial effect of DHNA was later confirmed *in vivo*, using mice with colitis induced by 2.0% dextran sodium sulphate (DSS). DHNA attenuated inflammation, through the modulation of intestinal bacterial microbiota and suppression of lymphocyte infiltration [72].

The bifidogenic growth stimulator derived from *P. freudenreichii* was also orally administrated to human patients in a pilot study, being promising for the treatment of ulcerative colitis [73]. Subsequent studies included optimizations of the production of bifidogenic growth stimulators, including an increased production by switching to aerobic growth conditions [74] and the use of lactic acid as a carbon source in a bioreactor system with a filtration device [75].

9. Immunomodulatory properties

There is mounting evidence, both *in vitro* and *in vivo*, that *P. freudenreichii* exerts immunomodulatory effects by several mechanisms, in a strain-dependent manner. For example, a screening for IL-10 induction in human peripheral blood mononuclear cells (PBMCs) was performed in 10 strains of *P. freudenreichii*, resulting in the selection of the two most anti-inflammatory strains: *P. freudenreichii* ITG P20 (equivalent to CIRM-BIA129) and SI48 [59]. In the same study, the strain *P. freudenreichii* SI48 was further tested *in vivo*, in mice with acute colitis induced by trinitrobenzenesulphonic acid (TNBS), lowering significantly inflammatory and histological markers of colitis [59]. Other studies also showed that the immunomodulatory properties were strain-dependent within the species *P. freudenreichii* [76]. An integrative strategy encompassing comparative genomics, surface proteomics, transcriptomics, assays of cytokines induction and genes inactivation, identified relevant proteins and strains specificities in immunomodulation [77]. Remarkably, surface proteins of the S-layer type were shown to be crucial in immunomodulation, but the immunomodulatory properties varied among strains, due to complex

Strain	Protein	Name/Description	Accession	Evidence level	Ref.
CIRM-BIA129 (ITG P20)	Ensemble of surface proteins			proteomic, *in vitro*	[82]
	GroL2	60 kDa chaperonin 2	CDP49125	genomic, proteomic	[77]
	HsdM3	Type I restriction-modification system DNA methylase	CDP48267	genomic, transcriptomic, mutant studies *in vitro*	[77]
	Lacl1	Arabinose operon repressor	CDP47860	transcriptomic	[77]
	MerA	Pyridine nucleotide-disulphide oxidoreductase	CDP48574	genomic, proteomic	[77]
	Pep	Hypothetical protein	CDP48241	genomic, mutant studies *in vitro*	[77]
	PFCIRM129_04790	Hypothetical protein	CDP48736	genomic, transcriptomic	[77]
	PFCIRM129_10785	Hypothetical protein	CDP49252	transcriptomic	[77]
	PFCIRM129_10930	Hypothetical protein	CDP48242	genomic, transcriptomic	[77]
	SlpB	Surface layer protein B	CDP48273	genomic, transcriptomic, proteomic, mutant studies *in vitro*	[77]
				mutant studies *in vitro* and *in vivo*	[83]
				mutant studies *in vitro*	[52]
	SlpE	Surface protein with SLH domain	CDP48858	genomic, transcriptomic, proteomic, mutant studies *in vitro*	[77]
	SlpF	Surface protein with SLH domain	CDP49687	proteomic, mutant studies *in vitro*	[77]
CIRM-BIA 121	Acn	Aconitase, Aconitate hydratase	CEG89374	transcriptomic	[77]
	DcuA	C4-dicarboxylate transporter	CEG91776	genomic	[77]
	Eno1	Enolase 1	CEG91483	proteomic, mutant studies *in vitro*	[77]
	HtrA4	Serine protease	CEG91080	genomic, transcriptomic, proteomic, mutant studies *in vitro*	[77]
	PFCIRM121_08235	Hypothetical protein/unknown function	CEG91253	genomic, mutant studies *in vitro*	[77]
	SlpC1	Surface layer protein C	CEG91216	genomic, transcriptomic	[77]
UF1	LspA	Large surface layer protein A	n.a.	proteomic, *in vivo*	[84]
	DlaT	Dihydrolipoamide acetyltransferase	n.a.	proteomic, mutant studies *in vivo*	[11]

Legend: Ref.: references, n.a.: not available.

Table 1.
Proteins from P. freudenreichii *related to its immunomodulatory properties.*

combinations of molecular features [77]. The strain-specific export of surface proteins, adhesins and moonlighting proteins was confirmed in a different subset of *P. freudenreichii* strains [78]. Additionally, acute colitis induced by dextran sodium sulfate (DSS) in rats was ameliorated by *P. freudenreichii* KCTC 1063, which stimulated in intestinal cells the expression of MUC2, a main component of mucus [79].

The roles of *P. freudenreichii* in the modulation of host immunological response became even more relevant when a human commensal strain was identified. *P. freudenreichii* UF1 was demonstrated to be a component of the gut microbiota of preterm infants that were fed with human breast milk and to mitigate intestinal inflammatory diseases [11]. Moreover, this strain modulated the intestinal immunity of mice against pathogen challenge, specifically against systemic *L. monocytogenes* infection, by regulating Th17 cells [80]. This beneficial effect was confirmed in newborn mice, which were susceptible to intestinal pathogenic infection, but had their defense enhanced by this strain, particularly by the increase in protective Th17 cells and regulatory T cells [81].

Regarding the bacterial factors involved in immunomodulation, evidence points out mainly to surface proteins (**Table 1**). The strain *P. freudenreichii* CIRM-BIA129 had its proteome investigated, with the identification of surface-exposed proteins and their role in induction of IL-10 and IL-6 release by PBMCs [82]. Among the identified proteins, there were cell wall-remodeling proteins, transport proteins, moonlighting proteins and other proteins involved in interactions with the host [82]. The multi-strain and multi-omics study conducted by Deutsch et al. [77] clarified that cytoplasmic proteins might also be relevant in immunomodulation, but confirmed the key role of surface-layer proteins B (SlpB) and E (SlpE), particularly in strain *P. freudenreichii* CIRM-BIA129. SlpB was then shown to be crucial for bacterial adhesion to epithelial intestinal cells [52], and a mutation in its gene had pleiotropic effects, suggesting this protein could have a central role in cellular processes [53]. Additionally, *in vivo* assays that were conducted in mice with mucositis induced by 5-Flourouracil (5-FU), showed that SlpB protein is crucial for the cytokine modulation triggered by *P. freudenreichii* CIRM-BIA129 [83]. Moreover, the glycosylated large surface layer protein A (LspA) of the commensal strain *P. freudenreichii* UF1 was shown to regulate the interaction with SIGNR1 receptor, which regulates dendritic cells and counteracts pathogenic-driven inflammation, maintaining gut homeostasis [84]. Interestingly, some of these immunomodulatory proteins, including SlpB and SlpE, were recently identified in association with extracellular vesicles produced by the strain *P. freudenreichii* CIRM-BIA129, which serve as an alternative export system [85].

In addition to surface proteins, DHNA was also associated to immunomodulation. Beside its bifidogenic properties, DHNA inhibited the production of proinflammatory cytokines in intestinal macrophages of IL-10(−/−) mice treated with piroxicam [86]. Moreover, DHNA was also described as an activator of aryl hydrocarbon receptor (AhR), which is involved in the detoxification of xenobiotics and inflammation regulation [87, 88].

10. Functional foods

Importantly, the immunomodulatory properties of *P. freudenreichii* were preserved when food matrices were used as delivery vectors, including cheese [18, 19, 42, 89] and fermented milk [90–92], indicating a great potential for developing probiotic-based functional foods with immunomodulatory properties. As an example, a dairy product fermented by strain CIRM-BIA129 reduced the secretion of pro-inflammatory cytokines by colonic mucosa, improved food intake and growth of piglets [92]. *P. freudenreichii* CIRM-BIA129 was also employed in the production of an immunomodulatory single-strain cheese, whose consumption by mice ameliorated colitis induced by TNBS, restoring the expression of tight-junction proteins and reducing the expression of markers of inflammation and of oxidative stress [89]. Similar protection, in the same colitis model, was observed using a two-strain model cheese containing *P. freudenreichii* and *L. delbrueckii* [20]. An industrial Emmental cheese was then produced using *S. thermophilus, P. freudenreichii* and *L. delbrueckii* [18] (**Figure 3**). Its consumption protected mice against colitis induced by DSS [18]. In healthy piglets, the consumption of the same CIRM-BIA129 strain associated to a cheese matrix was crucial in the preservation or enhancement of the immunomodulatory properties of the bacterium, including the induction of Th2 and Treg phenotypes [19]. The importance of the cheese matrix was also related to the protection of immunomodulatory protein SlpB against proteolysis in simulated gastrointestinal tract conditions [42]. These examples unveiled how appropriate food matrices protected or enhanced the beneficial properties of these traditional dairy propionibacteria, while establishing perspectives for the design of novel functional foods [91].

11. Safety assessments

The long history of safe production of fermented food, such as Emmental cheese, and the bacterium status of "generally recognized as safe" (GRAS) and "qualified presumption of safety" (QPS) assure the safety of *P. freudenreichii* consumption [5, 93]. However, additional assessments need to be conducted in different matrices and contexts. Probiotics included in humans trials are most frequently from genus *Lactobacillus* or *Bifidobacterium*; nevertheless, propionibacteria have also been tested [93]. For example, two clinical studies evaluated *P. freudenreichii* ET-3 culture medium safety in human adult subjects, the first one reported no differences in gastrointestinal symptoms between the groups and the other one reported differences in hematological parameters, although within the normal ranges [94]. *P. freudenreichii* strains SI 26 and SI 41 were given to adult healthy human volunteers without adverse effects, while a modulation of fecal bifidobacteria and of segmental colonic transit was observed [67]. In another study, *P. freudenreichii* strain SI 41 was given in capsules at the same dose to human volunteers without adverse effects, while an increase in fecal propionibacteria, concomitant with enhanced short chain fatty acids, was observed [95].

Moreover, several clinical trials tested multispecies probiotic supplementation containing propionibacteria. A complex formula that included *P. freudenreichii* JS, together with *L. rhamnosus* GG, *L. rhamnosus* Lc705, *B. breve* 99, and galacto-oligosaccharides prebiotics has been tested in several randomized, double-blind, placebo-controlled setups. The probiotic intervention was conducted in pregnant women and newborn infants, being safe and effective in the prevention of atopic eczema in children [96], increased children resistance to respiratory infections [97], protected Cesarean-delivered children from IgE-associated allergic disease [98], restored microbiota composition in children treated with antibiotics or born by cesarean procedure [99] and protected Cesarean-delivered children from allergic disease in a 13-year follow-up [100]. Finally, an integrative study analyzed adverse events associated with this probiotic combination in some of these trials, concluding that there was no association with adverse events in young and elderly subjects [101].

Importantly, probiotics supplementation is not recommended in cases of immunosuppression, such as during anticancer treatment [93]. Moreover, their beneficial effects and safety are conditioned to a complex interplay between peculiarities of the host and of the probiotic strain or strains, which both encourages further research and suggests caution in some of its applications [93].

12. Postbiotics and beyond

As previously detailed, *P. freurenreichii* probiotic effect has been associated to several factors, including cytoplasmic and surface-exposed proteins [52, 77, 82, 83], short chain fatty acids [62, 63], metabolites [71, 72, 75] and culture supernatants [58, 94] (**Figure 4**). These probiotic-derived factors, which exert a beneficial effect on the host, have been referred as postbiotics [102]. "Postbiotic" is an emerging denomination that encompasses probiotic-derived cell-free metabolic products with health-promoting properties, including proteins, lipids, organic acids, vitamins, supernatants, among others [102–104]. The advantages of postbiotics over probiotics include purity, easy production and storage, industrial scalability, higher specificity in the mechanism of action and less adverse effects [102, 103].

In the case of *P. freudenreichii*, a remarkable example of postbiotic is SlpB protein, which was purified and exerted an immunomodulatory effect, i.e. induction of IL-10, in cultured human intestinal epithelial cells [83]. Another example that would fit into postbiotics definition is extracellular vesicles, which are membranous spherical nanostructures that transport molecules between cells [105, 106]. In probiotic bacteria, such as several *Lactobacillus* and *Bifidobacteriaum* strains, extracellular vesicles have been reported as immunomodulatory [107]. In the case of *P. freudenreichii*, we recently described their production by the strain CIRM-BIA129, which has been the first report with physicochemical, proteomic and functional characterization of extracellular vesicles in the species [85]. We identified relevant proteins in their cargo, including SlpB, and demonstrated their anti-inflammatory activity via the modulation of NF-κB pathway in cultured human intestinal epithelial cells [85].

Postbiotics hold promising perspectives for developing novel probiotic-derived products with enhanced safety and functionality [107]. Moreover, yield and cargo loading optimization are promising for modulating their properties, enhancing their beneficial effect and biotechnological applications [108]. Finally, clinical trials should be conducted in the near future to assure the

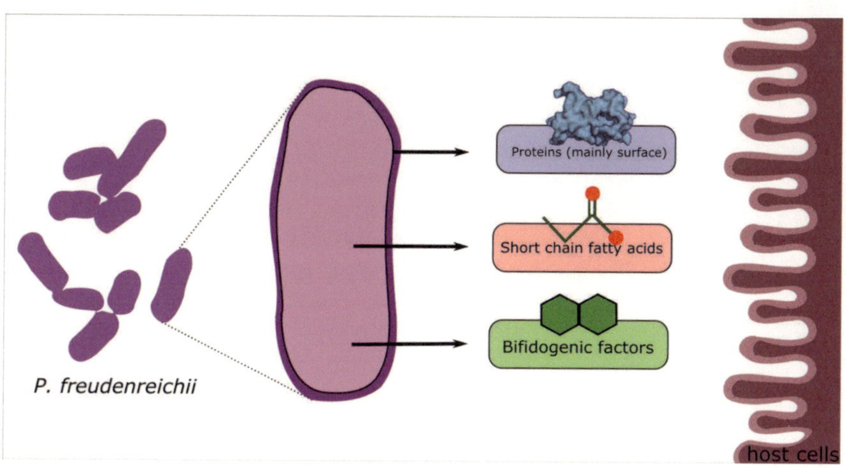

Figure 4.
Schematic summary of P. freudenreichii *probiotic traits at the molecular level.*

suitability of postbiotics and probiotics for therapy and prophylaxis, since they might exert a great impact in human health [93, 107, 109].

13. Conclusion

Overall, research on *P. freudenreichii* is consolidating its role as a probiotic, due to several outstanding features, such as the tolerance to stresses encountered in the gastrointestinal tract, adhesion to host cells, the anti-pathogenic activity, the anticancer potential and the immunomodulatory properties. Moreover, this species holds technological importance, due to long-established applications in the production of food, vitamin B12 and organic acids. Therefore, this is a promising 2-in-1 bacterium, with both fermentative and probiotic properties. New research on *P. freudenreichii* should allow the development of novel health-promoting fermented foods and should dive further into the characterization of strain diversity and of corresponding properties, as well as employ omics approaches to dissect the molecular mechanisms of its beneficial properties. Studies on this species hold a great potential for the development of novel technological approaches and therapeutic products directly impacting human health.

Acknowledgements

We are thankful to Houyem Rabah, who kindly supplied a photography of an Emmental cheese. We are also thankful to the financial support from INRAE (Rennes, France) and Institut Agro (Rennes, France). VRR was supported by the International Cooperation Program CAPES/COFECUB at the Federal University of Minas Gerais funded by CAPES – the Brazilian Federal Agency for the Support and Evaluation of Graduate Education of the Brazilian Ministry of Education (number 99999.000058/2017-2103).

Conflict of interest

The authors declare no conflict of interest.

Author details

Vinícius de Rezende Rodovalho[1,2], Diego Lucas Neres Rodrigues[1], Gwénaël Jan[2], Yves Le Loir[2], Vasco Ariston de Carvalho Azevedo[1] and Eric Guédon[2*]

1 Laboratory of Cellular and Molecular Genetics, Institute of Biological Sciences, Federal University of Minas Gerais, Belo Horizonte, Brazil

2 INRAE, Institut Agro, STLO, Rennes, France

*Address all correspondence to: eric.guedon@inrae.fr

References

[1] Ozen M, Dinleyici EC. The history of probiotics: The untold story. Benef Microbes 2015; 6: 159-165.

[2] Gasbarrini G, Bonvicini F, Gramenzi A. Probiotics History. J Clin Gastroenterol 2016; 50: S116–S119.

[3] de Melo Pereira GV, de Oliveira Coelho B, Magalhães Júnior AI, et al. How to select a probiotic? A review and update of methods and criteria. Biotechnology Advances 2018; 36: 2060-2076.

[4] Douillard FP, de Vos WM. Biotechnology of health-promoting bacteria. *Biotechnology Advances*; 37. Epub ahead of print 1 November 2019. DOI: 10.1016/j.biotechadv.2019. 03.008.

[5] Rabah H, Rosa do Carmo F, Jan G. Dairy Propionibacteria: Versatile Probiotics. *Microorganisms* 2017; 5: 24.

[6] Piwowarek K, Lipińska E, Hać-Szymańczuk E, et al. Propioni bacterium spp.-source of propionic acid, vitamin B12, and other metabolites important for the industry. Appl Microbiol Biotechnol 2018; 102: 515-538.

[7] Scholz CFP, Kilian M. The natural history of cutaneous propionibacteria, and reclassification of selected species within the genus Propionibacterium to the proposed novel genera Acidipropioni bacterium gen. nov., Cutibacterium gen. nov. and Pseudopropionibacterium gen. nov. Int J Syst Evol Microbiol 2016; 66: 4422-4432.

[8] Falentin H, Deutsch SM, Jan G, et al. The complete genome of propioni bacterium freudenreichii CIRM-BIA1T, a hardy actinobacterium with food and probiotic applications. *PLoS One*; 5. Epub ahead of print 2010. DOI: 10.1371/ journal.pone.0011748.

[9] Thierry A, Deutsch SM, Falentin H, et al. New insights into physiology and metabolism of Propionibacterium freudenreichii. International Journal of Food Microbiology 2011; 149: 19-27.

[10] Von Freudenreichii E, Orla-Jensen O. Uber die in Emmentalerkäse stattfindene Propionsäure-gärung. Zentralbl Bakteriol 1906; 17: 529-546.

[11] Colliou N, Ge Y, Sahay B, et al. Commensal Propionibacterium strain UF1 mitigates intestinal inflammation via Th17 cell regulation. J Clin Invest 2017; 127: 3970-3986.

[12] Ojala T, Laine PKS, Ahlroos T, et al. Functional genomics provides insights into the role of Propionibacterium freudenreichii ssp. shermanii JS in cheese ripening. Int J Food Microbiol 2017; 241: 39-48.

[13] Loux V, Mariadassou M, Almeida S, et al. Mutations and genomic islands can explain the strain dependency of sugar utilization in 21 strains of Propionibacterium freudenreichii. BMC Genomics 2015; 16: 296.

[14] Deborde C, Boyaval P. Interactions between Pyruvate and Lactate Metabolism in Propionibacterium freudenreichii subsp.shermanii: In Vivo 13C Nuclear Magnetic Resonance Studies. Appl Environ Microbiol 2000; 66: 2012-2020.

[15] Gagnaire V, Jardin J, Rabah H, et al. Emmental Cheese Environment Enhances Propionibacterium freudenreichii Stress Tolerance. PLoS One 2015; 10: e0135780.

[16] Poonam, Pophaly SD, Tomar SK, et al. Multifaceted attributes of dairy propionibacteria: A review. World Journal of Microbiology and Biotechnology 2012; 28: 3081-3095.

[17] Abeijón Mukdsi MC, Falentin H, Maillard MB, et al. The Secreted Esterase of Propionibacterium freudenreichii Has a Major Role in Cheese Lipolysis. Appl Environ Microbiol 2014; 80: 751-756.

[18] Rabah H, do Carmo FLR, Carvalho RD de O, et al. Beneficial propioni bacteria within a probiotic emmental cheese: Impact on dextran sodium sulphate-induced colitis in mice. *Microorganisms*; 8. Epub ahead of print 1 March 2020. DOI: 10.3390/microorganisms8030380.

[19] Rabah H, Ferret-Bernard S, Huang S, et al. The Cheese Matrix Modulates the Immunomodulatory Properties of Propionibacterium freudenreichii CIRM-BIA 129 in Healthy Piglets. Front Microbiol 2018; 9: 2584.

[20] Plé C, Breton J, Richoux R, et al. Combining selected immuno modulatory Propionibacterium freudenreichii and Lactobacillus delbrueckii strains: Reverse engineering development of an anti-inflammatory cheese. Mol Nutr Food Res 2016; 60: 935-948.

[21] Calderón-Ospina CA, Nava-Mesa MO. B Vitamins in the nervous system: Current knowledge of the biochemical modes of action and synergies of thiamine, pyridoxine, and cobalamin. CNS Neurosci Ther 2020; 26: 5-13.

[22] Takahashi-Iñiguez T, García-Hernandez E, Arreguín-Espinosa R, et al. Role of Vitamin B12 on methylmalonyl-CoA mutase activity. Journal of Zhejiang University: Science B 2012; 13: 423-437.

[23] Chamlagain B, Sugito TA, Deptula P, et al. In situ production of active vitamin B12 in cereal matrices using Propionibacterium freudenreichii. Food Sci Nutr 2018; 6: 67-76.

[24] Wang P, Shen C, Li L, et al. Simultaneous production of propionic acid and vitamin B12 from corn stalk hydrolysates by Propionibacterium freudenreichii in an expanded bed adsorption bioreactor. Prep Biochem Biotechnol 2020; 50: 763-767.

[25] Hajfarajollah H, Mokhtarani B, Mortaheb H, et al. Vitamin B12 biosynthesis over waste frying sunflower oil as a cost effective and renewable substrate. J Food Sci Technol 2015; 52: 3273-3282.

[26] Yu Y, Zhu X, Shen Y, et al. Enhancing the vitamin B12 production and growth of Propionibacterium freudenreichii in tofu wastewater via a light-induced vitamin B12 riboswitch. Appl Microbiol Biotechnol 2015; 99: 10481-10488.

[27] Assis DA de, Matte C, Aschidamini B, et al. Biosynthesis of vitamin B12 by Propionibacterium freudenreichii subsp. shermanii ATCC 13673 using liquid acid protein residue of soybean as culture medium. *Biotechnol Prog*. Epub ahead of print 2020. DOI: 10.1002/btpr.3011.

[28] Wang Z, Ammar EM, Zhang A, et al. Engineering Propionibacterium freudenreichii subsp. Shermanii for enhanced propionic acid fermentation: Effects of overexpressing propionyl-CoA: Succinate CoA transferase. Metab Eng 2015; 27: 46-56.

[29] Pillai V V, Prakash G, Lali AM. Growth engineering of Propionibacterium freudenreichii shermanii for organic acids and other value-added products formation. Prep Biochem Biotechnol 2018; 48: 6-12.

[30] Gaucher F, Bonnassie S, Rabah H, et al. Review: Adaptation of Beneficial Propionibacteria, Lactobacilli, and Bifidobacteria Improves Tolerance Toward Technological and Digestive Stresses. *Front Microbiol*; 10. Epub ahead

of print 24 April 2019. DOI: 10.3389/fmicb.2019.00841.

[31] Gaucher F, Gagnaire V, Rabah H, et al. Taking advantage of bacterial adaptation in order to optimize industrial production of dry propionibacterium freudenreichii. *Microorganisms*; 7. Epub ahead of print 1 October 2019. DOI: 10.3390/microorganisms7100477.

[32] Gaucher F, Rabah H, Kponouglo K, et al. Intracellular osmoprotectant concentrations determine Propionibacterium freudenreichii survival during drying. Appl Microbiol Biotechnol 2020; 104: 3145-3156.

[33] Gaucher F, Kponouglo K, Rabah H, et al. Propionibacterium freudenreichii CIRM-BIA 129 Osmoadaptation Coupled to Acid-Adaptation Increases Its Viability During Freeze-Drying. *Front Microbiol*; 10. Epub ahead of print 9 October 2019. DOI: 10.3389/fmicb.2019.02324.

[34] Deptula P, Laine PK, Roberts RJ, et al. De novo assembly of genomes from long sequence reads reveals uncharted territories of Propionibacterium freudenreichii. *BMC Genomics*; 18. Epub ahead of print 2017. DOI: 10.1186/s12864-017-4165-9.

[35] Jan G, Leverrier P, Pichereau V, et al. Changes in Protein Synthesis and Morphology during Acid Adaptation of Propionibacterium freudenreichii. Appl Environ Microbiol 2001; 67: 2029-2036.

[36] Leverrier P, Dimova D, Pichereau V, et al. Susceptibility and adaptive response to bile salts in Propionibacterium freudenreichii: Physiological and proteomic anlysis. Appl Environ Microbiol 2003; 69: 3809-3818.

[37] Leverrier P, Vissers JPC, Rouault A, et al. Mass spectrometry proteomic analysis of stress adaptation reveals both common and distinct response pathways in Propionibacterium freudenreichii. Arch Microbiol 2004; 181: 215-230.

[38] Huang Y, Adams MC. In vitro assessment of the upper gastrointestinal tolerance of potential probiotic dairy propionibacteria. Int J Food Microbiol 2004; 91: 253-260.

[39] Hervé C, Fondrevez M, Chéron A, et al. Transcarboxylase mRNA: A marker which evidences P. freudenreichii survival and metabolic activity during its transit in the human gut. Int J Food Microbiol 2007; 113: 303-314.

[40] Lan A, Bruneau A, Philippe C, et al. Survival and metabolic activity of selected strains of Propionibacterium freudenreichii in the gastrointestinal tract of human microbiota-associated rats. Br J Nutr 2007; 97: 714-724.

[41] Saraoui T, Parayre S, Guernec G, et al. A unique in vivo experimental approach reveals metabolic adaptation of the probiotic Propionibacterium freudenreichii to the colon environment. *BMC Genomics*; 14. Epub ahead of print 23 December 2013. DOI: 10.1186/1471-2164-14-911.

[42] Rabah H, Ménard O, Gaucher F, et al. Cheese matrix protects the immunomodulatory surface protein SlpB of Propionibacterium freudenreichii during in vitro digestion. Food Res Int 2018; 106: 712-721.

[43] Cousin FJ, Jouan-Lanhouet S, Dimanche-Boitrel MT, et al. Milk fermented by propionibacterium freudenreichii induces apoptosis of HGT-1 human gastric cancer cells. *PLoS One*; 7. Epub ahead of print 19 March 2012. DOI: 10.1371/journal.pone.0031892.

[44] Aburjaile FF, Rohmer M, Parrinello H, et al. Adaptation of Propionibacterium freudenreichii to long-term survival under gradual

nutritional shortage. *BMC Genomics*; 17. Epub ahead of print 8 December 2016. DOI: 10.1186/s12864-016-3367-x.

[45] Aburjaile FF, Madec MN, Parayre S, et al. The long-term survival of Propionibacterium freudenreichii in a context of nutrient shortage. J Appl Microbiol 2016; 120: 432-440.

[46] Cardoso FS, Castro RF, Borges N, et al. Biochemical and genetic characterization of the pathways for trehalose metabolism in Propionibacterium freudenreichii, and their role in stress response. Microbiology 2007; 153: 270-280.

[47] Dalmasso M, Aubert J, Even S, et al. Accumulation of intracellular glycogen and trehalose by Propionibacterium freudenreichii under conditions mimicking cheese ripening in the cold. Appl Environ Microbiol 2012; 78: 6357-6364.

[48] Huang S, Rabah H, Jardin J, et al. Hyperconcentrated Sweet Whey, a New Culture Medium That Enhances Propionibacterium freudenreichii Stress Tolerance. Appl Environ Microbiol 2016; 82: 4641-4651.

[49] Tuomola EM, Ouwehand AC, Salminen SJ. Human ileostomy glycoproteins as a model for small intestinal mucus to investigate adhesion of probiotics. Lett Appl Microbiol 1999; 28: 159-163.

[50] Ouwehand AC, Tölkkö S, Kulmala J, et al. Adhesion of inactivated probiotic strains to intestinal mucus. Lett Appl Microbiol 2000; 31: 82-86.

[51] Campaniello D, Bevilacqua A, Sinigaglia M, et al. Screening of Propionibacterium spp. for potential probiotic properties. Anaerobe 2015; 34: 169-173.

[52] do Carmo FLR, Rabah H, Huang S, et al. Propionibacterium freudenreichii surface protein SlpB is involved in adhesion to intestinal HT-29 cells. Front Microbiol 2017; 8: 1-11.

[53] do Carmo FLR, Silva WM, Tavares GC, et al. Mutation of the surface layer protein SlpB has pleiotropic effects in the probiotic propionibacterium freudenreichii CIRM-BIA 129. Front Microbiol 2018; 9: 1807.

[54] Collado MC, Meriluoto J, Salminen S. Development of new probiotics by strain combinations: Is it possible to improve the adhesion to intestinal mucus? J Dairy Sci 2007; 90: 2710-2716.

[55] Vesterlund S, Karp M, Salminen S, et al. Staphylococcus aureus adheres to human intestinal mucus but can be displaced by certain lactic acid bacteria. Microbiology 2006; 152: 1819-1826.

[56] Hajfarajollah H, Mokhtarani B, Noghabi KA. Newly Antibacterial and Antiadhesive Lipopeptide Biosurfactant Secreted by a Probiotic Strain, Propionibacterium Freudenreichii. Appl Biochem Biotechnol 2014; 174: 2725-2740.

[57] Nair DVT, Kollanoor-Johny A. Effect of Propionibacterium freudenreichii on Salmonella multiplication, motility, and association with avian epithelial cells. Poult Sci 2017; 96: 1376-1386.

[58] Nair DVTT, Kollanoor Johny A. Characterizing the Antimicrobial Function of a Dairy-Originated Probiotic, Propionibacterium freudenreichii, Against Multidrug-Resistant *Salmonella enterica* Serovar Heidelberg in Turkey Poults. *Front Microbiol*; 9. Epub ahead of print 12 July 2018. DOI: 10.3389/fmicb.2018.01475.

[59] Foligné B, Deutsch S-M, Breton J, et al. Promising Immunomodulatory Effects of Selected Strains of Dairy

Propionibacteria as Evidenced In Vitro and In Vivo. Appl Environ Microbiol 2010; 76: 8259-8264.

[60] Collado MC, Jalonen L, Meriluoto J, et al. Protection mechanism of probiotic combination against human pathogens: in vitro adhesion to human intestinal mucus. Asia Pac J Clin Nutr 2006; 15: 570-575.

[61] Myllyluoma E, Ahonen AM, Korpela R, et al. Effects of multispecies probiotic combination on Helicobacter pylori infection in vitro. *Clin Vaccine Immunol*; 15. Epub ahead of print September 2008. DOI: 10.1128/CVI.00080-08.

[62] Jan G, Belzacq A-SS, Haouzi D, et al. Propionibacteria induce apoptosis of colorectal carcinoma cells via short-chain fatty acids acting on mitochondria. Cell Death Differ 2002; 9: 179-188.

[63] Lan A, Lagadic-Gossmann D, Lemaire C, et al. Acidic extracellular pH shifts colorectal cancer cell death from apoptosis to necrosis upon exposure to propionate and acetate, major end-products of the human probiotic propionibacteria. Apoptosis 2007; 12: 573-591.

[64] Lan A, Bruneau A, Bensaada M, et al. Increased induction of apoptosis by Propionibacterium freudenreichii TL133 in colonic mucosal crypts of human microbiota-associated rats treated with 1,2-dimethylhydrazine. Br J Nutr 2008; 100: 1251-1259.

[65] Cousin FJ, Jouan-Lanhouet S, Théret N, et al. The probiotic Propionibacterium freudenreichii as a new adjuvant for TRAIL-based therapy in colorectal cancer. Oncotarget 2016; 7: 7161-7178.

[66] Casanova MR, Azevedo-Silva J, Rodrigues LR, et al. Colorectal Cancer Cells Increase the Production of Short Chain Fatty Acids by Propionibacterium freudenreichii Impacting on Cancer Cells Survival. Front Nutr 2018; 5: 44.

[67] Bouglé D, Roland N, Lebeurrier F. Effect of Propionibacteria Supplementation on Fecal Bifidobacteria and Segmental Colonic Transit Time in Healthy Human Subjects. Scand J Gastroenterol 1999; 34: 144-148.

[68] Hojo K, Yoda N, Tsuchita H, et al. Effect of Ingested Culture of Propionibacterium freudenreichii ET-3 on Fecal Microflora and Stool Frequency in Healthy Females. Biosci Microflora 2002; 21: 115-120.

[69] Kaneko T, Mori H, Iwata M, et al. Growth Stimulator for Bifidobacteria Produced by Propionibacterium freudenreichii and Several Intestinal Bacteria. J Dairy Sci 1994; 77: 393-404.

[70] Mori H, Sato Y, Taketomo N, et al. Isolation and Structural Identification of Bifidogenic Growth Stimulator Produced by Propionibacterium freudenreichii. J Dairy Sci 1997; 80: 1959-1964.

[71] Isawa K, Hojo K, Yoda N, et al. Isolation and identification of a new bifidogenic growth stimulator produced by propionibacterium freudenreichii ET-3. Biosci Biotechnol Biochem 2002; 66: 679-681.

[72] Okada Y, Tsuzuki Y, Miyazaki J, et al. Propionibacterium freudenreichii component 1.4-dihydroxy-2-naphthoic acid (DHNA) attenuates dextran sodium sulphate induced colitis by modulation of bacterial flora and lymphocyte homing. Gut 2006; 55: 681-688.

[73] Suzuki A, Mitsuyama K, Koga H, et al. Bifidogenic growth stimulator for the treatment of active ulcerative colitis: a pilot study. Nutrition 2006; 22: 76-81.

[74] Furuichi K, Hojo K ichi, Katakura Y, et al. Aerobic culture of Propionibacterium freudenreichii ET-3 can increase production ratio of 1,4-dihydroxy-2-naphthoic acid to menaquinone. J Biosci Bioeng 2006; 101: 464-470.

[75] Kouya T, Misawa K, Horiuchi M, et al. Production of extracellular bifidogenic growth stimulator by anaerobic and aerobic cultivations of several propionibacterial strains. J Biosci Bioeng 2007; 103: 464-471.

[76] Foligné B, Breton J, Mater D, et al. Tracking the microbiome functionality: Focus on Propionibacterium species. Gut 2013; 62: 1227-1228.

[77] Deutsch S-MM, Mariadassou M, Nicolas P, et al. Identification of proteins involved in the anti-inflammatory properties of Propionibacterium freudenreichii by means of a multi-strain study. *Sci Rep*; 7. Epub ahead of print 2017. DOI: 10.1038/srep46409.

[78] Frohnmeyer E, Deptula P, Nyman TA, et al. Secretome profiling of Propionibacterium freudenreichii reveals highly variable responses even among the closely related strains. Microb Biotechnol 2018; 11: 510-526.

[79] Ma S, Yeom J, Lim Y-HH. Dairy Propionibacterium freudenreichii ameliorates acute colitis by stimulating MUC2 expression in intestinal goblet cell in a DSS-induced colitis rat model. Sci Rep 2020; 10: 5523.

[80] Colliou N, Ge Y, Gong M, et al. Regulation of Th17 cells by P. UF1 against systemic Listeria monocytogenes infection. Gut Microbes 2018; 9: 279-287.

[81] Ge Y, Gong M, Colliou N, et al. Neonatal intestinal immune regulation by the commensal bacterium, P. UF1. Mucosal Immunol 2019; 12: 434-444.

[82] Le Maréchal C, Peton V, Plé C, et al. Surface proteins of Propionibacterium freudenreichii are involved in its anti-inflammatory properties. J Proteomics 2015; 113: 447-461.

[83] do Carmo FLR, Rabah H, Cordeiro BF, et al. Probiotic Propionibacterium freudenreichii requires SlpB protein to mitigate mucositis induced by chemotherapy. Oncotarget 2019; 10: 7198-7219.

[84] Ge Y, Gong M, Zadeh M, et al. Regulating colonic dendritic cells by commensal glycosylated large surface layer protein A to sustain gut homeostasis against pathogenic inflammation. Mucosal Immunol 2020; 13: 34-46.

[85] Rodovalho V de R, Luz BSR da, Rabah H, et al. Extracellular Vesicles Produced by the Probiotic Propionibacterium freudenreichii CIRM-BIA 129 Mitigate Inflammation by Modulating the NF-κB Pathway. Front Microbiol 2020; 11: 1544.

[86] Okada Y, Tsuzuki Y, Narimatsu K, et al. 1,4-Dihydroxy-2-naphthoic acid from Propionibacterium freudenreichii reduces inflammation in interleukin-10-deficient mice with colitis by suppressing macrophage-derived proinflammatory cytokines. J Leukoc Biol 2013; 94: 473-480.

[87] Fukumoto S, Toshimitsu T, Matsuoka S, et al. Identification of a probiotic bacteria-derived activator of the aryl hydrocarbon receptor that inhibits colitis. Immunol Cell Biol 2014; 92: 460-465.

[88] Cheng Y, Jin UH, Davidson LA, et al. Microbial-derived 1,4-Dihydroxy-2-naphthoic acid and related compounds as aryl hydrocarbon receptor agonists/antagonists: Structure-activity relationships and receptor modeling. Toxicol Sci 2017; 155: 458-473.

[89] Plé C, Richoux R, Jardin J, et al. Single-strain starter experimental cheese reveals anti-inflammatory effect of Propionibacterium freudenreichii CIRM BIA 129 in TNBS-colitis model. J Funct Foods 2015; 18: 575-585.

[90] Foligné B, Parayre S, Cheddani R, et al. Immunomodulation properties of multi-species fermented milks. Food Microbiol 2016; 53: 60-69.

[91] Moslemi M, Mazaheri Nezhad Fard R, Hosseini SM, et al. Incorporation of Propionibacteria in Fermented Milks as a Probiotic. Crit Rev Food Sci Nutr 2016; 56: 1290-1312.

[92] Cousin FJ, Foligné B, Deutsch SM, et al. Assessment of the probiotic potential of a dairy product fermented by propionibacterium freudenreichii in piglets. J Agric Food Chem 2012; 60: 7917-7927.

[93] Dudek-Wicher R, Junka A, Paleczny J, et al. Clinical Trials of Probiotic Strains in Selected Disease Entities. *Int J Microbiol*; 2020. Epub ahead of print 2020. DOI: 10.1155/2020/8854119.

[94] Uchida M, Tsuboi H, Takahashi Arita M, et al. Safety of high doses of Propionibacterium freudenreichii ET-3 culture in healthy adult subjects. Regul Toxicol Pharmacol 2011; 60: 262-267.

[95] Jan G, Leverrier P, Proudy I, et al. Survival and beneficial effects of propionibacteria in the human gut: in vivo and in vitro investigations. Lait 2002; 82: 131-144.

[96] Kukkonen K, Savilahti E, Haahtela T, et al. Probiotics and prebiotic galacto-oligosaccharides in the prevention of allergic diseases: A randomized, double-blind, placebo-controlled trial. J Allergy Clin Immunol 2007; 119: 192-198.

[97] Kukkonen K, Savilahti E, Haahtela T, et al. Long-term safety and impact on infection rates of postnatal probiotic and prebiotic (synbiotic) treatment: Randomized, double-blind, placebo-controlled trial. Pediatrics 2008; 122: 8-12.

[98] Kuitunen M, Kukkonen K, Juntunen-Backman K, et al. Probiotics prevent IgE-associated allergy until age 5 years in cesarean-delivered children but not in the total cohort. J Allergy Clin Immunol 2009; 123: 335-341.

[99] Korpela K, Salonen A, Vepsäläinen O, et al. Probiotic supplementation restores normal microbiota composition and function in antibiotic-treated and in caesarean-born infants. *Microbiome*; 6. Epub ahead of print 16 October 2018. DOI: 10.1186/s40168-018-0567-4.

[100] Kallio S, Kukkonen AK, Savilahti E, et al. Perinatal probiotic intervention prevented allergic disease in a Caesarean-delivered subgroup at 13-year follow-up. Clin Exp Allergy 2018; 49: 506-515.

[101] Tapiovaara L, Lehtoranta L, Poussa T, et al. Absence of adverse events in healthy individuals using probiotics - analysis of six randomised studies by one study group. Benef Microbes 2016; 7: 161-169.

[102] Żółkiewicz J, Marzec A, Ruszczyński M, et al. Postbiotics—A Step Beyond Pre- and Probiotics. Nutrients 2020; 12: 2189.

[103] Nataraj BH, Ali SA, Behare P V., et al. Postbiotics-parabiotics: the new horizons in microbial biotherapy and functional foods. Microb Cell Fact 2020; 19: 168.

[104] Tsilingiri K, Rescigno M. Postbiotics: what else? Benef Microbes 2013; 4: 101-107.

[105] Rohde M. The Gram-Positive Bacterial Cell Wall. Gram-Positive Pathog 2019; 3-18.

[106] Briaud P, Carroll RK. Extracellular Vesicle Biogenesis and Functions in Gram-Positive Bacteria. Infect Immun 2020; 88: 1-37.

[107] Molina-Tijeras JA, Gálvez J, Rodríguez-Cabezas ME. The Immunomodulatory Properties of Extracellular Vesicles Derived from Probiotics: A Novel Approach for the Management of Gastrointestinal Diseases. Nutrients 2019; 11: 1038.

[108] Liu Y, Alexeeva S, Defourny KA, et al. Tiny but mighty: bacterial membrane vesicles in food biotechnological applications. Curr Opin Biotechnol 2018; 49: 179-184.

[109] Rad AH, Abbasi A, Kafil HS, et al. Potential Pharmaceutical and Food Applications of Postbiotics: A review. *Curr Pharm Biotechnol*; 21. Epub ahead of print 17 May 2020. DOI: 10.2174/1389201021666200516154833.

Chapter 8

Probiotics from Fermented Fish

Nilofar Yasmin, Khusboo Kaur and Kaushal Sood

Abstract

The term 'Probiotics' is used to describe live microorganisms, which, when administered in adequate quantities, confer health benefits. The term probiotics was first introduced in 1965 by Lilly and Stillwell, who defined it to be microorganisms acting as growth promoters for other microorganisms. These microorganisms may include *Lactobacillus*, *Streptococcus*, *Bifidobacterium*, *Saccharomyces*, *Aspergillus*, *Enterococcus* etc., as well as a mixture of other microorganisms. The chapter focuses on providing a comprehensive and up-to-date review of probiotics that have been isolated from fermented fish-based products.

Keywords: probiotics, lactobacillus, fermented food, fermented fish

1. Introduction

The term 'Probiotics' conventionally refers to the substances produced by microorganisms that stimulated the growth of others. With the advancement of knowledge in the subject, the use of the term was later extended to describe the tissue extracts that stimulated microbial growth. This definition was further evolved to animal feed supplements which exerted a beneficial effect by contributing to intestinal flora [1]. With further advancement of knowledge in the field, the term *prebiotics* [2] was introduced to describe food supplements that were non-digestible by the host but were able to exert beneficial effects by selective stimulation of growth or activity of intestinal microorganisms. A combination of the two, probiotics and prebiotics, was referred to as *conbiotics* by certain authors while *synbiotics* by others [2, 3]. However, due to limited research in this field, the health benefits of prebiotics are yet to be verified. Over the recent years, functional foods have gained popularity due to their beneficial health effects, which have partly been attributed to their probiotic components [4]. Over the decades, the definition of probiotics has been refined by several workers. Vergin [5] suggested the action of the probiotic diet towards the intestinal microbiota in describing "the microbial balance of the body" [5]. Parker [6], defined probiotics as: "organisms and substances which contribute to intestinal microbial balance". This was the first time that probiotics were mentioned in the context of gut health. In 1989, Fuller [7] further refined the definition to "live microbial feed supplement which beneficially affects the host animal by improving its intestinal microbial balance". In the following years, the definition was extended to include mono- or mixed cultures of microorganisms that beneficially affected the host by improving the properties of the indigenous microbiota [8].

However, the widely accepted and currently in use definition is the one put forth by the World Health Organization:

"Probiotics are live microorganisms which, when administered in adequate amounts confer a health benefit on the host."

To summarize:

Prebiotic: A prebiotic is a non-viable food component that confers a health benefit by modulation of the gut microbiota.

Probiotics: These are live microorganisms, they confer health benefits to the host when administered in adequate doses.

Synbiotic: A product that contains both probiotics and prebiotics.

2. Probiotics: a brief history

Fermented dairy and other food products were produced and utilized for nutritional and therapeutic purposes long before the discovery of microorganisms. The discovery of fermentation was itself an incidence of serendipity. However, with the discovery of Lactic acid-producing bacteria by Pasteur in 1857, it was Pasteur and his successors who had a significant impact on the understanding of the microbiology involved in the process of fermentation [9]. The idea of using beneficial bacteria attracted interest along with the advances in microbiology and biotechnology in the following decades.

Research on the application of probiotic microorganisms in aquaculture started over two decades ago. Microorganisms, especially lactic acid bacteria (LAB), have long been associated with food fermentation. Dating back to 3200 BC, when the Egyptians produced fermented milk and dairy products during the Pharaonic period [10, 11]. Applications of probiotics in the field of animal husbandry gained popularity in the 1960s. In the 1980s, the most common probiotics for animal feeds belonged to three bacterial and one yeast genera: Lactobacillus, Streptococcus, Bacillus, and Saccharomyces spp. Lactobacillus sp. is recognized to produce potent antimicrobial compounds in order to establish their preservative and probiotic effects [12, 13] and have been consumed in the form of diverse food supplements through thousands of years and are "generally regarded as safe" (GRAS) [14, 15].

3. Probiotics: qualifying characteristics

Probiotics are an innate component of a healthy intestinal microbiota in humans and other animals. These colonize the gut through the diet or other non-dietary sources that are consumed by the organism. Novel species and strains of probiotic bacteria are being constantly identified with the exploration of previously unexplored sources. However, prior to incorporating such potential probiotic strains into products, their efficacy has to be carefully assessed based on a battery of criteria (**Figure 1**).

Foremost among such criteria is the safety of the host. Most of the probiotics in use today have been isolated from natural sources with a long history of safe use. Acid and bile salt stability of such strains are self-evident properties as these were able to colonize the intestinal tract. The development of probiotic products requires that the strains should also have antimicrobial activity and antibiotic resistance to the commonly administered drugs. Adhesion to intestinal cells and colonization of the gut are among the other primary requisites [3–5, 7, 16–19].

Acidic conditions ($pH < 3.0$) in the stomach act as a natural barrier to microorganisms and prevents most of them from passing into the intestine. Acid tolerance

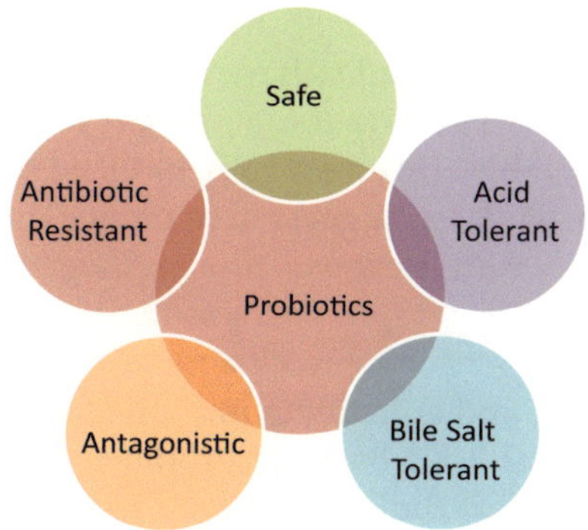

Figure 1.
Probiotics: Characteristic criteria.

is, hence, a preliminary character for any strain that is expected to have probiotic effects [16, 20]. Resistance to pH 3.0 for 2 h is one standard test to determine the low pH tolerance of potential probiotic isolates [21]. The exact mechanism of tolerance to low pH conditions is not yet known. The next barrier for a potential probiotic to survive is the bile salt in the intestine, the normal level of which is around 0.3%, but may range up to the extreme 2.0% during the first hour of digestion. In conjunction with acid tolerance, it has been used widely as a selection criterion of potential probiotics [22]. Bile resistance of potential probiotic strains is related to the activity of the enzyme- bile salt hydrolase (BSH) which catalyzes the hydrolysis of conjugated bile, hence reducing its toxic effects [23]. In addition, according to Ganzle et al. [24] bile resistance can be increased due to the protective effect of some food components.

The potential of lactic acid bacteria and probiotic yeast to inhibit the growth of other microorganisms in the intestine is a valuable feature for considering their application in the development of functional foods. The antagonistic property of the probiotic strains against pathogenic bacteria may be exerted by either competitive exclusion, a decrease of redox potential, inter-bacterial aggregation, or production of antimicrobial substances including organic acids, other inhibitory primary metabolites such as hydrogen peroxide, and special compounds like bacteriocins and antibiotics [25, 26]. This property enables the probiotics to alter the resident intestinal flora and modify it for the benefit of the host [27].

The ability of probiotic strains to endure and survive in the presence of antibiotics ensures the maintenance of healthy intestinal microbiota during the treatment of microbial infections. LAB has been shown to exhibit susceptibility to a broad spectrum of antibiotics. Although isolates of lactobacilli with strong resistance to penicillin, cephalosporins, and bacitracin have been recovered from the human gastro-intestinal tract and dairy products, in most of these cases, this resistance is not transmissible and represents an intrinsic characteristic of the organism [17, 28].

4. Probiotics: health benefits

The health benefits of probiotics were proposed over a century ago by Eli Metchnikoff when he postulated that manipulating the intestinal microbiome could enhance health and delay senescence [29]. There is now sufficient scientific evidence supporting the incorporation of probiotics in the diet for health benefits. The best documented benefits include- relief from bowel disorders such as lactose intolerance, antibiotic-associated diarrhea, and infectious diarrhea, and allergy. Emerging evidence has indicated the potential role of probiotics in managing different kinds of cancers as well. Multiple *in vivo* studies have indicated that the administration of specific strains of lactic acid bacteria could prevent the establishment, growth, and metastasis of transplantable and chemically induced tumors [30]. In human subjects, probiotic therapy has been suggested to reduce the risk of colon cancer through the inhibition of transformation of procarcinogen to active carcinogens, binding/inactivating mutagenic compounds, producing antimutagenic compounds, suppressing the growth of pro-carcinogenic bacteria, reducing the absorption of mutagens from the intestine, and enhancing immune function [31, 32]. However, evidence is still lacking to establish a basis for probiotic therapy in cancer prevention.

Probiotics are known to exert their effects by influencing the intestinal microflora and protecting against infections, alleviating lactose intolerance, reducing blood cholesterol levels, improving weight gain and feed conversion ratio, and also stimulating the immune system [33]. Lactic acid bacteria (LAB) are a part of normal gut microflora in humans and some other animals and are known to produce lactic acid, hydrogen peroxide, diacetyl, acetaldehyde, and bacteriocins which are able to inhibit the growth of harmful microorganisms [34, 35].

Probiotics are mostly administered as live supplements in diet and exert diverse effects on the host. These influence the intestinal luminal environment and the innate and adaptive immune response systems [34, 36].

The use of probiotics for enhancing bio-growth parameters and in improving disease resistance ability has been well documented in aquaculture of fish for human consumption [37–41] but research on the effect of feeding probiotics in ornamental fishes is still an under-explored research territory.

Although most probiotics known so far are Gram-positive, with lactobacillus and bifidobacterium being the main species used for treatments of intestinal dysfunctions [42], some Gram-negative bacteria, such as *Escherichia coli* Nissle 1917 (EcN) [43], also known as "Mutaflor," have also been reported to function as probiotics. Mutaflor has been used in Germany for many years in the treatment of chronic constipation [44] and colitis [45]. Probiotic bacteria have been shown to modulate intestinal microbiota through the modulation of luminal pH and the production of antimicrobial compounds [46, 47]. In addition to the foregoing, probiotics have also been reported to enhance the intestinal barrier function [48]. These effects collectively contribute to the management of inflammatory bowel disease [46].

There is strong evidence that the administration of probiotics is able to downregulate over-expressed immune responses in subjects with autoimmune/immune-inflammatory disorders and enhance specific aspects of immune function in healthy subjects. Schiffrin and colleagues reported enhanced phagocytic capacity of peripheral blood leucocytes (polymorphonuclear and monocytes) in healthy human adults administered with specific strains of probiotics [49–52]. The effectiveness of probiotics in enhancing the immunogenicity of mucosal and systemic vaccines has also been reported. It has been reported that probiotic administration could induce antibody responses to completely unrelated antigens and to themselves [53, 54].

5. Probiotics from fermented fish

Probiotics have been obtained from a wide variety of traditionally fermented and preserved products that include dairy-based items like fermented milk, cheese, buttermilk, milk powder, and yogurt [55, 56]. Non-dairy food sources like soy-based products, cereals, and a variety of fermented juices have also proved to be promising [57, 58]. With more and more sources being explored, new strains and species of probiotics are being added to the list.

Fish and their products have emerged to be a potential source of novel probiotics that can be utilized to enhance the value of human nutrition [59]. Fish gut confers a congenial environment for colonization of bacteria abundant in the aquatic environment. Most of the probiotic bacteria isolated from the fish gut are either aerobes or facultative anaerobes. Worldwide, fishes have been consumed in diverse formats. Among some ethnic groups, there has been a tradition to preserve fish by drying and fermenting for enhanced shelf-life. In the North-eastern states of India, freshwater fish have been fermented by traditional practices into products such as Utonga-kupsu, Hentak, and Ngari. Workers have studied the bacterial communities in these products and isolated *Lactococcus lactis* subsp. *cremoris*, *L. plantarum*, *Enterococcus faecium*, *Lactobacillus fructosus*, *Lactobacillus amylophilus*, *Lactobacillus coryniformis*, *Bacillus subtilis* and *B. pumilus*, *B. cereus*, *Staphylococcus aureus* and Enterobacteriaceae population. Most of these have been characterized as probiotics [60, 61]. Similar explorations have reported several strains of probiotics from a variety of other fishes. The table in the following section (**Table 1**) summarizes various such sources and probiotic strains isolated from them.

Country/state/region	Fish species	Bacteria isolated	Accession No.	References
Manipur (India)	*Puntius sophore*	*Lactococcus plantarum*		[60, 62]
		Lactobacillus fructosus		
		Lactobacillus amylophilus		
		Enterococcus faecium	JX 847611	
		Lactobacillus coryniformis subsp. *torquens*		
		Lactobacillus lactis subsp. *cremoris*		
		L.brevis	KU945827	[63]
		Bacillus coagulans	JX847608	[64]
		Bacillus subtilis	KX953135	[65]
Meghalaya (India)	*Danio* spp.	*Lactobacillus rossiae* isolate LS6	JN680708	[66]
		L. plantarum isolate LS5	JN680707	
		L. rossiae isolate LS4	JN680706	
		Lactobacillus pentosus isolate LS3	JN680705	
		Lactobacillus pobuzihii isolate TTp4	HQ141620	
		L. pobuzihii isolate TTp6	HQ141621	
		L. pobuzihii isolate TTp12	H Q141622	
		L. pobuzihii isolate TTp13	H Q141623	
		L. pobuzihii isolate TTp14	HQ141624	
Assam (India)	*Puntius* spp.	*Staphylococcus sp.*	KR706310	[67]
NE India	*Puntius* sp.	*Staphylococcus piscifermentans*		[68]
		Staphylococcus arlettae		
		S. condiment		
		Staphylococcus sciuri		
		Staphylococcus warneri		
		S. nepalensis		
		Staphylococcus hominis		

Country/state/ region	Fish species	Bacteria isolated	Accession No.	References
Malaysia	*Parastromateus niger* BLOCH	*Pediococcus pentosaceus*		[69]
		Lactobacillus plantarum		
		L. pentosus		
	Stolephorus spp.	*Lactobacillus casei*		[8]
		Lactobacillus plantarum		
		Lactobacillus paracasei		
Thailand	*Chitala ornata*	*Lactobacillus plantarum*		[7]
	Channa micropeltes	*L. pentosus*		
		Staphylococcus simulans	MG798679.1	[70]
Phillipines	*Chanos chanos*	*Leuconostoc mesenteroides*		[71]
		P.cerevisiae		
		Enterococcus faecalis		
		P.acidilactici		
		Leu.paramesenteroides		
		L. plantarum		
	Loriculus philippensis	*P. pentosaceus*		
		Streptococcus equinus		
		Leuconostoc sp.		
		Lactobacillus sp.		
	Eleutheronema tetradactylum	*P. halophilus.*		

Table 1.
Probiotics isolated from fish.

The processes like fermentation, salting, drying, and smoking are the popularly followed traditional methods of preservation of fish [72, 73]. As evident from the list (**Table 1**) lactic acid bacteria have been found to be predominant in most of the fermented fish products. However, the microbial diversity of these products also encompasses some species of *Micrococcus*, *Lactococcus*, *Enterococcus*, *Bacillus*, *Staphylococcus,* and *Enterobacteriaceae*. Conventionally, culture-based methods have been employed to identify LAB in food samples, and isolates are evaluated for probiotic properties under controlled conditions. With the advances in molecular techniques, the isolation and identification of microorganisms missed by culture-dependent methods have now been achieved. Consequently, as new microbial metabolites, such as bacteriocins, defensins, and other antimicrobial compounds are being reported, an extensive database for identification and comparison of potential novel products is now available [71]. Several strains of probiotic bacteria were isolated from various fish species (African catfish, European eel, Bream, Perch, Rudd) and most of these were reported to be *Lactobacillus* isolates which were able to inhibit pathogens by acid productions [75]. Various probiotic strains of *Bacillus subtilis* have been reported from the gastrointestinal tract of carps [75], coastal fishes [76], bivalves [77], shrimp culture ponds [78], and shrimp larvae-rearing medium [79]. Multiple studies supported that *B. subtilis* could reduce pathogenic bacteria in aquaculture. The *Lactobacillus* species associated with the traditionally fermented fish product—Tungtap (a fermented product of ethnic tribes of the state of Meghalaya in India) were found to possess many health-promoting probiotic properties [66]. Alcaligenes sp. isolated from the gastrointestinal tract of *Tor tambroides*, function as an important probiotic that promote gut microbiota composition, improve gut health including bacterial nutritional enzyme activity, volatile short-chain fatty acids (VSCFA) production and gut morphology, and enhance production performance of Malaysian Mahseer (*T. tambroides*) [80].

The fish gut microbiota embodies diverse enzyme-producing microorganisms capable of producing multiple hydrolytic enzymes that aid in the digestion of carbohydrates, proteins, and lipids [81, 82]. *Bacillus* spp. has been reported from Utonga-kupsu, Hentak, and Ngari (traditional fermented fish of Manipur, North-East India) alongside *Staphylococcus*. These have also been reported from other fermented fish products such as Namplaa and Kapi (from Thailand) and have been shown to exhibit amylase, protease, and cellulase activities that can improve the quantity, availability, and digestibility of dietary nutrients in the body in addition to other probiotic effects [65, 83]. *S. simulans* PMRS35 isolated from *budu*, a traditional Thai salt-fermented fish-based product, possessed high lipase and protease activities and a vast array of desirable probiotic characteristics [70]. In any fermented food, the diverse microorganisms are capable of producing many useful enzymes like oxidase, β-galactosidase, amylase, *etc.* which are essential for aesculin hydrolysis, starch hydrolysis, nitrate to nitrite reduction, and other important biochemical conversions and can hence be useful in bioremediation as well [84].

Although the above list is not comprehensive, it represents the potential of fish and their products as a source of novel probiotics. The knowledge of the health benefits of fermented fish products has been utilized by many cultures worldwide and this information can be utilized for the development of probiotic products for human consumption.

6. Future prospects

The incorporation of probiotics from fish and fish products into the development of functional foods containing known probiotic strains can provide alternatives in therapeutics and ensure food security. Isolation and standardization of bacteriocins and other metabolites from probiotics can lead to the development of functional foods for individuals surviving on a vegan diet.

7. Conclusions

The host- probiotic relationship can be regarded as evolutionarily one of the most primitive associations. It represents a dynamic relationship that is influenced by dietary and other intrinsic and extrinsic factors. The kind of diet consumed by the host plays an important role in the maintenance of the probiotic microbiome in the body. On the other hand, a healthy probiotic microbiome in the host ascertains good growth and health of the host. The various health benefits and the potential role of probiotics in various human diseases have been highlighted in this chapter. As the kind of diet consumed influences the gut microbiome significantly, it, therefore, becomes essential to explore this intricate food-host-probiotic relationship in order to understand human health and diseases. The traditional food- preparation practices evolved through close observation of the effect of food on human and animal health. Hence, exploration of such traditionally prepared foods can reveal some novel probiotics with potential therapeutic applications. In this chapter, some of such sources of probiotics have been listed. However, there is an urgent need to study these in detail as most of them have not been completely characterized to the extent of their utilization for human applications.

Conflict of interest

The authors declare no conflict of interest.

Author details

Nilofar Yasmin[1], Khusboo Kaur[2] and Kaushal Sood[3]*

1 Center for Biotechnology and Bioinformatics, Dibrugarh University, Dibrugarh, Assam, India

2 Department of Life Sciences, Dibrugarh University, Dibrugarh, Assam, India

3 Department of Zoology, Tinsukia College, Tinsukia, Assam, India

*Address all correspondence to: kaushalsood@gmail.com

References

[1] Fuller R. Probiotics for farm animals. In: Tannock GW, editor. Probiotics: A Critical Review. Wymondham, UK: Horizon Scientific Press; 1998

[2] Gibson GR, Roberfroid MB. Dietary modulation of the human colonic microbiota: Introducing the concept of prebiotics. The Journal of Nutrition. 1995;**125**(6):1401-1412

[3] Berg RD. Probiotics, prebiotics or 'conbiotics'? Trends in Microbiology. 1998;**6**(3):89-92

[4] Ziemer CJ, Gibson GR. An overview of probiotics, prebiotics and synbiotics in the functional food concept: perspectives and future strategies. International Dairy Journal. 1998; **8**(5-6):473-479

[5] Vergin F. Antibiotics and probiotics. Hippokrates. 1954;**25**(4):116-119

[6] Parker RB. Probiotics, the Other Half of Antibiotic Story. Animal Nutrition & Health; 1974;**29**:4-8

[7] Fuller R. Probiotics in man and animals. The Journal of Applied Bacteriology. 1989;**66**(5):365-378

[8] Havenaar R, Ten Brink B, JHJ H. Selection of strains for probiotic use. In: Probiotics: The Scientific Basis. London: Chapman and Hall; 1992. pp. 209-224

[9] Ozen M, Dinleyici E. The history of probiotics: The untold story. Beneficial Microbes. 2015;**6**(2):159-165

[10] Abou-Donia S. Origin, history and manufacturing process of Egyptian dairy products: An overview. Alexandria Journal of Food Science and Technology. 2008;**5**(1):51-62

[11] Tannock GW. Probiotics: time for a dose of realism. Current Issues in Intestinal Microbiology. 2003;**4**(2): 33-42

[12] Abo-Amer AE. Characterization of a bacteriocin-like inhibitory substance produced by Lactobacillus plantarum isolated from Egyptian home-made yogurt. Science Asia. 2007;**33**:313-319

[13] Vijayakumar M et al. In-vitro assessment of the probiotic potential of Lactobacillus plantarum KCC-24 isolated from Italian rye-grass (Lolium multiflorum) forage. Anaerobe. 2015;**32**:90-97

[14] De Vries MC et al. Lactobacillus plantarum—Survival, functional and potential probiotic properties in the human intestinal tract. International Dairy Journal. 2006;**16**(9):1018-1028

[15] Haghshenas B et al. Different effects of two newly-isolated probiotic Lactobacillus plantarum 15HN and Lactococcus lactis subsp. Lactis 44Lac strains from traditional dairy products on cancer cell lines. Anaerobe. 2014;**30**:51-59

[16] Salminen S et al. Development of selection criteria for probiotic strains to assess their potential in functional foods: A Nordic and European approach. Bioscience and Microflora. 1996;**15**(2):61-67

[17] Mattila-Sandholm T, Mättö J, Saarela M. Lactic acid bacteria with health claims—Interactions and interference with gastrointestinal flora. International Dairy Journal. 1999; **9**(1):25-35

[18] Gibson GR, Fuller R. Aspects of in vitro and in vivo research approaches directed toward identifying probiotics and prebiotics for human use. The Journal of Nutrition. 2000;**130**(2): 391S-395S

[19] Sanders ME. Considerations for use of probiotic bacteria to modulate human health. The Journal of Nutrition. 2000;**130**(2):384S-390S

[20] Marteau P et al. Survival of lactic acid bacteria in a dynamic model of the stomach and small intestine: Validation and the effects of bile. Journal of Dairy Science. 1997;**80**(6):1031-1037

[21] Arihara K et al. Lactobacillus acidophilus group lactic acid bacteria applied to meat fermentation. Journal of Food Science. 1998;**63**(3):544-547

[22] De Smet I et al. Significance of bile salt hydrolytic activities of lactobacilli. Journal of Applied Bacteriology. 1995;**79**(3):292-301

[23] Du Toit M et al. Characterisation and selection of probiotic lactobacilli for a preliminary minipig feeding trial and their effect on serum cholesterol levels, faeces pH and faeces moisture content. International Journal of Food Microbiology. 1998;**40**(1-2):93-104

[24] Gänzle MG et al. Effect of bacteriocin-producing lactobacilli on the survival of Escherichia coli and Listeria in a dynamic model of the stomach and the small intestine. International Journal of Food Microbiology. 1999;**48**(1):21-35

[25] Vaughan E, Mollet B. Probiotics in the new millennium. Food/Nahrung. 1999;**43**(3):148-153

[26] Kalantzopoulos G. Fermented products with probiotic qualities. Anaerobe. 1997;**3**(2-3):185-190

[27] Gilliland SE. Health and nutritional benefits from lactic acid bacteria. FEMS Microbiology Reviews. 1990;**7**(1-2):175-188

[28] Salminen S et al. Demonstration of safety of probiotics—A review. International Journal of Food Microbiology. 1998;**44**(1-2):93-106

[29] Anukam KC, Reid G. Probiotics: 100 years (1907-2007) after Elie Metchnikoff's observation. Communicating Current Research and Educational Topics and Trends in Applied Microbiology. 2007;**1**:466-474

[30] Rafter J. Lactic acid bacteria and cancer: Mechanistic perspective. British Journal of Nutrition. 2002;**88**(S1): S89-S94

[31] van't Veer P et al. Consumption of fermented milk products and breast cancer: A case-control study in The Netherlands. Cancer Research. 1989;**49**(14):4020-4023

[32] Gill, HS, Cross, ML. Probiotics and immune function. In: Calder, PC, Field, CJ and Gill, HS, editors. Nutrition and Immune Function. Wallingford, UK: CABI International. pp. 251-272

[33] Agrawal R. Probiotics: An emerging food supplement with health benefits. Food Biotechnology. 2005;**19**(3):227-246

[34] Gatesoupe FJ. The use of probiotics in aquaculture. Aquaculture. 1999;**180**(1-2):147-165

[35] Ringø E, Gatesoupe F-J. Lactic acid bacteria in fish: A review. Aquaculture. 1998;**160**(3-4):177-203

[36] Holzapfel WH et al. Overview of gut flora and probiotics. International Journal of Food Microbiology. 1998;**41**(2):85-101

[37] Gatesoupe F-J. Lactic acid bacteria increase the resistance of turbot larvae, Scophthalmus maximus, against pathogenic Vibrio. Aquatic Living Resources. 1994;**7**(4):277-282

[38] Bogut I et al. Influence of probiotic (Streptococcus faecium M74) on growth and content of intestinal microflora in carp (Cyprinus carpio). Czech Journal of Animal Science-UZPI (Czech Republic). 1998:231-235

[39] Gildberg A, Mikkelsen H. Effects of supplementing the feed to Atlantic cod

(Gadus morhua) fry with lactic acid bacteria and immuno-stimulating peptides during a challenge trial with Vibrio anguillarum. Aquaculture. 1998;**167**(1-2):103-113

[40] Naik ATR, Ramesha T. Effect of graded levels of G-probiotic on growth, survival and feed conversion of tilapia, Oreochromis mossambicus. Fishery Technology. 1999;**36**(1):63-66

[41] Robertson P et al. Use of Carnobacterium sp. as a probiotic for Atlantic salmon (Salmo salar L.) and rainbow trout (Oncorhynchus mykiss, Walbaum). Aquaculture. 2000;**185**(3-4):235-243

[42] Marco ML, Pavan S, Kleerebezem M. Towards understanding molecular modes of probiotic action. Current Opinion in Biotechnology. 2006;**17**(2):204-210

[43] Nissle A. Explanations of the significance of colonic dysbacteria & the mechanism of action of E. coli therapy (mutaflor). Die Medizinische. 1959;**4**(21):1017-1022

[44] Möllenbrink M, Bruckschen E. Treatment of chronic constipation with physiologic Escherichia coli bacteria. Results of a clinical study of the effectiveness and tolerance of microbiological therapy with the E. coli Nissle 1917 strain (Mutaflor). Medizinische Klinik (Munich, Germany: 1983). 1994;**89**(11):587-593

[45] Schütz E. The treatment of intestinal diseases with Mutaflor. A multicenter retrospective study. Fortschritte der Medizin. 1989;**107**(28):599-602

[46] Ng SCMRCP, Hart AL, Kamm MA, Stagg AJ, Knight SC. Mechanisms of action of probiotics: Recent advances. Inflammatory Bowel Diseases. 2009;**15**(2):300-310

[47] Asahara T, Shimizu K, Nomoto K, et al. Probiotic bifidobacteria protect mice from lethal infection with Shiga toxin-producing Escherichia coli O157:H7. Infection and Immunity. 2004;**72**:2240-2247

[48] Meddings J. The significance of the gut barrier in disease. Gut. 2008;**57**:438-440

[49] Schiffrin E et al. Immunomodulation of human blood cells following the ingestion of lactic acid bacteria. Journal of Dairy Science. 1995;**78**(3):491-497

[50] Arunachalam K, Gill H, Chandra R. Enhancement of natural immune function by dietary consumption of Bifidobacterium lactis (HN019). European Journal of Clinical Nutrition. 2000;**54**(3):263-267

[51] Sheih Y-H et al. Systemic immunity-enhancing effects in healthy subjects following dietary consumption of the lactic acid bacterium Lactobacillus rhamnosus HN001. Journal of the American College of Nutrition. 2001;**20**(2):149-156

[52] Donnet-Hughes A et al. Modulation of nonspecific mechanisms of defense by lactic acid bacteria: Effective dose. Journal of Dairy Science. 1999;**82**(5):863-869

[53] Link-Amster H et al. Modulation of a specific humoral immune response and changes in intestinal flora mediated through fermented milk intake. FEMS Immunology and Medical Microbiology. 1994;**10**(1):55-63

[54] Yasui H, Mike A, Ohwaki M. Immunogenicity of bifidobacterium breve and change in antibody production in Peyer's patches after oral administration. Journal of Dairy Science. 1989;**72**(1):30-35

[55] Stanton C et al. Market potential for probiotics. The American Journal of Clinical Nutrition. 2001;**73**(2):476s-483s

[56] Food Processing. Modest Growth for Global Probiotic Market. 2009. Available from: http://www.foodprocessing.com/articles/2008/383.html

[57] Ewe J-A, Wan-Abdullah W-N, Liong M-T. Viability and growth characteristics of Lactobacillus in soymilk supplemented with B-vitamins. International Journal of Food Sciences and Nutrition. 2010;**61**(1):87-107

[58] Sheehan VM, Ross P, Fitzgerald GF. Assessing the acid tolerance and the technological robustness of probiotic cultures for fortification in fruit juices. Innovative Food Science and Emerging Technologies. 2007;**8**(2):279-284

[59] Prado R et al. The herbicide paraquat induces alterations in the elemental and biochemical composition of non-target microalgal species. Chemosphere. 2009;**76**(10):1440-1444

[60] Thapa N, Pal J, Tamang JP. Microbial diversity in ngari, hentak and tungtap, fermented fish products of North-East India. World Journal of Microbiology and Biotechnology. 2004;**20**(6):599-607

[61] Thapa N. Ethnic fermented and preserved fish products of India and Nepal. Journal of Ethnic Foods. 2016;**3**(1):69-77

[62] Abdhul K et al. Antioxidant activity of exopolysaccharide from probiotic strain Enterococcus faecium (BDU7) from Ngari. International Journal of Biological Macromolecules. 2014;**70**:450-454

[63] Aarti C et al. In vitro studies on probiotic and antioxidant properties of Lactobacillus brevis strain LAP2 isolated from Hentak, a fermented fish product of North-East India. LWT. 2017;**86**:438-446

[64] Abdhul K et al. Bacteriocinogenic potential of a probiotic strain Bacillus coagulans [BDU3] from Ngari. International Journal of Biological Macromolecules. 2015;**79**:800-806

[65] Singh SS et al. Antimicrobial, antioxidant and probiotics characterization of dominant bacterial isolates from traditional fermented fish of Manipur, North-East India. Journal of Food Science and Technology. 2018;**55**(5):1870-1879

[66] Rapsang GF, Joshi S. Molecular and probiotic functional characterization of Lactobacillus spp. associated with traditionally fermented fish, Tungtap of Meghalaya in northeast India. Proceedings of the National Academy of Sciences, India Section B: Biological Sciences. 2015;**85**(4):923-933

[67] Borah D et al. Isolation and characterization of the new indigenous Staphylococcus sp. DBOCP06 as a probiotic bacterium from traditionally fermented fish and meat products of Assam state. Egyptian Journal of Basic and Applied Sciences. 2016;**3**(3):232-240

[68] Majumdar RK, Gupta S. Isolation, identification and characterization of Staphylococcus sp. from Indian ethnic fermented fish product. Letters in Applied Microbiology. 2020;**71**(4): 359-368

[69] Muryany IM et al. Identification and characterization of the lactic acid bacteria isolated from Malaysian fermented fish (Pekasam). International Food Research Journal. 2017;**24**(2):868

[70] Kanjan P, Sakpetch P. Functional and safety assessment of Staphylococcus simulans PMRS35 with high lipase activity isolated from high salt-fermented fish (Budu) for starter development. LWT. 2020;**124**:109183

[71] Banaay CGB, Balolong MP, Elegado FB. Lactic acid bacteria in Philippine traditional fermented foods. In: Lactic Acid Bacteria-R & D for Food,

Health and Livestock Purposes. Rijeka: IntechOpen; 2013

[72] Cooke RD, Twiddy DR, Reilly PA. Lactic fermentation of fish as a low-cost means. Fish Fermentation Technology. 1993:291

[73] Tamang JP. Food culture in the Eastern Himalayas. Journal of Himalayan Research and Cultural Foundation. 2001;**5**(3-4):107-118

[74] Bairagi A, Ghosh KS, Sen SK, Ray AK. Enzyme producing bacterial flora isolated from fish digestive tracts. Aquaculture International. 2002;**10**(2):109-121

[75] Bucio A, Hartemink R, Schrama JW, Rombouts FM. Screening of lactobacilli from fish intestines to select a probiotic for warm freshwater fish. Bioscience and Microflora. 2004;**23**(1):21-30

[76] Kumar R, Mukherjee SC, Prasad KP, Pal AK. Evaluation of Bacillus subtilis as a probiotic to Indian major carp Labeo rohita (Ham.). Aquaculture Research. 2006;**37**(12):1215-1221

[77] Sugita H, Hirose Y, Matsuo N, Deguchi Y. Production of the antibacterial substance by Bacillus sp. strain NM 12, an intestinal bacterium of Japanese coastal fish. Aquaculture. 1998;**165**(3-4):269-280

[78] Sugita H. Bacterial flora of coastal bivalves. Nippon Suisan Gakkaishi. 1981;**47**:655-661

[79] Vaseeharan BA, Ramasamy P. Control of pathogenic Vibrio spp. by Bacillus subtilis BT23, a possible probiotic treatment for black tiger shrimp Penaeus monodon. Letters in Applied Microbiology. 2003;**36**(2): 83-87

[80] Rengpipat S, Phianphak W, Piyatiratitivorakul S, Menasveta P. Effects of a probiotic bacterium on black tiger shrimp Penaeus monodon survival and growth. Aquaculture. 1998;**167**(3-4):301-313

[81] Asaduzzaman MD, Iehata S, Akter S, Kader MA, Ghosh SK, Khan MN, et al. Effects of host gut-derived probiotic bacteria on gut morphology, microbiota composition and volatile short chain fatty acids production of Malaysian Mahseer Tor tambroides. Aquaculture Reports. 2018;**9**:53-61

[82] Gutowska MA, Drazen JC, Robison BH. Digestive chitinolytic activity in marine fishes of Monterey Bay, California. Comparative Biochemistry and Physiology Part A: Molecular and Integrative Physiology. 2004;**139**(3):351-358

[83] Tanasupawat S, Ezaki T, Suzuki KI, Okada S, Komagata K, Kozaki M. Characterization and identification of Lactobacillus pentosus and Lactobacillus plantarum strains from fermented foods in Thailand. The Journal of General and Applied Microbiology. 1992;**38**(2):121-134

[84] Majumdar RK, Basu S. Characterization of the traditional fermented fish product Lona ilish of Northeast India. Indian Journal of Traditional Knowledge. 2010; **9**(3):453-458

Chapter 9

Food Health with Increased Probiotic Survival During Storage

Fatemeh Shoaei

Abstract

In recent years, due to the increasing concern of consumers about their food health. Pay attention to foods not only as a source of nutrients but also as promoters of health and wellness-hence the increase in demand for foods that have active or functional ingredients (especially natural ingredients). They increase nutritional value and nutritional health. Changes in food consumption, disorder the intestinal microbial system. Maintaining the health benefits of consuming beneficial bacteria that are present in the intestinal system. Probiotics are essential for improving intestinal microbial homeostasis. Probiotics are living microorganisms that, if recommended in sufficient quantities, can have positive effects on human health. Lowers cholesterol, improves lactose intolerance, increases nutritional value and prevents cancer. Probiotics are unstable during storage and the gastrointestinal tract (pH and bile salts). For this reason, the survival of probiotic cells and the absence of changes in the sensory properties of the product during storage are of have fundamental importance. Encapsulation and co-encapsulation with prebiotics are often a good way to increase the resistance of probiotic bacteria to difficult conditions and their survival. This leads to improved production of probiotic products and increased food health in the world.

Keywords: probiotic, encapsulation, survival, functional foods, intestine

1. Introduction

Probiotics are living microbes that must be in the number of 10^6 log Cfu/gr at the time of entering the intestinal environment to have their beneficial effects on human health [1]. Probiotics are usually one or mixture of several microorganisms, when consumed by humans or animals, they have many beneficial effects on the body. Therefore, researchers are trying to add it to food the survival of probiotics. Since dairy products are Suitable for the transmission and survival of probiotic bacteria, most probiotic bacteria enter dairy products such as yogurt, Dough and various dairy desserts [2]. Due to the presence of animal cholesterol, lactose intolerance and sensitivity of some people to dairy products, it is necessary to study probiotic products with new flavors and non-dairy products, especially herbal [2]. Researchers are always looking for ways to improve the survival of probiotic bacteria to increase the survival of probiotics in Unfavorable environmental conditions, including during the production and storage of food products, as well as acidic and biliary conditions in the gastrointestinal tract [3, 4]. it is recommended that probiotic foods contain at least 108 log Cfu / gr at the time of consumption [1]. One of the newest methods that has had significant effects in this regard is the microencapsulation of bacteria in different ways by different coatings. From a microbiological point of view, microencapsulation is the monopoly of bacterial cells with hydrocolloid coatings that are used to separate and protect it from the external environment. The main purpose of microencapsulation is to increase the survival of bacterial cells during storage, passage and release in the gastrointestinal tract [5]. Symbiotic, on the other hand, are a mixture of probiotics and prebiotics that affect the health of the host, selectively stimulating probiotic growth. And activate, metabolize beneficial intestinal bacteria, thus improving beneficial effects on the host [5]. By adhering to intestinal epithelial cells, probiotics can improve micro biota and digestion. Provides protection against pathogens and carcinogenic properties [1]. In this chapter, a brief description of probiotics and their increase in survival in different ways are depicted.

2. Definition and role of probiotics

The word probiotic, meaning to live, is derived from the Greece language. For more than 4,000 years, lactic acid bacteria have been used to increase the shelf life of various foods through fermentation processes. In 1857, Pasteur discovered that microorganisms were responsible for fermenting milk and play role in the production of lactic acid, which was eliminated by boiling milk. The Clinton Processing Company (USA), for first in 1881, produced lactic acid by fermentation Process. The idea of using one-way primer cultures in the decades 1940 and 1950 consisting of lactic acid bacteria was evolving and becoming commercially available [3]. Researchers have observed widespread in the decades 1980, use of lactic acid bacteria in biomedicine, food preservation, food processing, and fermentation and animal husbandry [3]. In 2002, the World Health Organization provided a comprehensive definition of probiotics: Probiotics are living microorganisms that, if taken in sufficient amounts, have beneficial effects on host health [6, 7].

The gastrointestinal tract contains millions of bacteria, the balance of which is very important for the gastrointestinal tract and the functioning of the immune system. During the day, the intestinal microflora is exposed to various stresses (use of antibiotics, anxiety and food poisoning). Which can create an imbalance between the so-called (good) and (bad) bacteria. However, eating foods that contain extra probiotics can increase the level of healthy or "good" bacteria in the gut which can change the microbial balance in this way [8]. Probiotics are classified as "safe" bacteria because their metabolism is saccharolytic. Probiotics are classified as "safe" bacteria because their metabolism is saccharolytic, (That is, they break down carbohydrates in the large intestine to produce short-chain fatty acids). This process is also known as fermentation and is beneficial to the host [8].

3. Selection criteria and requirements for probiotic strains

In the process of selecting probiotic strains for consumption, it must be approved by the WHO, FAO and the European Food Safety Authority (EFSA) for their safe status (GRAS) and (QPS) [4]. Recommended properties for a probiotic bacterium that have shown good and prominent effects on human health include [9]:

3.1 Having a safe status, probiotic bacteria

Bacterial lactic acid has been used to produce commercial probiotic products such as *Lactobacillus casei* and *L. plantarum* isolated from cheese and has shown good and prominent effects on human health [3].

3.2 Survive and have resistance to low pH and bile salts

Grosu-Tudor et al observed in Species (*L. citreum, L. brevis, Leuconostoc mesenteroides, L. plantarum*) isolated from fermented vegetables. have acceptable resistance in the presence of stomach acid and bile salts [3]. with the viability rates of 105 .10^8 CFU/ml after 24 hours of incubation [3].

3.3 Ability to adhere to and colonize the gastrointestinal tract (GIT)

Adherence to intestinal surfaces is one of the most important criteria for selecting strong probiotic isolates. Some probiotic strains are isolated from fermented foods that have significant adhesion by producing intestinal mucosa. Such as *Lactococcus lactis IS.16183, L. plantarum and Lactobacillus rhamnosus IS.7257* and inhibits the binding of *Escherichia coli* [3].

3.4 Ability to survival during storage and fermentation process in food

Probiotic products are usually recommended for storage in 4 to 5°C and should be used before the expiration date [3]. The criteria and requirements of probiotic strains are listed in detail in the **Table 1** below:

Criteria	Required specifications
Immunomodulatory effects	• Animal or human origin. • Isolated from the gastrointestinal tract of healthy individuals. • Accurate identification and matching (phenotype and genotype traits). • Lack of relevant information related to infectious diseases. • No side effects.
Function	• Competing with intestinal bacteria. • Ability to survive and maintain metabolic growth activity at the site. • Resistant to bile salts and enzymes. • Resistance to bile salt and low pH environment • Antagonistic activity against pathogens (For example: *Helicobacter pylori*, Salmonella sp., *Listeria monocytogenes*, Clostridium
Technological capability	• Easy production at high inoculation rates • vSurvival and stability of probiotic bacteria during the process (freezing and freeze-drying under vacuum • Preparation and distribution of probiotic products. • Increase survival in final products (in aerobic and aerobic conditions) • Ensure the optimal sensory properties of the final products • Resistance to bacteriophages

Table 1.
Criteria for selection of probiotic species.

4. Strategies to improve the survival of probiotics in food products and the digestive system

Probiotics are now recognized as the top pragmatic food products, and these health benefits are enhanced by prebiotics and short-chain oligosaccharides; because these substances help increase the growth of beneficial bacteria in the intestinal tract [5]. Processing conditions in food products such as oxidation and temperature are important for the preservation and survival of bacterial cells. High temperatures during the survival process are harmful to microorganisms. Reduction of oxygen during fermentation plays an important role in the elimination of aerobic microorganisms. Storage conditions such as packaging such as moisture, oxygen, temperature should be appropriate. Microencapsulation techniques to protect bacterial cells cause high

Food product	Compound added	Research Findings	References
Semi- hard cheese	Fructo- oligosaccharide	viability of probiotic strains	Langa el al., 2019
Wheat bread	Microbial polysaacharide- Pullalan	digestibility and fermentation of wheat bread samples	Nithyabalasundari et al., 2019
Yogurt	Chitoologosaccharide		
Orange juice	Xylooligosaccharide	Preservation of chemical stability in ultrasound treatment	Eric et al., 2019
Edible starch film	Nystose	growth of probiotic organisms and formation of organic acids	Gabrielly et al., 2019
Fermented milk	Inulin	Improves the growth of lactic acid bacteria and improves sensory and physical properties	Ozturkuglu et al., 2019
Apple by-product	homogalacturonan and rhamnogalacturonan	Consumption of carbon source by probiotics and production of short chain fatty acids and increase the level of HDL in rats.	Inmaculada et al., 2020
Whole wheat grain flour	Arabinoxylan	increase the growth of intestinal microbiota and reduce the growth of pathogenic organisms	Candela et al., 2020
Stirred bio yogurt	Chickpea flour	Improves bacterial growth and our sensory, antioxidant and tissue properties	Hend et al., 2020
The Human Body	arabinoxylan and arabinoxylan oligosaccharides	Effected in adiposity reduction	Kerry et al., 2018
Green coffee spent	Mono- oligosaccharide with mannose and galactose	Stimulates the growth of *Lactobacillus casei* andLactobacillus fermentum, Resistance to stomach environment	Nivas et al., 2019

Table 2.
The effect of prebiotics on food.

survival of these microorganisms in food products as well as in the gastrointestinal tract (low pH in gastric salt and bile in the small intestine) (**Table 2**) [5].

5. Prebiotic

Probiotics are indigestible foods that are by beneficial bacteria and promote the growth and activity of probiotics in the gut, therefore probiotics can be used as functional foods. Prebiotics increase the body's immune system by increasing intestinal microbial activity and the production of short-chain fatty acids [10]. The presence of prebiotics in the large intestine causes energy to be created by some bacteria during sugar consumption and fermentation. The most common hosts for prebiotics are Bifidobacterium bacteria and Lactobacillus. Which improves the growth of these two bacterial species and leads to the production of bacteriocins, which are a potential inhibitor of the growth of pathogenic bacteria [11]. Some of the prebiotics available in the inulin market are fructoo oligosaccharides (FOS) and galacto oligosaccharides (GOS), arabinoxylan [11]. Prebiotics can be obtained naturally from sources such as vegetables, fruits and grains. Prebiotics can reduce the incidence and duration of diarrhea, relieve inflammation, prevent colon cancer, and absorb minerals [11]. In a study by Anirban et al., Prebiotics such as fructoligosac (FOS) and inulin were used for stimulate the growth of Bifidobacterium in food [6]. The combination of probiotics and prebiotics leads to the formation of synbiotics. They increase the life and efficiency of probiotic bacteria in the intestine. Research has shown the effect of synbiotics on human health.

6. Effective level of probiotic microorganisms

In order of probiotic to survive, in the gastrointestinal tract, they must be able to tolerate low pH, gastric pepsin, bile salts, pancreatic, and the ability to attach to the intestinal mucosa [7, 8]. Probiotic survival in product is affected by various factors such as pH, acidity, hydrogen peroxide and storage temperature [12, 13] The efficiency of probiotic bacteria in the product depends on the dose, and their survival during storage, its survival in the intestinal environment [14]. Therefore, bacteria cannot survive due to unfavorable conditions during food processing and storage [15]. If probiotics survive, they will change the taste of the final product during storage [16]. Survival means the presence of at least a sufficient number of viable probiotic cells at the time of food consumption [17]. The general agreement on the recommended levels for the amount of probiotics in the product at the time of consumption should contain at least 10^8 (CFU) / ml or gr [18]. The International Dairy Federation recommends that the minimum concentration of probiotics be around $10^6.10^7$ CFU / ml at the end of the shelf life [10].

7. Common genera and species of probiotic microorganisms

Probiotic products may contain one or more selected microbial strains. Human probiotic microorganisms mostly belong to the genera *Lactobacillus, Bifidobacterium, Lactococcus, Streptococcus* and *Enterococcus*. In addition, gram-positive bacteria belonging to the genus *Bacillus* and some yeast species belonging to the genus *Saccharomyces* are commonly used in probiotic products. The largest group of lactic acid bacteria belongs to the genus *Lactobacillus,* which includes more than 50 different species. Lactic acid bacteria are gram-positive, spore-free, anaerobic fermentative bacteria that grow anaerobically and they are traditionally used in preserving a variety of fermented foods. Inoculated in the food industry as a fermente. Because they play a role in preserving the taste and texture of fermented foods. While the conversion of fermented sugars in raw materials to lactic acid is their main function, the production of antimicrobial peptides, exopolysaccharides and other metabolites is another important feature [9].

8. Functional foods

In many countries today, the role of food in human health and nutrition is very important. So that most of the importance of food, instead of the primary role of food as a source of energy and growth has changed to the biological role of food on functional food. The food production and consumption market has shifted more towards the production of healthy foods. Functional foods are foods that, in addition to their normal nutritional properties, have health benefits for the consumer. They have medicinal value beyond nutritional value and have positive effects on human health. Demand for healthy food products is growing rapidly due to increasing consumer awareness of the benefits of these products. Functional foods include a wide range of dietary supplements, special foods for children, foods enriched with vitamins and minerals, probiotic products, foods containing antioxidants, fiber, protein and soy [8].

8.1 Property of functional foods

The amount of food consumed is important to achieve the beneficial effect of the added nutrient. Identify quality components in the food composition and optimal intake of nutrients in the diet; they reduced diseases and increased the level of health in the human body. In order to achieve the benefits of a healthy food, it must be possible to use it as part of a balanced diet [8]. The gut microflora can face daily challenges such as poor diet, antibiotic use, stress, or food poisoning, leading to an imbalance between "good" and "bad" bacteria. However, eating foods containing probiotics can increase the amount of healthy bacteria in the gut [8]. Probiotics are a group of beneficial microorganisms that, if consumed in sufficient doses of 10^6 log Cfu/gr, can lead to health.promoting properties in humans [8]. The majority of probiotics belong to the genera *Lactobacillus*, *Bifidobacterium* and *Lactococcus,* which are the natural inhabitants of the large intestine [7, 19]. Their beneficial effects have been extensively studied [4, 20]. Probiotic bacteria can be used in pure culture (as found in supplements) or added to dairy products or other foods. Due to the special conditions that probiotic bacteria need to grow, their survival in most foods will face many problems. One of the methods that can increase the survival of these bacteria and protect them against adverse conditions is the use of encapsulation techniques [13, 21, 22]. This technology refers to a physical and chemical process that inserts the desired bacteria into a coating to produce particles with diameters ranging from a few nanometers to a few micrometers [5]. The purpose of microencapsulation is to create a small environment in which bacteria survive during production and storage and are released in appropriate places (such as the small intestine) in the gastrointestinal tract [21].

9. Microencapsulation of probiotic bacteria

Microencapsulation technologies can be used in many applications in the food industry, such as controlling the oxidative reaction, coating flavors, colors and odors, stable and controlled release of the desired substance, extending the useful life, etc. [5]. Techniques to reduce the lethal effects of the gastrointestinal tract on probiotic microorganisms have been developed and evaluated. Among these, the microencapsulation technique is one of the most appropriate solutions. Microencapsulation is a physicochemical or mechanical process for trapping probiotic bacteria in an emulsion to produce particles with a diameter of a few nanometers to a few millimeters [5].

Technology The microencapsulation of living probiotic cells is covered by other preservatives or mixtures thereof in different techniques [23]. Protection of microcapsules when passing through the stomach can be increased by the use of insoluble wall materials [23]. Microencapsulation protects bacterial cells from environmental pressures such as oxygen, high acidity, and gastric conditions and can be used to pass through the stomach with little damage [24]. In recent years, many studies have been conducted on the preservation of probiotic microorganisms by microencapsulation during food processing and storage [23]. The purpose of microencapsulation is to create an environment in which bacteria survive during processing and storage and are released into, Suitable places the gastrointestinal tract (eg the small intestine) [23].

10. Structure and characteristics of microencapsulation

The first and foremost step in all microencapsulation methods is to select a suitable material as a wall or membrane for the stability and properties of the particles produced in the microencapsulation [25]. These materials are used alone or in combination to form a layer. Covering microencapsulation with a double membrane can act as a barrier against external conditions [26]. The most important choice for the coating material is the Yield of the coatings. The finely coated probiotic in the final product must be degradable and create a boundary between the internal phase and the environment (permeability) and also be evaluation in opinion of cost [4]. The properties of the coating materials and their placement are the main determinants of the functional properties of the microencapsulation [26]. The materials used as coatings for bead can contain two or more layers of base materials [5, 26]. The properties of the coating materials and their shape are the main determinants of the functional properties of the coatings [5]. Microencapsulation must be soluble in water to maintain the coherence of their structure in the food matrix and the digestive tract [5]. Therefore, the materials used as coatings in the microencapsulation should have the following properties. Chemically with the main substance. Ability to form membranes around bacterial cells. Be able to protect bacterial cells against adverse environmental conditions. Be stable and economically viable [26]. To date, there has been no ideal coverage that fits all goals. Therefore, obtaining suitable coatings to create a balance point between the optimal properties, such as protection against moisture, acidity, high temperature, gas exchange (oxygen and carbon dioxide) [26]. The encapsulating agent should not be toxic, as it can directly affect the morphology, diameter and permeability of the particles. Selecting the right material for probiotic microencapsulation is essential for the stability and properties of the particles produced [25]. There is a wide range of natural or synthetic polymers, including: proteins (such as zein, soy protein, collagen, and gelatin), polysaccharides (such as cellulose, starch, alginate, and chitosan), and fats [26].

10.1 Polysaccharide

Polysaccharides are biopolymers composed of monosaccharaides. They have hydroxyl groups that may be intramolecular hydrogen bonded with water or other molecules. They are also influenced by the nature of the monomers of their substituent groups, which alter the molecular and functional properties [26].

10.1.1 Anionic polysaccharides

Alginate, gum Arabic, carrageenan, xanthan, carboxymethylcellulose, gelan are natural anionic polysaccharides that tend to be negative at pH values above pKa. And when they are lower than pKa, they are neutralized [26]. Ionic chemical elements such as Ca^{+2} change the electrical charge properties of all ions. Such as alginate gel, which interacts with opposing groups on the polymer chain [27].

10.1.1.1 Alginate

Alginates are natural marine polysaccharides that are extracted from seaweed [28]. The most important applications of alginate are its stabilizing, gelling and water retaining properties [28]. Alginates are natural polymer chains consisting of 100.3000 monomer units in a chain rigid and somewhat flexible [26]. The ability to connect polymer alginate chains with polyatomic ions such as Ca^{+2}, Ba^{+2}, $Sr.^{+2}$ is through electrostatic bonding and hydrogel formation [26]. When a cation such as Ca^{+2} participates in an interchain bond. It creates a three-dimensional network of gel and micro-and Nano-sized hydrogel bead in the microencapsulation of materials. Which has received much attention in recent studies [26]. One of the benefits of alginate is the formation of gels around bacterial cells. It is also safe and inexpensive. Some of the disadvantages attributed to alginate beads. The resulting beads are highly porous, which reduces the protection of bacterial cells in adverse environmental conditions. Another disadvantage of alginate bead is that it is sensitive to the effects of acid and is not compatible with the resistance of bead in gastric conditions [29, 30]. However, defects can be remedied by combining alginate with other polymer compounds, coating the bead with another compound, or structural modification of alginate using various additives [31].

10.1.1.2 Gum Arabic

Acacia trees are the main source of Gum Arabic. The chemical composition of Gum Arabic is complex and consists of a group of macromolecules composed of a large proportion of carbohydrates (97%) [32]. Gum Arabic (GA) is highly soluble in water and also has a relatively low viscosity compared to other gums [26]. The functional properties of gum Arabic are closely related to its structure, for example, solubility, viscosity, interaction with water and oil in an emulsion, determine the ability of fine coating in Gum Arabic [32]. Some researchers tested Gum Arabic as an indigestible polysaccharide, finding that Gum Arabic reached the large intestine without digestion in the small intestine [33]; Gum Arabic is gradually fermented by the bacterial flora of the large intestine, which produces short-chain fatty acids [34]. Therefore, it can be taken in large daily doses without side effects. Daily consumption of 25 and 30 grams of Gum Arabic for 21 to 30 days reduces total cholesterol by 6 and 10.4%, respectively [32]. Arabic gum is used as a stabilizer, emulsifier and as a coating in the food industry [33]. Solubility and properties of low viscosity emulsions by Gum Arabic enables the ability to retain and transfer the Trapped material in fine encapsulation. Gum Arabic with maltodextrin is a good choice for coating in microencapsulation [35].

10.1.1.3 Carrageenan

Carrageenans are extracted from red seaweed (*Rhodophyta*) and are composed of various mixtures of sulfated polysaccharides. Carrageenan is a neutral polysaccharide polymer that requires high temperatures to dissolve in large quantities. Potassium chloride is used to preserve and stabilize Carrageenan is a suitable coating material in encapsulation that contain flavorings and aromatic compounds. Forms a brittle, hard gel that melts when heated to low temperatures, forming soft, elastic gels in cold water while carrageenan is soluble. At present, carrageenan has not been widely studied for use in probiotic encapsulation [36, 37]. The properties of carrageenan gel are improved by mixing it with other coating materials such as vegetable oils, calcium alginate, and gums such as xanthan, gelan and locust bean gums by emulsion method [26].

10.1.1.4 Xanthan

Xanthan gum is a microbial exo polysaccharide with a cellulosic structure and a chain of two mannose and a glucuronic acid. They are produced from plant pathogens *Sphingomonas elodea* and *Xanthomonas campestris*. Despite its high molecular weight, it dissolves easily in hot and cold water and even in small amounts, it produces a very concentrated solution. as a result of stirring, its viscosity decreases. XG has been shown to be an excellent coating for probiotic microencapsulation, protecting probiotic cells against simulated digestive conditions and high temperatures [26]. Also, XG was successful when used with other coatings such as alginate, chitosan, gelan and cyclodextrin to improve the coating properties of probiotics microencapsulation and increased the viability of microencapsulated probiotics in simulated gastric conditions and intestinal bile salts [26]. Therefore, the addition of chitosan to the alginate-xanthan complex improved the viability of microencapsulation *L. plantarum* at high temperature and low pH [38]. Other studies using XG in combination with other substances such as protein and alginate improved the survival of *Lactobacillus acidophilus* in microencapsulation added to yogurt [39].

10.1.1.5 Carboxymethylcellulase

Carboxymethyl cellulose are also called semi-synthetic anionic polysaccharides. The properties of carboxymethylcellulose include; Concentration, adhesion, strength building, water retaining agent, colloidal state, stabilizer, emulsion and layer formation. Due to their diverse properties, they are widely used in the food industry, among them is their use as a coating material in encapsulation of probiotics. In one study, CMC and chitosan were used as coatings for *L. acidophilus* microencapsulation. They found that the ability of the probiotic to survive during transmission from the simulated gastrointestinal tract was improved [40].

10.1.2 Cationic polysaccharides

Cationic polysaccharides are those that tend to be positive below their pKa value, while remaining much higher than the neutral pKa value. Chitosan is the only naturally Extracted cationic polysaccharide [27]. Other synthetic cationic polysaccharides have been previously described, for example, cation hydroxyethylcellulose and cation hydroxypropyl, that have cosmetic applications [26]. However, despite their potential and benefits as cationic materials, none of them have yet been reported as a coating material for probiotic microencapsulation.

10.1.2.1 Chitosan

Chitosan is a semi-synthetic polymer. Due to its low cost, non-toxicity and adhesion to the outer surface of the particle, it increases the stability of the particles. Which is often used for probiotic microencapsulation [25]. In addition, it provides resistance to the gastrointestinal tract simulator. It has an electrostatic interaction with sodium alginate [10]. The use of chitosan as a capsule for probiotic bacteria can have disadvantages. Because this polysaccharide has an inhibitory effect against microorganisms [25], including lactic acid bacteria [25], Despite the antimicrobial properties of chitosan, it has been used in combination with other encapsulating agents to microencapsulated probiotics [41]. Chitosan coating improves the survival of encapsulated *Bifidobacterium longum* in the gastrointestinal tract and high temperature [42]. Also, *L. rhamnosus ASCC 290* and *L. casei ATCC 334* were microencapsulated by alginate-chitosan using extrusion method was observed, 76% microencapsulation efficiency [25].

10.1.3 Non-ionic polysaccharides

Non-ionic polysaccharides are macromolecules that have no formal charge. However, other neighboring species and / or environmental conditions may affect their loading characteristics Natural, non-ionic polysaccharides such as starch, maltodextrins, cyclodextrins and guar gum have been used as coatings for probiotic microencapsulation [43].

10.1.3.1 Starch

Starch is produced by plants and is mostly composed of two different polysaccharides of D-glucose: linear and spiral amylose and highly branched amylopectin. Starch due to its high amylose leads to the formation of flexible and strong coatings. Corn starch is also known as resistant starch (RS) due to its high amylose content, which is the most common type of starch [44]. Starch films are: odorless, tasteless, colorless, non-toxic and semi-permeable to carbon dioxide, moisture, oxygen as well as fat and flavoring components [44]. Modified starch such as (actinyl-succinate starch) is a food additive. It was successfully optimized as a coating material for microencapsulation of *Bifidobacterium* by spray drying method. Actinyl-succinate starch is preferred because it is suitable for spray drying.

10.1.3.2 Maltodextrin

Maltodextrins H2o {(c6H10o5) n} starch is hydrolyzed. It is a natural, non-ionic polysaccharide that binds glucose units together mainly by glycoside bonds (4 → 1). Its macromolecules do not have a specific charge [26]. Unlike starch, they have high solubility and low viscosity in the formation of encapsulation, moisture control, reduced wall permeability to oxygen, reduced adhesion problems, easy digestibility and easy drying are the properties of gel formation in maltodextrin [26]. Equivalent dextrose (DE) indicates the reduced number of aldehyde groups relative to pure glucose (constant concentration), so that high DE indicates lower weight, higher solubility. Due to having a hydrophilic group, it increases the moisture in the final product. Due to their low cost, neutral flavor and aroma, as well as their role in protecting bacterial cells, resistant to thermal degradation during drying, maltodextrins are used as Coating material in encapsulation [26, 45]. In general, in maltodextrins, the solubility and stability dependence of the high molecular mass and the viscosity, adhesion, and crystallization depend on the low molecular weight [35].

10.1.3.3 Guar gum

Guar gum is structurally a type of polysaccharide whose main chain is mannose and the sidelong groups attached to it are galactose. This substance is extracted from

Guar plant and in combination with water, creates a concentrated solution, and due to this property has many applications in the food industry. According to the US Food and Drug Administration, the use of appropriate amounts of guar gum in various food products is safe. It has recently been *described as a coating agent for probiotic encapsulation. Amita et al.* [46] *found that a* mixture of fructooligosaccharide and guar gum improved the viability of microencapsulation probiotics in a simulated gastrointestinal tract during heat treatment. In another study by Muzzafar et al. On the bacteria *L. acidophilus*, *L. rhamnosus* and *B. longum* with guar gum *and xanthan gum, they observed an improvement in probiotic survival in the preparation of* cream biscuits [47]. Recent studies have found that microencapsulation of *Lactobacillus* by alginate and guar gum coatings increased the viability of chocolate milk, and that microencapsulation had no effect on the flavor of the final product.

10.1.3.4 Cyclodextrin

Cyclodextrins are annular oligosaccharides containing glucose units with alpha 1 and 4 glucopyranose bonds. Cyclodextrins are produced through starch by enzymatic conversion. The spatial structure of cyclodextrin forms a hydrophilic surface and a hydrophobic cavity. Its benefits include the ability to remove cholesterol from many foods (eg eggs and dairy); inhibits the increase of plasma cholesterol and triacylglycerol [26]. Cyclodextrin coatings are also used more for controlled release in drugs [48]. Therefore, not many studies have been performed on encapsulation of probiotics. In recent studies, microencapsulation of *Saccharomyces boulardii*, *L. acidophilus*, and *Bifidobacterium bifidum* by cyclodextrin and gum arabic increased survival in gastric and intestinal cloning conditions and thermal resistance compared to free cells [26].

10.2 Lipids

Lipids are made up of fats, fatty acids, waxes and phospholipids. Lipids are used as coatings in microencapsulation. Due to their relatively low polarity, they prevent moisture transfer. The hydrophobicity of lipids makes the microencapsulation coatings brittle [49]. Therefore, lipids are combined with other coatings such as proteins and polysaccharides to improve the microencapsulation properties. In previous reports, polysaccharide coatings and proteins have been found to cause structural cohesion and selective permeability to gases (so2, o2) [50]. The addition of fat also made the coatings resistant to water vapor. Most lipid coatings are fats: their source-dependent fats include vegetable and animal fats. The chemical structure of fats is composed of fatty acids and glycerol. Hence, their properties largely depend on the composition of fatty acids. Vegetable fats are widely used as concurrent encapsulation materials in microencapsulation of probiotics by method emulsification or by spry drying [26]. Silva et al., On the other hand, microencapsulated probiotics using vegetable oil as a coating alone or covered with gum Arabic and gelatin. Microencapsulated bacteria showed greater protection than free bacteria in simulated gastrointestinal conditions (eg, pH, temperature, sodium chloride, and sucrose) [51].

Waxes are GRAS materials and have been widely used in the food industry, for example as food additives or as a protective coating for fruits, vegetables and cheese. Nevertheless, waxes are less commonly used as coatings for microencapsulation probiotics. For example, Mandal et al. [52] reported the use of wax, stearic acid, or poly-L-lysine as the outer coating of probiotic microcapsules prepared with resistant starch and alginate, that wax and stearic acid showed improved survival of *L. casei* encapsulated probiotic cells under simulated gastrointestinal conditions.

In particular, stearic acid coatings provide better protection. Contrary to the results of the previous study, Rao et al. [53], evaluated the use of wax or stearic acid as the outer coating of probiotic microcapsules prepared with cellulose acetate phthalate (CAP). They found that wax-coated microcapsules the highest survival rate of *Bifidobacterium pseudolongum* in simulated gastric juice.

Phospholipids are a large group of lipids commonly used in the food industry and have the ability to form emulsions, micelles and liposomes. These lipids contain phosphorus and play an important role in the construction and metabolism of living cells. Phospholipids are more complex than simple lipids (fats and waxes). Examples of phospholipids are phosphatidic acid (phosphatidate) (PA), phosphatidyl ethanolamine (cephalin) (PE), phosphatidylcholine (PC) and phosphatidylserine (PS). In this regard, phospholipids are the main components of liposomes. When phospholipids are dispersed in water, the molecules come together to form a distinct bilayer. Such interactions cause the formation of vesicles, also called liposomes [53]. Liposomes have been used extensively as systems to transport active compounds such as drugs, vitamins, enzymes, and so on.

Although liposomes have shown great potential for controlled encapsulation and release of nutrients, their use in food has not yet been fully utilized [26]. Despite the high potential of liposomes for encapsulation and controlled release of nutrients, their use in food has not yet been fully utilized [26]. For example, up to now, microencapsulation of probiotics by liposomes has not been reported, which may be due to the cost of the process and materials as well as the large size of the probiotic microorganisms [54]. However, the resistance of liposomes to the gastrointestinal tract as well as the survival of probiotics in the intestinal there are issues that need to be review.

10.3 Protein

Proteins are excellent materials for microencapsulation of probiotics; however, they are often used in combination with other coating agents. To date, few proteins have been used as coatings [26]. Due to their properties, many proteins are used as a good barrier against O2 permeability and CO2 as a coating agent. Each protein has a unique set of physicochemical properties [55]. Proteins used as coating agents for probiotic microcapsules, on their nature, can be classified as plant or animal proteins based. Examples of animal origin proteins include gelatin, casein, whey protein concentrate (WPC), whey protein isolate (WPI), egg whites, and caseinates. Examples of plant origin proteins, on the other hand, include corn (saddle), pea, wheat, and soy. Gelatin is one of the oldest and most widely used proteins in the food industry, as an ideal coating material in the preparation of microencapsulation in probiotics [56]. Recent studies have shown that gelatin provides a suitable coating by interacting with a wide range of polysaccharides in a variety of ways [26].

Some of the other proteins used in probiotic microencapsulation are egg white (albumin), soy protein and whey protein. These proteins have good emulsifying and gelling properties that are considered as ideal materials for microencapsulation [26]. In the study, soy protein isolates and alginate were used as a coating material for microencapsulation of *L. plantarum* and *L. acidophilus* by spray drying. Also in the study, Pitigraisorn et al. Used egg albumin coatings and stearic acid to protect *L. acidophilus* by electro spraying and fluidized bed drying [57]. Soy plant protein isolate is suitable in the microencapsulation of probiotics, for vegetarians and Milk sensitive people, which is a source of high quality proteins [58]. The synergistic effects of soy protein isolate with other nutrients enhance the final properties of microcapsule coatings. In addition, previous studies have found that the jelly properties of soy protein isolate are deformed in the presence of CaSO4, MgCl2 or

MgSO4. And can be useful for future applications in the food industry, including the microencapsulation process [26]. Sodium caseinate (SC) is the most common form of casein, which is used as a suitable coating material in microencapsulation due to its physicochemical properties, increased denaturation and heat resistance.

Whey proteins in concentrate (WPC) and isolated (WPI) contain 35%. 85% and > 95% protein, respectively. WPCs are low in fat and cholesterol and high in lactose and total fats, while WPIs are high in protein and low in lactose and fat [59]. Whey proteins, in its various forms, have recently been studied as coatings for microencapsulation of probiotics [26]. In some studies, it has been shown that the ability and elasticity and strength of the gel increase in the presence of the main components of whey protein (beta-lactoglobin and alpha-lactoalbumin).

Sweet whey (SW) is an example of a product that contains casein and whey proteins. In recent studies, sweet whey was used to microencapsulation *B. lactis* with spray dryer method [60].

11. Microencapsulation of methods

Microencapsulation methods for encapsulate bioactive compounds have been proposed in several ways. To increase their ability release and stability under conditions product process and storage [26]. The attention of the food industry to the low cost of the method used is also worth considering. However, the final quality of the product should not be affected. The method used in forming the beads affects indicators such as the diameter and moisture of the beads [26]. Successful methods used in microencapsulating such as spray drying, spray freeze drying, electro spraying, fluidized bed drying; extrusion, Emulsification and coacervation [26].

11.1 Fluidized bed drying

Fluidized bed technology was patented by Dr. Wurster et al. And developed between 1957 and 1966 [5]. Proper air circulation in the atomic nozzle ensures that all particles in the fluidized bed achieve a uniform coating. This nozzle atomizes the selected coating (an aqueous solution) at low temperature by evaporating the solid solvent [5]. Air turbulence allows the coated particles to be suspended and coated evenly. The wall materials used in this method include cellulose derivatives, dextrin, emulsifiers, lipids, protein derivatives and starch which is used dissolved in an evaporative solvent. Fluidized bed technology is suitable for microencapsulation probiotic bacteria using cell layering with various preservatives such as glucose, maltodextrin, trehalose or sucrose, preferably skim milk to improve bacterial dehydration [5]. Recent studies have shown the effectiveness of fluidized bed drying for probiotic microencapsulation [25, 26].

11.2 Freeze drying

This method of drying is called lyophilization. In this method, probiotics are frozen in the presence of a coating material. It works by reducing the ambient pressure and creating a vacuum at low temperatures to sublimate frozen water directly. The most common uses of wall materials include proteins, maltodextrins, disaccharides, and gums. One of the most important benefits of freeze drying is water phase conversion and prevention of oxidation. It has the highest survival rate after drying and the lowest loss during storage. In any case, freeze-drying is a very expensive technology. Therefore, in further studies, spray drying [61], is used to dry probiotics. The freeze drying process provides maximum stability during storage. For this reason, this technique is used as a second method during microencapsulation. In this way, the stability of probiotic bacteria can be improved in the gastrointestinal tract and the beneficial effect of probiotic [45].

11.3 Spray drying

Spray drying is a common method for producing microencapsulation in food because it has been proven to be suitable for large-scale industrial applications [62]. The first spray dryer was made in 1878 and is therefore a relatively old method compared to rival technologies [62]. This is probably the most economical and effective drying method in the industry, first used to preserve a flavor in the decade of 1930. However, the industrial production of encapsulated probiotics using hot air dryers is not very useful in food, due to the reduced viability when bacteria dry and the reduced stability during storage. The bacterial cell is transferred to an emulsion that acts as a microencapsulation. The encapsulate is usually a hydrocolloid such as gelatin, vegetable gum, modified starch, dextrin or non-gelling protein. The resulting solution dries and acts as a barrier to oxygen and aggressive substances. In the spray drying process, a liquid mixture in a container with a single-fluid nozzle, a two-liquid nozzle is atomized, and the solvent is evaporated by contact with hot air [62].

11.4 Extrusion

It is a physical method of trapping probiotic living cells and uses hydrocolloids (alginates and carrageenan) as encapsulates. Tiny droplets from inside a nozzle device under air pressure or a syringe, dropped out inside a hardening solution such as calcium. Extrusion is a simple and inexpensive method that uses a gentle operation. It does not damage probiotic cells and increases the survival of probiotic bacteria. This technology does not contain harmful solvents and can be done under aerobic and anaerobic conditions. The most important disadvantage of this method is that due to the slow formation of bead, it is very difficult to use in industry [63]. Gel granules can be added to a second polymer solution as a coating. The second layer is used to protect the cell or improve the organoleptic properties of the cell [63].

11.5 Emulsion

It is a chemical technique for trapping probiotic cells. Most hydrocolloids (alginate, carrageenan and pectin) are used as encapsulates. An emulsifier and a surfactant are needed to form the bead. A hardening solution such as calcium chloride is then added to the emulsion [63]. Its main disadvantage is the large diameter of the bead.

11.6 Electro spraying

The electrospray technology used for microencapsulation is based on the principle of electro-hydrodynamics. This process includes a high voltage electric field. Which enters capillary liquid containing the main substance and is sprayed where the spherical droplets precipitates. Freezing occurs through various methods, for example by chemical hardening or by solvent evaporation. This method is combined with other microencapsulation techniques to increase the microencapsulation efficiency. So far, the electrospray extrusion technique has been used successfully for probiotic microencapsulation [64].

11.7 Coacervation

Drops are rich in organic matter that are formed through the separation of the liquid phase. It is mainly due to the association of oppositely charged molecules (polyelectrolytes, polysaccharides) or hydrophobic proteins (elastin polypeptides) [65]. A phenomenon produced by the accumulation of colloidal droplets that causes the simultaneous separation of two liquid phases. A dense phase is rich in polymer and a very dilute phase. Particle diameters range from 1 to 100 micrometers [65].

12. Application of microencapsulation bacteria

The efficiency of microencapsulated bacteria can be evaluated from different angles. Such as increasing the survival of probiotics, increasing the resistance of microcapsules to bacteriophage invasion, increasing their resistance to toxic and lethal chemical agents, as well as the ability to produce probiotic foods by improving the survival and stability of probiotic cells during production, storage and passage of the digestive system-Finally, it preserves the sensory properties of the product, which contains microencapsulation bacteria [23, 66].

13. Adding probiotic microencapsulation to food products

Dairy products have traditionally been the best producer of probiotics. They showed excellent conditions for the survival of probiotic bacteria. Because milk has a physicochemical composition rich in protein and with a significant amount of lipids. As a result, it creates a protective matrix for probiotics [23]. Microencapsulation is important to increase probiotic The addition of bead should not affect the sensory properties of food products. The addition of bead should not affect the sensory properties of food products [63]. Most of the research has been done and the products that are marketed in the food industry as probiotics. Dairy products are probiotics. Due to the problems of lactose intolerance in some people in the community (about 70% in Asia), sensitivity to milk proteins and the prevalence of high cholesterol require foods other than dairy that are good carriers for probiotic bacteria. Non-dairy foods provide a variety of substrates of antioxidants, dietary fiber, minerals, and vitamins [23]. The development of non-dairy probiotic products such as fruits, vegetables and grains has been shown to be one of the best choices and has increased the demand for non-dairy probiotics [23]. Properties and structural compounds (nutrients such as minerals, vitamins, dietary fiber and antioxidants, including the right amount of sugar) Fruits, vegetables and grains are suitable and ideal substrates for probiotic microbes [67]. Various factors such as protein concentration, sugar, fat and pH level in the food product can affect the growth and survival of probiotics [63].

14. Release of probiotic bacteria from microencapsulation

Scientific sources related to the probiotic microencapsulation emphasize on its destruction, in the large intestine. The microencapsulated bacteria can resist acidic conditions in the stomach. Depending on the processing conditions and the type of coated material used, it regulates the release rate of microencapsulation bacteria in the presence of bile salts [5]. In this way, probiotic bacteria are protected and as a result, high concentrations of living cells can be achieved [5]. The finely coated must have selective permeability to support the environmental conditions that keep cells live, so that it can be designed to release probiotic cells in a specific area of the body [5].

Author details

Fatemeh Shoaei
Department of Nutrition and Food Safety, School of Medicine, Nutrition Health Research Center, Hamadan University of Medical Sciences, Hamadan, Iran

*Address all correspondence to: fatemeshoaei92@gmail.com

References

[1] Ganguly N, Bhattacharya S, Sesikeran B, Nair G, Ramakrishna B, Sachdev H, et al. ICMR-DBT guidelines for evaluation of probiotics in food. The Indian Journal of Medical Research. 2011;**134**(1):22

[2] da Silva MN, Tagliapietra BL, da Silva TM, da Cruz Carpes A, do Amaral Flores V, Steffler B, et al. Probióticos Comerciais: Simulação Gastrointestinal. 1-388-416

[3] Gupta R, Jeevaratnam K, Fatima A. Lactic acid bacteria: Probiotic characteristic, selection criteria, and its role in human health (a review). International Journal of Emerging Technologies and Innovative Research. 2018;**5**(10)

[4] Rokka S, Rantamäki P. Protecting probiotic bacteria by microencapsulation: Challenges for industrial applications. European Food Research and Technology. 2010;**231**(1):1-12

[5] Chávarri M, Marañón I, Villarán MC. Encapsulation technology to protect probiotic bacteria. In: Probiotics. IntechOpen; 2012

[6] Anirban M, Wheeler D, Susmita D, Ajanta D, Istiak S. Mangrove spatial distribution in the Indian Sundarbans: Predicting salinity-induced migration in a changing climate. Journal of Management and Sustainability. 2019;**9**(1):1-13

[7] Vivek K. Use of encapsulated probiotics in dairy based foods. International Journal of Food, Agriculture & Veterinary Sciences. 2013;**3**(1):188-199

[8] Williamson C. Functional foods: What are the benefits? British Journal of Community Nursing. 2009;**14**(6):230-236

[9] Markowiak P, Śliżewska K. Effects of probiotics, prebiotics, and synbiotics on human health. Nutrients. 2017;**9**(9):1021

[10] Chen L, Yang T, Song Y, Shu G, Chen H. Effect of xanthan-chitosan-xanthan double layer encapsulation on survival of Bifidobacterium BB01 in simulated gastrointestinal conditions, bile salt solution and yogurt. LWT-Food Science and Technology. 2017;**81**:274-280

[11] Priya B. A role of prebiotics in food and health: A review. Journal of Critical Reviews. 2020;7:782-785

[12] Gbassi GK, Vandamme T. Probiotic encapsulation technology: From microencapsulation to release into the gut. Pharmaceutics. 2012;**4**(1):149-163

[13] Peredo A, Beristain C, Pascual L, Azuara E, Jimenez M. The effect of prebiotics on the viability of encapsulated probiotic bacteria. LWT. 2016;**73**:191-196

[14] Kailasapathy K, Chin J. Survival and therapeutic potential of probiotic organisms with reference to *Lactobacillus acidophilus* and Bifidobacterium spp. Immunology and Cell Biology. 2000;**78**(1):80-88

[15] Hasani S, Khodadadi I, Heshmati A. Viability of lactobacillus acidophilus in rice bran-enriched stirred yoghurt and the physicochemical and sensory characteristics of product during refrigerated storage. International Journal of Food Science & Technology. 2016;**51**(11):2485-2492

[16] Bansal S, Mangal M, Sharma SK, Yadav DN, Gupta RK. Optimization of process conditions for developing yoghurt like probiotic product from peanut. LWT. 2016;**73**:6-12

[17] Korbekandi H, Mortazavian A, Iravani S. Stability and technology of

probiotic in fermented milks. In: Probiotic and prebiotic foods: Technology, stability and benefits to the human health. USA: Nova Science Publishing Ltd; 2011. pp. 131-169

[18] Arepally D, Reddy RS, Goswami TK. Studies on survivability, storage stability of encapsulated spray dried probiotic powder. Current Research in Food Science. 2020;**3**:235-242

[19] Mattia A, Merker R. Regulation of probiotic substances as ingredients in foods: Premarket approval or "generally recognized as safe" notification. Clinical Infectious Diseases. 2008;**46**(Suppleme nt_2):S115-S1S8

[20] Saranya S, Hemashenpagam N. Antagonistic activity and antibiotic sensitivity of lactic acid bacteria from fermented dairy products. Advances in Applied Science Research. 2011;**2**(4):528-534

[21] Anal AK, Singh H. Recent advances in microencapsulation of probiotics for industrial applications and targeted delivery. Trends in Food Science & Technology. 2007;**18**(5):240-251

[22] Champagne CP, Fustier P. Microencapsulation for the improved delivery of bioactive compounds into foods. Current Opinion in Biotechnology. 2007;**18**(2):184-190

[23] Lebaka VR, Wee YJ, Narala VR, Joshi VK. Development of new probiotic foods—A case study on probiotic juices, Therapeutic, Probiotic, and Unconventional Foods2018. pp. 55-78

[24] Huq T, Khan A, Khan RA, Riedl B, Lacroix M. Encapsulation of probiotic bacteria in biopolymeric system. Critical Reviews in Food Science and Nutrition. 2013;**53**(9):909-916

[25] Rodrigues F, Cedran M, Bicas J, Sato H. Encapsulated probiotic cells: Relevant techniques, natural sources as encapsulating materials and food applications—a narrative review. Food Research International. 2020;**137**:109682

[26] AdlC P-C, Ortega D, García-Triana A, González-Silva N, Solis-Oviedo RL. A brief review of edible coating materials for the microencapsulation of probiotics. Coatings. 2020;**10**(3):197

[27] Matalanis A, Jones OG, McClements DJ. Structured biopolymer-based delivery systems for encapsulation, protection, and release of lipophilic compounds. Food Hydrocolloids. 2011;**25**(8):1865-1880

[28] Meng Y, Cloutier S. Gelatin and other proteins for microencapsulation. In: Microencapsulation in the Food Industry. Elsevier; 2014. pp. 227-239

[29] Mortazavian A, Azizi A, Ehsani M, Razavi S, Mousavi S, Sohrabvandi S, et al. Survival of encapsulated probiotic bacteria in Iranian yogurt drink (Doogh) after the product exposure to simulated gastrointestinal conditions. Milchwissenschaft. 2008;**63**(4):427

[30] Weinbreck F, De Vries R, Schrooyen P, De Kruif C. Complex coacervation of whey proteins and gum arabic. Biomacromolecules. 2003;**4**(2):293-303

[31] Krasaekoopt W, Bhandari B, Deeth H. Evaluation of encapsulation techniques of probiotics for yoghurt. International Dairy Journal. 2003;**13**(1):3-13

[32] Montenegro MA, Boiero ML, Valle L, Borsarelli CD. Gum arabic: More than an edible emulsifier. Products and Applications of Biopolymers. 2012;**51**:953-978

[33] Verbeken D, Dierckx S, Dewettinck K. Exudate gums: Occurrence, production, and applications. Applied Microbiology and Biotechnology. 2003;**63**(1):10-21

[34] Annison G, Trimble RP, Topping DL. Feeding Australian acacia gums and gum arabic leads to non-starch polysaccharide accumulation in the cecum of rats. The Journal of Nutrition. 1995;**125**(2):283-292

[35] Takeiti C, Kieckbusch T, Collares-Queiroz F. Morphological and physicochemical characterization of commercial maltodextrins with different degrees of dextrose-equivalent. International Journal of Food Properties. 2010;**13**(2):411-425

[36] Chakraborty S. Carrageenan for encapsulation and immobilization of flavor, fragrance, probiotics, and enzymes: A review. Journal of Carbohydrate Chemistry. 2017;**36**(1):1-19

[37] Setijawati D, Nursyam H, Salis H, editors. Carrageenan: The difference between PNG and KCL gel precipitation method as *Lactobacillus acidophilus* encapsulation material. In: IOP Conference Series: Earth and Environmental Science. IOP Publishing; 2018

[38] Fareez IM, Lim SM, Lim FT, Mishra RK, Ramasamy K. Microencapsulation of lactobacillus sp. using chitosan-alginate-xanthan gum-β-cyclodextrin and characterization of its cholesterol reducing potential and resistance against pH, temperature and storage. Journal of Food Process Engineering. 2017;**40**(3):e12458

[39] Khorshidi M, Heshmati A, Taheri M, Karami M, Mahjub R. Effect of whey protein-and xanthan-based coating on the viability of microencapsulated *Lactobacillus acidophilus* and physiochemical, textural, and sensorial properties of yogurt. Food Science & Nutrition. 2021

[40] Priya AJ, Vijayalakshmi S, Raichur AM. Enhanced survival of probiotic *Lactobacillus acidophilus* by encapsulation with nanostructured polyelectrolyte layers through layer-by-layer approach. Journal of Agricultural and Food Chemistry. 2011;**59**(21):11838-11845

[41] Călinoiu L-F, Ştefănescu BE, Pop ID, Muntean L, Vodnar DC. Chitosan coating applications in probiotic microencapsulation. Coatings. 2019;**9**(3):194

[42] Ji R, Wu J, Zhang J, Wang T, Zhang X, Shao L, et al. Extending viability of *Bifidobacterium longum* in chitosan-coated alginate microcapsules using emulsification and internal gelation encapsulation technology. Frontiers in Microbiology. 2019;**10**(1389)

[43] Gruber JV. Polysaccharide-based polymers in cosmetics. In: Cosmetic Science and Technology Series. 1999. pp. 325-390

[44] Shah U, Naqash F, Gani A, Masoodi F. Art and science behind modified starch edible films and coatings: A review. Comprehensive Reviews in Food science and Food Safety. 2016;**15**(3):568-580

[45] Ozdal T, Yolci-Omeroglu P, Tamer E. Role of encapsulation in functional beverages. In: Biotechnological Progress and Beverage Consumption. Elsevier; 2020. pp. 195-232

[46] Salaria A, Thompkinson D, Kumar SM, Sabikhi L. Prebiotics in the microencapsulating matrix enhance the viability of probiotic *Lactobacillus acidophilus* LA1. International Journal of Fermented Foods. 2013;**2**(1):33

[47] Muzzafar A, Sharma V. Microencapsulation of probiotics for incorporation in cream biscuits. Journal of Food Measurement and Characterization. 2018;**12**(3):2193-2201

[48] Leghari AA, Shahid S, Farid MS, Saeed M, Hameed H, Anwar S, et al.

Beneficial aspects of probiotics, strain selection criteria and microencapsulation using natural biopolymers to enhance gastric survival: A review. Life Science Journal. 2021;**18**(1):30-47

[49] Shit SC, Shah PM. Edible polymers: Challenges and opportunities. Journal of Polymers. 2014;**2014**:427259

[50] Vargas M, Pastor C, Chiralt A, McClements DJ, Gonzalez-Martinez C. Recent advances in edible coatings for fresh and minimally processed fruits. Critical Reviews in Food Science and Nutrition. 2008;**48**(6):496-511

[51] Silva MP, Tulini FL, Matos-Jr FE, Oliveira MG, Thomazini M, Fávaro-Trindade CS. Application of spray chilling and electrostatic interaction to produce lipid microparticles loaded with probiotics as an alternative to improve resistance under stress conditions. Food Hydrocolloids. 2018;**83**:109-117

[52] Mandal S, Hati S, Puniya AK, Khamrui K, Singh K. Enhancement of survival of alginate-encapsulated *Lactobacillus casei* NCDC 298. Journal of the Science of Food and Agriculture. 2014;**94**(10):1994-2001

[53] Rao A, Shiwnarain N, Maharaj I. Survival of microencapsulated *Bifidobacterium pseudolongum* in simulated gastric and intestinal juices. Canadian Institute of Food Science and Technology Journal. 1989;**22**(4):345-349

[54] Sarao LK, Arora M. Probiotics, prebiotics, and microencapsulation: A review. Critical Reviews in Food Science and Nutrition. 2017;**57**(2):344-371

[55] Pavli F, Tassou C, Nychas G-JE, Chorianopoulos N. Probiotic incorporation in edible films and coatings: Bioactive solution for functional foods. International Journal of Molecular Sciences. 2018;**19**(1):150

[56] Gómez-Guillén M, Giménez B, Ma L-C, Montero M. Functional and bioactive properties of collagen and gelatin from alternative sources: A review. Food Hydrocolloids. 2011;**25**(8):1813-1827

[57] Pitigraisorn P, Srichaisupakit K, Wongpadungkiat N, Wongsasulak S. Encapsulation of *Lactobacillus acidophilus* in moist-heat-resistant multilayered microcapsules. Journal of Food Engineering. 2017;**192**:11-18

[58] Rizzo G, Baroni L. Soy, soy foods and their role in vegetarian diets. Nutrients. 2018;**10**(1):43

[59] Morr CV, Ha E. Whey protein concentrates and isolates: Processing and functional properties. Critical Reviews in Food Science & Nutrition. 1993;**33**(6):431-476

[60] Pinto SS, Verruck S, Vieira CR, Prudêncio ES, Amante ER, Amboni RD. Influence of microencapsulation with sweet whey and prebiotics on the survival of Bifidobacterium-BB-12 under simulated gastrointestinal conditions and heat treatments. LWT-Food Science and Technology. 2015;**64**(2):1004-1009

[61] Chávez B, Ledeboer A. Drying of probiotics: Optimization of formulation and process to enhance storage survival. Drying Technology. 2007;**25**(7-8):1193-1201

[62] Boonanuntanasarn S, Ditthab K, Jangprai A, Nakharuthai C. Effects of microencapsulated *Saccharomyces cerevisiae* on growth, hematological indices, blood chemical, and immune parameters and intestinal morphology in striped catfish, *Pangasianodon hypophthalmus*. Probiotics and Antimicrobial Proteins. 2019;**11**(2):427-437

[63] Burgain J, Gaiani C, Linder M, Scher J. Encapsulation of probiotic

living cells: From laboratory scale to industrial applications. Journal of Food Engineering. 2011;**104**(4):467-483

[64] Coghetto CC, Brinques GB, Ayub MAZ. Probiotics production and alternative encapsulation methodologies to improve their viabilities under adverse environmental conditions. International Journal of Food Sciences and Nutrition. 2016;**67**(8):929-943

[65] Frakolaki G, Giannou V, Kekos D, Tzia C. A review of the microencapsulation techniques for the incorporation of probiotic bacteria in functional foods. Critical Reviews in Food Science and Nutrition. 2021;**61**(9):1515-1536

[66] Esmaeili SSS, Mortazavin S, Nematollahi A, Shadnoush M, Eivani M. Microencapsulation effectiveness of probiotics. Teb va Tazkiyeh. 2016;**24**:9-22

[67] Reddy KBPK, Madhu AN, Prapulla SG. Comparative survival and evaluation of functional probiotic properties of spray-dried lactic acid bacteria. International Journal of Dairy Technology. 2009;**62**(2):240-248

Chapter 10

Natural Probiotics and Nanomaterials: A New Functional Food

Ilza Fernanda Barboza Duarte,
Naianny Lívia Oliveira Nascimento Mergulhão,
Valdemir da Costa Silva, Laisa Carolina Gomes de Bulhões,
Irinaldo Diniz Basílio Júnior and Anielle C.A. Silva

Abstract

Natural probiotics are functional foods with several biological properties and nutritional value inherent to their chemical composition and can play a potentially beneficial role in reducing the risk of chronic degenerative diseases. In order to improve the stability of these compounds, increase the encapsulating power, delay oxidation, increase their effectiveness, control their release and improve the bioavailability of their combination with nanomaterials is a potential tool in the food area enabling the development of new products with functional and nutraceutical characteristics. In addition, the study of nanomaterials in natural probiotics is rarely reported in the literature, being an area of paramount importance in the development of new functional foods. Therefore, in this chapter, a review of nanomaterials' use in natural probiotics will be addressed to specify their advantages and methodologies of preparation and characterization.

Keywords: natural probiotics, nanomaterials, new functional foods, nutraceutical characteristics, nanobiotecnology

1. Introduction

The consumer's interest in a healthier lifestyle has led to the development of foods that meet nutritional and health needs and that at the same time are attractive, tasty, and with good acceptance in the market. Products that support positive health effects or ingredients with these characteristics, claimed or proven, are called "emitted foods" [1].

The relationship between food and health is one of the keys to disease prevention and well-being promotion. As a result, industries have started to enrich foods with specific ingredients, differentiating them about the benefits offered to health compared to foods in their traditional forms [2–4].

In the present century, the scientific literature reports functional foods as allies in the treatment of obesity [5], prevention of cardiovascular diseases [1], plasma cholesterol balance [6], and cancer prevention [7]. Among functional foods, the literature reports prebiotics (added with non-digestible fibers), fortified (with vitamins, omega-3), altered (removing harmful components), and probiotics [8].

According to Resolution No. 19, of April 30, 1999, on the claim of functional property of food, it is that related to the metabolic or physiological role that the nutrient or non-nutrient has in the growth, development, maintenance, and other normal functions of the human organism [9]. Among the functional compounds most investigated by science, we have probiotics, which according to RDC n° 241, of July 26, 2018, are defined as live microorganisms that confer benefits to the individual's health [10, 11].

The word probiotic has a Greek derivation in which it means "for the sake of life", that term was first introduced by Lilly; Stillwel in 1965 to describe substances secreted by a microorganism, which stimulates the growth of another [12–14]. Fuller (1989) defined probiotics as a supplement composed of live microorganisms that benefit the host's health through the balance of the intestinal microbiota. The term probiotic can be complemented as a pure culture or composed of living microorganisms that supplied to man or animals benefit the host by stimulating the properties existing in the natural microbiota [15].

Probiotics, after ingested, must be able to survive the stress conditions present in the gastrointestinal tract, such as gastric juice, the presence of bile salts, and digestive enzymes, and maintain their viability and metabolic activity in the intestine to exert beneficial effects on the hosts. As for the technological challenges for the industrial production of cells, they must remain stable and viable at satisfactory levels throughout the product's validity period [16–18]. Based on this assumption, there is a recent and growing scientific interest in improving the stability, bioavailability, and shelf life of products with probiotic sources using nanotechnology as an enhancement technique, since nanostructured systems may be able to control stability, improve solubility, bioavailability, and controlling the release of bioactive compounds [19–21].

The reduction of materials to the nanoscale leads to new and exciting properties and the increase of the surface volume ratio, increasing its reactivity. This characteristic of nanoparticles has attracted commercial interest in the manufacture of nano-ingredients, supplements, and nutraceuticals. Several types of nanoparticles can be found in the literature, such as metallic, semiconductor, carbon-based, metallic, and polymeric oxides, which can be applied in various sectors, predominantly personal care, health care, and cosmetics. The benefits of nanotechnology in the food sector go through the entire food chain, starting from production to processing, transportation, security, storage, and delivery [22, 23]. Based on the above, we will cover in this chapter a review on the use of natural probiotics and nanomaterials, aiming to specify their advantages and methodologies of preparation and characterization.

2. Natural probiotics

Probiotics can be defined as food supplements that contain live microorganisms or microbial components that, when ingested in a certain number, have a beneficial effect on the health and well-being of the host [17].

Among these benefits include antimicrobial activity; control of pathogenic microorganisms [24]; lactose hydrolysis; modulation of constipation; antimutagenic and anticarcinogenic activity [25, 26]; reduction of blood cholesterol, improvement of patients with type 2 diabetes (insulin resistance) and obesity [27–29]; modulation of the immune system; improvement in inflammatory bowel disease; and suppression of *Helicobacter pylori* infection [30–32]. Some of these benefits are already well established, such as constipation and lactose hydrolysis modulation, while other benefits have shown promising results in animal models, requiring further clinical studies [33].

Probiotics can be incorporated into a wide variety of food products, mainly in dairy products, such as milk, ice cream, yogurt, and cheese. Its application has also grown in other types of foods, such as soy milk, mayonnaise, pates, meats, baby food, confectionery, sweets, cakes, and chewing gum [34–37].

The selection of probiotic bacteria is based on the following criteria: gender, origin (which must be human), stability against stomach acid and bile salts, the ability to adhere to the intestinal mucosa, the ability to colonize, at least temporarily, the human gastrointestinal tract, the ability to produce antimicrobial compounds and metabolic activity in the intestine [38–40].

In order for the microorganism to be able to promote the aforementioned beneficial effects, a minimum intake of 10^8–10^9 colony-forming units (UFC) per day is recommended [41]. In addition, the minimum concentration of live bacteria should not be less than 10 CFU/g of food since many cells die during passage through the gastrointestinal tract (TGI) [1, 42].

2.1 Types of probiotics

Specific probiotic strains give the benefits transmitted to health, and not by specific species or genus. However, that each strain is related to a specific benefit. In this way, no strain will provide all of the proposed benefits. For example, *Lactobacillus casei* lineage Shirota, in which evidence supports the view that its oral administration can assist in the digestion and absorption of nutrients and restore the normal balance of the intestinal microbiota [43]. Other relevant factors are the addition of mixtures of probiotic cultures instead of individual strains [44] and the number of viable cells of these microorganisms in the marketed product.

In a healthy adult intestine, the predominant microbiota is composed of health-promoting microorganisms (**Table 1**), mostly belonging to the genera *Lactobacillus* and *Bifidobacterium* [45]. Other lactic acid bacteria with probiotic properties are:

Lactobacilli	Bifidobacteria	Other bacteria	Fungus
Lactobacillus acidophillus sp	*Bifidobacteirum bifidum*	*Enterococcus faecium*	*Saccharomyces boulardii*
L. acidophilus LA-1*	*B. lactis* Bb-12	*Enterococcus faecalis*	*Saccharomyces cerevisiae*
L. casei sp.*	*B. breve*	*Escherichia coli* Nissle 1917	
L. rhamnosus GG*	*B. infantis*	*Streptococcus salivarius* subsp. *Termophilus*	
*L. reuteri**	*B. longum*	*Sporolactobacillus inulinus*	
L. delbrueckii subs.* *bulgaricus*			
L. plantarum sp			
L. plantarum 299 V			
L. fermentum KLD			
L. johnsonii			

**Strains that have been used in the prevention and treatment of allergic diseases [45].*

Table 1.
Main microorganisms used for their probiotic properties, in the form of drugs or added to foods.

Ent. faecalis, *Ent. faecium*, and *Sporolactobacillus inulinus*, while the microorganisms *Bacillus cereus, Escherichia coli Nissle, Propionibacterium freudenreichii,* and *Saccharomyces cerevisiae* have been cited as non-lactic microorganisms associated with probiotic activities mainly for pharmaceutical or animal use [32, 33, 46].

Some individuals may experience little of the side effects related to the ingestion of probiotics due to the death of pathogens in the intestinal environment since they release toxic cellular products, a reaction called a "die-off reaction". In such cases, the use of probiotics should be persisted in order to improve symptoms. There is a slight increase in gas production, abdominal discomfort, and even diarrhea, which resolves over time [12].

2.2 Mechanism of action

Three possible mechanisms of action are attributed to probiotics: the suppression of the number of viable cells through the production of compounds with antimicrobial activity, competition for nutrients, and competition for adhesion sites. The second of these mechanisms would be the alteration of microbial metabolism by increasing or decreasing enzyme activity. The third would be to stimulate the host's immunity by increasing the levels of antibodies and increasing the activity of macrophages. The spectrum of activity of probiotics can be divided into nutritional, physiological, and antimicrobial effects [47, 48]. The direct modulation of the immune system may be secondary to the induction of anti-inflammatory cytokines or by the increase in the production of secretory IgA [45].

Despite the scientific evidence regarding the mechanisms of action of probiotics, there is still a lack in the literature on biochemical and molecular pathways that fully explain these effects, such as, for example, increasing the function of the intestinal barrier. Despite the scientific evidence regarding the mechanisms of action of probiotics, there is still a lack in the literature on biochemical and molecular pathways that fully explain these effects, such as, for example, increasing the function of the intestinal barrier [49].

Currently, the mechanisms of action of probiotics for anticarcinogenic effects have been studied. These are believed to occur through (1) inhibition of bacteria responsible for converting pre-carcinogenic substances (such as polycyclic aromatic hydrocarbons and nitrosamines) into carcinogens; (2) direct inhibition in the formation of tumor cells; and (3) the ability to bind and/or inactivate carcinogenic substances [25]. Several mechanisms of action have been suggested, including the stimulation of the host's immune response (by increasing phagocytic activity, IgA synthesis, and the activation of T and B lymphocytes), the binding and degradation of compounds with carcinogenic potential, qualitative changes and/or quantitative in the intestinal microbiota involved in the production of carcinogens and promoters (ex: bile acid degradation), production of antitumor or antimutagenic compounds in the colon (such as butyrate), alteration of the metabolic activity of the intestinal microbiota, alteration of the physical- colon chemicals with decreased pH and effects on host physiology [33, 50].

The use of probiotics represents a promising and rapidly growing area for the development of functional foods. Probiotic cultures are successfully applied to different food matrices. However, the development of non-dairy products represents a challenge for the industry, as each food matrix has unique characteristics, and it is necessary to optimize and standardize each type of product [51].

In this context, nanomaterials have been widely studied as a technique to improve the stability of these microorganisms and functional foods, protecting them from unfavorable environments, improving the uptake, absorption, and bioavailability of nutrients for the body (**Table 2**) [19].

Documented effects on humans and/or animals		Possible immunomodulation mechanism
Local effects		
Mucous barrier	Maintenance and repair of the intestinal barrier and intercellular junctions	Reduced permeability and decreased systemic absorption of allergens/antigens
Enterocytes	Increased production of TGF-β and prostaglandin E2 responsible for promoting tolerance of antigen-presenting cells	Reduction of local inflammation and promotion of tolerance
Receivers enterocytes (toll-like)	Anti-inflammatory effects of probiotics mediated by toll-like receptors 9	Inhibition of allergic responses, type Th2: mechanism not yet clarified
Cells presenting antigens (dendritic cells)	Increased activity of dendritic cells in the intestine	Promotion of tolerogenic effect by dendritic cells
Auxiliary (or effector) T cells	Increased Th1-type response	Inhibition of Th2 response differentiation
Regulatory T cells	Production of Il-10 and TGF-β associated with oral tolerance. Increased TGF-β (Th3)	TGF-β produced locally (including by enterocytes) promotes tolerogenic effect by dendritic cells, local IgA, and increased Treg activity
B cells and antibodies	Colonization: enlarged lymphoid tissue	Promotion of a tolerogenic environment
Systemic effects		
T cells	Increased Th1 differentiation	Secondary to the effects of T cells in the gastrointestinal tract
B/IGA cells	Increased production of IgA in other tissues (respiratory tract)	Secondary to the effects of B cells in the tract gastrointestinal

Adapted from Souza et al. [45].

Table 2.
Immune mechanisms of action associated with probiotics.

3. Nanomaterials

Technological advances aimed at developing imaging equipment and techniques for characterization make it possible to develop and characterize systems on a nanoscale through scanning electron microscopy and transmission electron microscopy. Nanotechnology in the food area is designed to encapsulate, carry, and release bioactive ingredients to incorporate and modify the food structure. In addition, they make it possible to study the structures in detail, make it possible to understand their properties and facilitate their handling to obtain new, high-quality and safe foods [52].

Nanotechnology involves the characterization, fabrication and/or manipulation of structures, devices, or materials that have at least a dimension of about 1–100 nm in length [53, 54] and has emerged as one of the most promising scientific areas of research. Numerous companies are currently specialized in the manufacture of new forms of materials (nanometric size) with typical applications in medical therapy, diagnostics, energy production, molecular computing, and structural materials [55]. This technology in food introduces new opportunities for innovation in the food industry with immense speed. Thus, some of the applications result in the presence of nanoparticles or nanostructured materials in the food. This innovation can be applied to the macroscale characteristics of foods, such as texture, taste, other sensory attributes, color intensity, processability, and stability during shelf life, leading to many new products. In addition, nanoencapsulation technology can also improve water solubility, thermal stability, and oral bioavailability of bioactive compounds [14, 56].

One of the biggest focuses of nanotechnology in the food industry is encapsulation systems and the controlled release of nutrients. The use of nanomaterials has shown improved properties for the encapsulation of probiotics. Due to their unique physical and chemical properties, nanostructured encapsulating materials show great promise of protecting microorganisms from acidic stomach conditions, increasing absorption and, therefore, allowing the successful release of probiotic cells trapped in the intestinal lumen with natural pH [57, 58].

The clinical efficacy of oral administration of probiotic bacteria is still diminished due to loss of viability during the gastrointestinal passage, resulting in poor intestinal distribution. Microencapsulation technology using nanomaterials is a successful strategy to solve this problem, maintaining the viability of probiotics, thus improving their effectiveness after oral administration [58]. In recent years, the production of probiotic and functional foods using nanotechnology represents one of the main current challenges [59].

The most basic nanomaterials used are nanoparticles. These can be presented in different forms, such as spherical nanoparticles (three nanometric dimensions); nanotubes and nanofibers (elongated structures with two dimensions on a nanoscale), and nanoplates (only have the nanometric thickness). Several examples of nanoparticles are cited in the literature, such as nano-clay, silver (Ag), titanium dioxide (TiO2), and zinc oxide (ZnO) nanoparticles [22].

Different types of nanoformulations can be used, which requires the adequate formulation and timely processing conditions. Among them, polymeric nanoparticles, nanocomposites, solid lipid nanoparticles (NLS), liposomes, and nanoemulsions are suitable for food applications [57, 60].

3.1 Types of systems for encapsulation of bioactive compounds

Nanoparticles (NPs) and nanostructured materials (NSMs) represent an active area of research with application in several domains. They are exciting nanoscale systems due to the ease with which they can be produced in different ways. NPs and NSMs arouse interest due to their adjustable physicochemical characteristics, such as melting point, wettability, electrical and thermal conductivity, catalytic activity, light absorption, and dispersion, resulting in improved performance compared to their mass counterparts [61]. NPs and nanosystems are broadly divided into several categories, depending on their morphology, size, and chemical properties [62]. Currently, some of the most studied nanostructured delivery systems are nanoemulsions, nanoliposomes, nanohydrogels, lipid nanoparticles, and coacervates with application in food (**Figure 1**) [63].

3.1.1 Polymeric nanoparticles

Polymeric nanoparticles are formed by a polymeric matrix (nanospheres) or a reservoir system in which the main content is hydrophobic or oily surrounded by a polymeric wall (nanocapsule) [64]. They are among the delivery systems for bioactive compounds most accepted and approved by GRAS [65]. In addition, they gained considerable attention in nanomedicine due to the potential for surface modification, pharmacokinetic control, suitability for targeted delivery of therapies [66], mechanical properties [67], and design flexibility. More specifically, size, surface morphology, chemistry and charge, porosity and diffusivity of the drug,

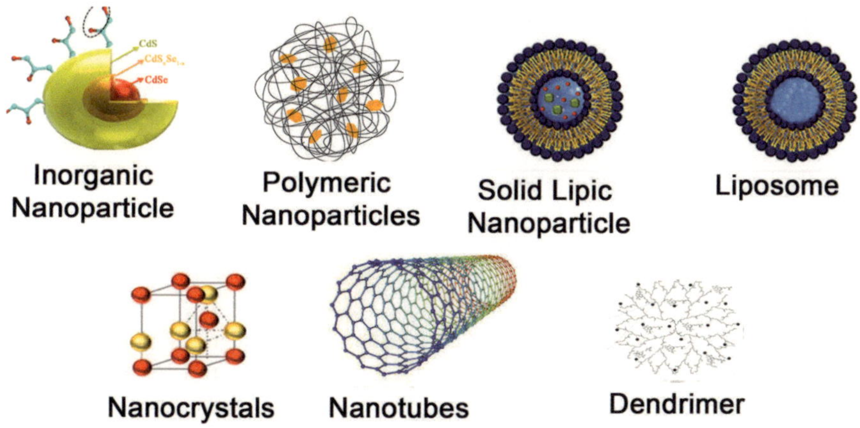

Figure 1.
Types of nanoparticles. Inorganic nanoparticles, polymeric nanoparticles, solid lipid nanoparticles, nanosomes, nanocrystals or quantum dots, carbon nanotubes, and dendrimers.

and encapsulation efficiency are properties that push polymeric nanoparticles to the forefront of nanomedicine applications [68] and may behave similarly when incorporated into food.

The chemical and biocompatibility properties of polymeric nanoparticles have been studied extensively in recent years and allow these nanometric delivery systems formed by natural or synthetic polymers to be helpful in the controlled release of natural bioactive compounds, hormones, genes, and anticancer drugs with greater effectiveness than micrometric systems such as microparticles [69]. Due to a high surface contact area occur an intense interaction between the matrix in which they are inserted and the nanoparticles [70].

Currently, the most used polymers for the formation of the nanometric system are poly (lactic acid) (PLA), poly (glycolic acid) (PGA), poly (lactic-co-glycolic acid) - (PLGA), and polycaprolactone (PCL). Nanoparticles and microparticles can be obtained through different techniques that can be classified into four categories. Category 1: a traditional method based on the formation of an emulsion consisting of single emulsion, double emulsion, and multiple emulsions, followed by evaporation of the solvent. Category 2: methods based on nanoprecipitation, the rapid expansion of supercritical fluid in liquid, salting, and dialysis. Category 3: direct composition methods, such as fusion technique, spray-drying, supercritical fluid. Category 4: new approaches, including microfluidic and mold/mold-based techniques [65, 69].

The main active substances used for encapsulation by the methods of obtaining nanoparticles are isolated substances. However, some authors, such as Nascimento et al. [71] and Azevedo et al. [65], developed polymeric nanoparticles of Brazilian red propolis extract contributing to the development of nanostructured technologies for natural products.

3.1.2 Nanoliposomes

Nanoliposomes are defined as spherical lipid bilayer vesicles, resemble the lipid bilayer of cell membranes, and maintain nanometric or submicronic bands during storage and applications [72–74]. Its bilayer structure, formed by one-half of the lipid bilayer, contains a hydrophilic head and a lipophilic acyl chain. Thus, its amphipathic nature allows it to encapsulate hydrophilic and hydrophobic compounds individually or simultaneously due to its bifunctional physicochemical properties and, consequently, it presents interaction with a wide range and variety of molecules [75]. Nanosystems are drug-carrying structures with potential for application in the medical field and food industry. However, they have low robustness regarding physical and thermal stability and pH variations, being considered significant challenges for their intended commercialization [76].

The most common method used for the production of nanoliposomes is to obtain a double emulsion followed by a microfluidization process at room temperature after the previous removal of the solvent. It is possible to produce nanoliposomes using low-cost natural ingredients (for example, soy, egg yolk, sunflower, milk), optimizing the cost-effectiveness of the final product [72]. The literature reports several clinical trials using nanoliposomes, and studies reveal that they are excellent candidates for various distribution systems, such as anticancer, antifungal and antibiotic drugs, administration of genetic drugs, and administration of anesthetics and anti-inflammatory drugs [77]. Similarly, it will have application in the food area, allowing the incorporation and simultaneous release of two or more bioactive compounds with different solubilities, as is the case of medium-chain liposomes and vitamin C, enhancing food functionality [74].

3.1.3 Solid lipid nanoparticles

Lipid nanoparticles are similar to nanoemulsions in which the oil phase was totally or partially solidified [56]. It is a colloidal carrier system that makes it possible to encapsulate, protect and distribute functional lipophilic components, such as bioactive lipids and drugs [70]. The size and structure of the lipid nanoparticles are similar to nanoemulsions, with a size that usually ranges from 50 to 1000 nm. The lipid nucleus in nanoemulsions is liquid, but the lipid nucleus is in a solid-state [78].

Solid lipid nanoparticles can be classified as solid lipid nanoparticles (SLNs) and nanostructured lipid transporters (NLCs). In general, homogenization techniques of cold or hot high pressure and double emulsions are currently being used more to produce SLNs and NLCs to encapsulate bioactive oils [79]. The composition of SLNs is usually lipids such as triglycerides (tristearin), partial glycerides (glyceryl monostearate), fatty acids (stearic acid), sterols (cholesterol), and waxes (cetyl palmitate) [70].

There is a great difficulty associated with lipophilic bioactive agents in food matrices in the food industry, one of the main problems for manufacturers in the development of nutraceutical and functional foods [80]. Thus, SLNs and NLCs aim to assist as a nanoparticle carrier of bioactive compounds with a lipophilic character. SLNs are nanometric lipid matrices between 50 nm and 1 mm in diameter, and these nanostructured systems are capable of effectively encapsulating active, sensitive molecules that must be protected from different environmental conditions, such as light, moisture, and oxidation. In addition, the solid matrix allows a controlled release and a high capacity to reach the target organ [79]. NLCs, whose matrix consists of a mixture of lipids with different physicochemical properties instead of just one type of lipid, were initially synthesized to avoid SLN problems with loading. They can form physical lipid mixtures through the mixture of solid and liquid lipids (oil), but without crystallization, presenting a more unstructured (entropic) matrix that allows the control of the molecular load [74, 79].

3.1.4 Nanohydrogels

Nanohydrogels are defined as an infinite network of hydrophilic three-dimensional polymers swollen by water without losing their interconnected porous structure, expanding, and disintegrating [81–83]. For application in food, they must be composed of non-toxic, biodegradable, and biocompatible biopolymers to deliver bioactive compounds in / or through the mucosa of the gastrointestinal tract. Nanohydrogels are soft materials widely used by the food and nutraceutical industries [83].

Generally, hydrogels are formed by chemical or physical cross-linking polymers. They are basically formed by three integral parts: monomer, initiator, and cross-linker [84]. Different techniques can be adapted to obtain the nanohydrogels such as mass polymerization, solution, and suspension, taking into account that the impurities, including unreacted monomer, initiators, crosslinkers, and unwanted products generated, need to be removed after their preparation [81].

Nanohydrogels formed by biopolymeric proteins or polysaccharides are the best alternatives for application in food since they can offer improved functional properties compared to native proteins. The size, structure, load, permeability, porosity, and stability to environmental and solution conditions are essential and fundamental characteristics for nanohydrogels and depend in general on the physicochemical properties of the biopolymers chosen to obtain the gel. [85]. The proper adjustment of these variables allows the functional compounds to be loaded and then released from the polymeric matrix [86]. The choice of the type of polymeric matrix must be adequate considering that hydrophilic compounds can be released from a protein matrix by diffusion, while lipophilic compounds are released mainly by enzymatic degradation of the protein matrix in the GI tract [21, 81, 85].

3.1.5 Nanoemulsion

The definition of nanoemulsion consists of an excellent dispersion composed of an oily phase (triglycerides or hydrocarbons) and an aqueous phase (water or water with some electrolyte or polyol), which appears as spherical drops with a diameter less than 100 nm [70]. The nanoemulsion droplets most often have a core of lipophilic material, which one or more non-polar components may form. The surrounding contents of the nucleus are formed by the material of opposite polarity [81].

There is a wide variety of methods for making stable nanoemulsion. The nanoemulsion preparation is divided according to the energy level adopted in the system as the high and low energy method [87]. The main methods used to obtain a nanoemulsion include high-pressure homogenizers and ultrasound generators representing the high energy method, including microfluidization [88]. Low-energy emulsification methods are cost-effective, in which nanoemulsions with tiny droplets are prepared using low amounts of energy, which stand out the methods of spontaneous emulsification, reverse phase technique, membrane emulsification method, and solvent displacement method [89].

Nanoemulsions offer a wide range of applications due to their composition flexibility in several fields, including food, beverage, and pharmaceutical industries for product storage and delivery. Currently, it can be used to encapsulate lipophilic components, such as vitamins, substances that impart flavors, colors, preservatives, nutraceuticals, and medicines. In addition, it can be applied to preserve food and bioactive compounds, increasing bioavailability and shelf life. Another essential application aimed at the food industry is the possibility of masking unpleasant odors and flavors and protecting bioactive molecules from oxidation and hydrolysis by the action of air and water, respectively [89].

4. Conclusion

Nanotechnology is a potential new technology in food, being one of the primary resources for development and innovation. Reducing the particle size of bioactive compounds can improve bioavailability, release control, delivery targeting, and solubility. The choice of the preparation technique for the nanostructured systems depends on the characteristics of the bioactive compound, such as hydrophilic or lipophilic, solubility, stability, and the desired properties for the product, such as particle size and bioavailability, among others. Thus, it is possible to verify some of the nanoencapsulation techniques that can be used in bioactive compounds, and many undesirable characteristics can be circumvented with nanotechnology.

Acknowledgements

This work was supported by grants of CNPq, CAPES, FAPEAL, and FAPEMIG.

Conflict of interest

The authors declare no conflict of interest.

Author details

Ilza Fernanda Barboza Duarte[1,3],
Naianny Lívia Oliveira Nascimento Mergulhão[1], Valdemir da Costa Silva[1],
Laisa Carolina Gomes de Bulhões[2], Irinaldo Diniz Basílio Júnior[2]
and Anielle C.A. Silva[1,3]*

1 Programa de Pós-Graduação da Rede Nordeste de Biotecnologia (RENORBIO), Federal University of Alagoas, Maceió, AL, Brazil

2 Laboratory of Pharmaceutical Technology, Research Program Post-Graduation in Pharmaceutical Sciences, Institute of Pharmaceutical Sciences, Maceió, AL, Brazil

3 Laboratory of New Nanostructured and Functional Materials, Physics Institute, Federal University of Alagoas, Maceió, AL, Brazil

*Address all correspondence to: acalmeida@fis.ufal.br

References

[1] Farias, TGS, Stamford, TCM, Ribeiro, VMS, Ladislau, HFL, Medeiros, JAC, Arnaud, TMS, Stamford, TLM. Mint: Alimentos simbióticos: uso da coencapsulação como forma de veiculação de probióticos e prebióticos. Ed. Científica digital - Avanços em Ciência e Tecnologia de Alimentos. 2021; 4: 39-58.

[2] Bagchi, D. Mint: Nutraceuticals and functional foods regulations in the United States and around the world. Toxicology. 2006; 221: 1-3.

[3] Salgado, J. In: Alimentos funcionais. 1 ed., São Paulo: Oficina de textos, 2017.

[4] Wildman, REC. Mint: Handbook of Nutraceuticals and Functional Foods. Boca Raton: CRC Press, 2000.

[5] Souza, FCA, et al. Mint: Alimentos Funcionais No Manejo Do Diabetes Melitus Tipo 2: Uma Abordagem Bibliográfica. Ciência & Saberes. 2017; 3.

[6] Reis, SA, Conceição, LL, Rosa, DD, Siqueira, NP, Peluzio, MG. Mint: Mechanisms responsible for the hypocholesterolaemic effect of regular consumption of probiotics. Nutrition Research Reviews. 2017; 30: 36-49.

[7] Reis, FS, et al. Functional foods based on extracts or compounds derived from mushrooms. Trends in Food Science & Technology. 2017; 66: 48-62.

[8] Bigliardi, B.; Galati, F. Mint: Innovation trends in the food industry: The case of functional foods. Trends in Food Science & Technology. 2013; 31: 118-129.

[9] AGÊNCIA NACIONAL DE VIGILÂNCIA SANITÁRIA - ANVISA. Resolução n° 19, de 30 de abril de 1999. Aprova o Regulamento Técnico de Procedimentos Para Registro de Alimento com Alegação de Propriedades Funcionais e ou de Saúde em sua Rotulagem [Internet]. Diário Oficial da União, Brasília, 03 mai. 1999. Disponível em: http://portal.anvisa.gov.br/documents/10181/2718376/RES_18_1999_COMP.pdf/dd30fd35-e7ea-4f8d-be72-ae2e439191b. Acessado em: 28 de julho de 2020. [Accessed: 2021-05-08]

[10] AGÊNCIA NACIONAL DE VIGILÂNCIA SANITÁRIA - ANVISA. Resolução n° 241 de 26 de julho de 2018. Dispõe sobre os requisitos para comprovação da segurança e dos benefícios à saúde dos probióticos para uso em alimentos [Internet]. Diário Oficial da União, Brasília, 27 de julho de 2018. Disponível em: http://www.in.gov.br/materia/- /asset_publisher/Kujrw0TZC2Mb/content/id/34379910/do1-2018-07-27-resolucao-dadiretoria-colegiada-rdc-n-241-de-26-de-julho-de-2018-34379900. [Accessed: 2021-05-08]

[11] Filho, WFSB, Torres, LN, Barros, MCLB, Sousa, SF. Mint: Alimentos funcionais probióticos, um novo estilo de vida. Congresso internacional da agroindústria (CIAGRO) – Ciência, tecnologia e inovação: do campo à mesa, 25 a 27 de setembro, 2020.

[12] Raizel, R, Santini, E, Kopper1, AM, Filho, ADR. Mint: Efeitos do consumo de probióticos, prebióticos e simbióticos para o organismo humano. Revista Ciência & Saúde. 2011; 4: 66-74.

[13] Santos, FL, Silva, MR, Pitangueira, BS, Conceição, CFA. Mint: Utilização de Probióticos na Redução da Anemia Ferropriva. Diálogos e CiênciaRevista da Rede de Ensino FTC. 2008; 7: 13-18.

[14] Silva, ASS, Haas, P, Sartori, NT. Anton, AA, Francisco, A. Mint: Fruooligossacarídeos: Fibras alimentares ativas. Revista saúde e Ambiente. 2007; 25: 259-304.

[15] Fuller, R. Probiotics in man and animals. The Journal of Applied Bacteriology. 1989;03 66: 365-78.

[16] Araújo, EA. Mint: Desenvolvimento e caracterização de queijo tipo Cottage adicionado de Lactobacillus Delbrueckii UFV H2b20 e de Inulina [Thesis] - Universidade Federal de Viçosa. Viçosa; 2007.

[17] Badaró, ACL, Guttierres, APM, Rezende, ACV, Stringheta, PC. Mint: Alimentos probióticos: Aplicações como promotores da saúde humana. Nutrir Gerais. Revista Digital de Nutrição. 2008; 2.

[18] Saad, SMI. Mint: Probióticos e prebióticos: o estado da arte. Revista Brasileira de Ciências Farmacêuticas. 2006; 42: 1-16.

[19] Abbas, S, Karangwa, E, Bashari, M, Hayat, K, Hong, X, Sharif, HR, Zhang, X. Mint: Fabrication of polymeric nanocapsules from curcumin-loaded nanoemulsion templates by self-assembly. Ultrasonics Sonochemistry. 2015; 23: 81-92.

[20] Neves, MA, Hashemi, J, Prentice, C. Mint: Development of novel bioactives delivery systems by micro/ nanotechnology. Current Opinion in Food Science. 2015; 1: 7-12.

[21] Wang, S, Marcone, MF, Barbut, S, Lim, LT. Mint: Fortification of dietary biopolymersbased packaging material with bioactive plant extracts. Food Research International. 2012; 49: 80-91.

[22] Banjare, J. Application of nanotechnology in food technology and targeted drug therapy for prevention of obesity: an overview. J Crit Rev. 2017; 4: 7-11.

[23] Ranjan, S, Dasgupta, N, Chakraborty, AR, Samuel, SM, Ramalingam, C, Shanker, R, et al. Mint: Nanoscience and nanotechnologies in food industries: opportunities and research trends. J Nanoparticle Res. 2014; 16: 1-23.

[24] Lahtinen, SJ, Forssten, S, Ako, J, Granlund, L, Rautonen, N, Salminen, S, Viitanen, M, Ouwehand, AC. Mint: Probiotic cheese containing Lactobacillus rhamnosus HN001 and Lactobacillus acidophilus NCFM modifies subpopulations of fecal lactobacilli and Clostridium difficilein the elderly. Age (Dordr). 2012; 34: 133-143.

[25] Denipote, FG, Trindade, EBSM, Burini, RC. Mint: Probióticos e prebióticos na atenção primária ao câncer de cólon. Arq. Gastroenterol. 2010; 47.

[26] Kumar, M, Verma, V, Nagpal, R, Kumar, A, Behare, PV, Singh, B, Aggarwal, PK. Mint: Anticarcinogenic effect of probiotic fermented milk and Chlorophyllin on aflatoxin-B1 induced liver carcinogenesis in rats. Br. J. Nutr. 2011; 107: 1006-1016.

[27] An, HM, Park, SY, Lee, K, Kim, JR, Cha, MK, Lee, SW, Lim, HT, Kim, KJ, Ha, NJ. Mint: Anti-obesity and lipid lowering effects of Bifidobacterium spp. in high fat diet induced obese rats. Lipids Health Dis. 2011; 10: 116.

[28] Aronsson, L, Huang, Y, Parini, P, Korach-André, M, Håkansson, J, Gustafsson, J, Pettersson, S, Arulampalam, V, Rafter, J. Mint: Decreased fat storage by Lactobacillus paracasei is associated with increased levels of angiopoietin-like 4 protein (ANGPTL4). PLoS ONE. 2010; 5.

[29] Naito, E, Yoshida, Y, Makino, K, Kounoshi, Y, Kunihiro, S, Takahashi, R, Matsuzaki, T, Miyazaki, K, Ishikawa, F. Mint: Beneficial effect of oral administration of Lactobacillus casei strain Shirota on insulin resistance in

dietinduced obesity mice. J. Appl. Microbiol. 2011; 110: 650-657.

[30] Myllyluoma, E, Veijola, L, Ahlroos, T, Tynkkynen, S, Kankuri, E, Vapaatalo, H, Rautelin, H, Korpela, R. Mint: Probiotic supplementation improves tolerance to Helicobacter pylorieradication therapy - a placebo-controlled, doubleblind randomized pilot study. AP&T. 2005; 21: 1263-1272.

[31] Salminen, S, Nybom, S, Meriluoto, J, Collado, MC, Vesterlund, S, El-Nezami, H. Mint: Interaction of probiotics and pathogens—benefits to human health? Curr. Opin. Biotechn. 2010; 21: 157-167.

[32] Shah, NP. Mint: Probiotic bacteria: selective enumeration and survival in dairy foods. J. Dairy Sci. 2000; 83: 894-907.

[33] Costa, MP, Balthazar, CF, Moreira, RVBP, Cruz, AG, Júnior, CAC. Mint: Leite fermentado: Potencial alimento funcional. Enciclopédia biosfera, Centro Científico Conhecer. 2013; 9: 13.

[34] Champagne, CP, et al. Mint: Effects of storage conditions, microencapsulation and inclusion in chocolate particles on the stability of probiotic bacteria in ice cream. International Dairy Journal. 2015; 47: 109-117.

[35] Garcia-Ceja, A et al. Mint: Viability during refrigerated storage in selected food products and during simulated gastrointestinal conditions of individual and combined lactobacilli encapsulated in alginate or alginate-chitosan. Food Science and Tecnology. 2015; 63: 482-489.

[36] Kingwatee, N, et al. Mint: Spray drying Lactobacillus casei 01 in Lychee juice varied carrier materials. Food Science and Technology. 2015; 62: 847-853.

[37] Shaikh, A. Demanda por probióticos cresce significativamente. [Internet] Disponível em: https://www.milkpoint.com.br/artigos/espaco-aberto/demanda-por-probioticos-cresce-significativamente-207775/. [Accessed: 2021-05-11].

[38] Brizuela, MA, Serrano, P, Perez, Y. Mint: Studies on probiotics properties of two Lactobacillus strains. Braz. arch. biol. technol. 2001; 44: 95-99.

[39] Oliveira, MN, Sivieri K, Alegro JHA, Saad SMI. Mint: Aspectos tecnológicos de alimentos funcionais contendo probióticos. Rev Bras de Ciên Farm. 2002; 38: 1-21.

[40] Santos, MS, Ferreira, CLLF, Gomes, PC, Santos, JL, Pozza, PC, Teshima, E. Mint: Influência do fornecimento de probiótico à base de Lactobacillus sp. Sobre a microbiota intestinal de leitões. Ciência. agrotec. 2003; 27: 1395-1400.

[41] BRASIL. Agência Nacional de Vigilância Sanitária. RDC n° 2, de 7 de janeiro de 2002. Regulamento Técnico de Substâncias Bioativas e Probióticos Isolados com alegação de propriedades funcional e/ou de saúde. Disponível em: http://portal.anvisa.gov.br/wps/wcm/connect/1c77370047457bcc8888dc3fbc4c6735/RDC_02_2002.pdf?MOD=AJPERES. [Accessed: 2021-05-11]

[42] Fao/Who. Guidelines for the evaluation of probiotics in food. Report of a joint FAO/WHO working group on drafting guidelines for the evaluation of probiotics in food. 2002.

[43] Cats, A, Kuipers, EJ, Bosschaert, MA, Pot, RG, Vandenbrouckegrauls, CM, Kusters, JG. Mint: Effect of frequent consumption of a Lactobacillus casei-containing Milk drink in Helicobacter pylori-colonized subjects. AP&T. 2003; 17: 429-435.

[44] Chapman, CMC, Gibson, GR. Mint: Health benefits of probiotics: are

mixtures more effective than single strains? Eur. J. Nutr. 2011; 50: 1-17.

[45] Souza, FS, Cocco, RR, Sarni, ROS, Mallozi, MC, Solé, D. Mint: Prebióticos, probióticos e simbióticos na prevenção e tratamento das doenças alérgicas. Rev Paul Pediatr. 2010; 28: 86-97.

[46] Moraes, FP, Colla, LM. Mint: Alimentos funcionais e nutracêuticos: definições, legislação e benefícios à saúde. Revista Eletrônica de Farmácia. 2006; 3: 99-112.

[47] Serviço Brasileiro de Respostas Técnicas – SBRT. Probióticos, prebióticos e simbióticos: definição, benefícios e aplicabilidade industrial, Dossiê técnico, 2014.

[48] Varavallo, MA, et al. Mint: Aplicação de bactérias probióticas para profilaxia e tratamento de doenças gastrointestinais. Semina: Ciências Biológicas e da Saúde. 2008; 29: 83-104.

[49] Bermudez-Brito, M, Plaza-Díaz, J, Muñoz-Quezada, S, Gómezllorente, C, Angel Gil, A. Mint: Probiotic Mechanisms of Action. Ann. Nutr. Metab. 2012; 61: 160-174.

[50] Rafter, J. Mint: Probiotics and colon cancer. Best Pract. Res. Clin. Gastroenterol. 2003; 17: .849-859.

[51] Maciel, MIS, Souza, MMB. Mint: Prebióticos e probióticos - benefícios potenciais na nutrição e saúde humana. IntechOpen. 2019.

[52] Livney, YD. Mint: Nanostructured delivery systems in food: latest developments and potential future directions. Current Opinion in Food Science. 2015; 3: 125-135.

[53] Cambrussi, ANCO, et al. Mint: O papel da nanotecnologia na redução do estresse oxidativo: uma revisão. Boletim Informativo Geum. 2018; 9: 1.

[54] Ferreira, AS. In: Ciência E Tecnologia De Alimentos: Conceitos E Aplicações. Eduft. 2019. p. 109-122.

[55] Bazana, MT, Codevilla CF, Silva, CB, Menezes, CR. Mint: Nanoencapsulação de licopeno em alimentos. Ciência e Natura. 2015; 37: 38-48.

[56] McClements, DJ. Mint: Edible nanoemulsions: fabrication, properties, and functional performance. Soft Matter. 2011; 7: 2297-2316.

[57] Martins, VC, Braga, ECO, Godoy, RLO, Borguin, RG, Pacheco, S, Santiago, MCPA, Nascimento, LSM. Mint: Nanotecnologia em alimentos: Uma breve revisão. Perspectivas da Ciência e Tecnologia. 2015; 7: 25-42.

[58] Razavi, S, Janfaza, S, Tasnim, N, Gibson, DL, Hoorfar, M. Mint: Nanomaterial-based encapsulation for controlled gastrointestinal delivery of viable probiotic bactéria. Nanoscale Adv. 2021.

[59] Silva, Vs, Orlandelli, Rc. Mint: Desenvolvimento de alimentos funcionais nos últimos anos: Uma Revisão. Rev. Uningá. 2019; 56: 182-194.

[60] Codevilla, CF, Bazana, MT, Silva, CB, Barin, JS, Menezes, CR. Mint: Nanoestruturas contendo compostos bioativos extraídos de plantas. Ciência e Natura. 2015; 37: 142– 151.

[61] Jeevanandam, J, Barhoum, A, Chan, YS, Dufresne, A, Danquah, MK. Mint: Review on nanoparticles and nanostructured materials: history, sources, toxicity and regulations. Beilstein Journal of Nanotechnology. 2018; 9: 1050-1074.

[62] Khan, I, Saeed, K, Khan, I. Mint: Nanoparticles: properties, applications and toxicities. Arabian Journal Of Chemistry. 2019; 12: 908-931.

[63] Figueira, CS, Santos, RP. Mint: Biossíntese de nanopartículas de ouro utilizando vegetais. Nanocell News. 2017; 4.

[64] Barratt, GM. Mint: Therapeutic applications of colloidal drug carriers. Pharmaceutical Science & Technology Today. 2000; 3: 163-171.

[65] Azevedo, LF, et al. Polymeric nanoparticle systems loaded with red propolis extract: a comparative study of the encapsulating systems, PCL-Pluronic versus Eudragit®E100-Pluronic. Journal Of Apicultural Research 2018; 57: 255-270.

[66] Faraji, AH, Wipf, P. Mint: Nanoparticles in cellular drug delivery, Bioorg. Med. Chem. 2009; 17: 2950-2962.

[67] Doshi, N, Mitragotri, S. Mint: Designer biomaterials for nanomedicine, Adv. Funct. Mater. 2009; 19: 3843-3854.

[68] Kumari, A, Yadav, SK, Yadav, SC. Mint: Biodegradable polymeric nanopar¬ticles based drug delivery systems, Colloids Surf. B. 2010; 75: 1-18.

[69] Lee, BK, Yun, Y, Park, K. Mint: PLA micro- and nano-particles. Advanced Drug Delivery Reviews. 2016; 107: 176-191.

[70] Assis, LM, Zavareze, ER, Prentice-Hernández, C, Souza-Soares, LA. Mint: Revisão: características de nanopartículas e potenciais aplicações em alimentos. Brazilian Journal Of Food Technology. 2012; 15: 99-109.

[71] Nascimento, TG, et al. Mint: Polymeric Nanoparticles of Brazilian Red Propolis Extract: Preparation, Characterization, Antioxidant and Leishmanicidal Activity. Nanoscale Research Letters. 2016; 11: 1-16.

[72] Khorasani, S, Danaei, M, Mozafari, MR. Mint: Nanoliposome technology for the food and nutraceutical industries. Trends Food Sci. Technol. 2018; 79: 106-115.

[73] Pathakoti, K, Manubolu, M, Hwang, HM. Mint: Nanostructures: current uses and future applications in food science. Journal of Food and Drug Analysis. 2017; 25: 245-253.

[74] Santiago, LG, Castro, GR. Mint: Novel technologies for the encapsulation of bioactive food compounds. Current Opinion in Food Science. 2016; 7: 78-85.

[75] Zhang, HY, Tehrany, EA, Kahn, CJF, Ponçot, M, Linder, M, Cleymand, F. Mint: Effects of nanoliposomes based on soya, rapeseed and fish lecithins on chitosan thin films designed for tissue engineering. Carbohydrate Polymers. 2012; 88: 618-627.

[76] Milani, D, Athiyah, U, Hariyadi, DM, Pathak, YV. Mint: "Surface modification of nanoparticles for targeted drug delivery," in Surface Modification of Nanoparticles for Targeted Drug Delivery. 2019; 207-220.

[77] Allen, TM, Cullis, PR. Mint: Liposomal drug delivery systems: from concept to clinical applications. Adv. Drug Deliv. Rev. 2013; 65: 36-48.

[78] Farhang, B. Mint: Nanotechnology and lipids. Lipid Technology. 2007; 19: 132-135.

[79] Rodríguez, J, Martín, MJ, Ruiz, MA, Clares, B. Mint: Current encapsulation strategies for bioactive oils: from alimentary to pharmaceutical perspectives. Food Research Inter*national. 2016; 83: 41-59.

[80] Weiss, J, Decker, EA, McClements, J, Kristbergsson, K, Helgason, T, Awad, T. Mint: Solid lipid nanoparticles as delivery systems for bioactive food

components. Food Biophisics. 2008; 3: 146-154.

[81] Artiga-Artigas, M, Odriozola-Serrano, I, Oms-Oliu, G, Martín-Belloso, O. Mint: Nanostructured Systems to Increase Bioavailability of Food Ingredients. Nanomaterials For Food Applications. 2019; 13-33.

[82] Fuciños, C, Fuciños, P, Amado, IR, Míguez, M, Fajardo, P, Pastrana, LM, Rðа, ML. Mint: Smart Nanohydrogels for Controlled Release of Food Preservatives. Antimicrobial Food Packaging. 2016; 349-362.

[83] Ji, N, Qin, Y, Li, M, Xiong, L, Qiu, L, Bian, X, Sun, Q. Mint: Fabrication and Characterization of Starch Nanohydrogels via Reverse Emulsification and Internal Gelation. Journal Of Agricultural And Food Chemistry. 2018; 66: 9326-9334.

[84] Ahmed, EM. Mint: Hydrogel: preparation, characterization, and applications: a review. Journal of Advanced Research. 2015; 6: 105-121.

[85] Bourbon, AI, Pinheiro, AC, Carneiro-da-Cunha, MG, Pereira, RN, Cerqueira, MA, Vicente, AA. Mint: Development and characterization of lactoferrin-GMP nanohydrogels: evaluation of pH, ionic strength and temperature effect. Food Hydrocolloids. 2015; 48: 292-300.

[86] Cal, OE, Khutoryanskiy, VV. Biomedical applications of hydrogels: a review of patents and commercial products. European Polymer Journal. 2015; 65: 252-267.

[87] Tadros, T, Izquierdo, R, Esquena, J, Solans, C. Mint: Formation and stability of nano-emulsions. Adv. Colloid Interf. Sci. 2004; 108-109, 303-318.

[88] Kentish, S, Wooster, TJ, Ashokkumar, M, Balachandran, S, Mawson, R, Simons, L. Mint: The use of ultrasonics for nanoemulsion preparation. Innovative Food Science and Emerging Technologies. 2008; 9: 170-175.

[89] Borthakur, P, Boruah, PK, Sharma, B, Das, MR. Mint: Nanoemulsion: preparation and its application in food industry. Emulsions. 2016: 153-191.

Chapter 11

Prebiotics, Probiotics and Synbiotic for Bone Health

Bolaji Lilian Ilesanmi-Oyelere and Marlena Cathorina Kruger

Abstract

Prebiotics, probiotics and synbiotics has been shown to enhance calcium absorption, gut and bone health. Probiotics are also known to ferment prebiotics to produce the fermentative substrates such as short chain fatty acids (SCFAs), mainly acetate, butyrate and propionate with the help of beneficial micro-organisms in the gut. The expression of these SCFAs has been associated with the inhibition of osteoclast differentiation and bone resorption both *in vitro* and *in vivo.* In this review, we discuss the benefits of SCFAs and ways in which prebiotics and probiotics affect bone health by the reduction of inflammation in the gut and the bone.

Keywords: prebiotic, probiotic, synbiotic, gut microbiota, bone metabolism

1. Introduction

Prebiotics and probiotics have been proven to confer multiple health benefits to animals and humans alike when consumed either singly or in combination. Consumption of prebiotics and probiotics modulates the gut microbiota and the colonization of the gastrointestinal tract which is now known as the second gene pool of the human body. Evidence shows the health benefits of synbiotic intake in many aspects of human health including metabolic functions, gastrointestinal diseases, and bone health. Some of these documented evidence-based benefits include their immunomodulatory effect [1], improvement of diarrhea, lactose metabolism, digestive health and metabolic syndrome [2], antidiabetic and hypocholestrolemic [3], anticarcinogenic [4] and hypotensive attributes/features [5]. In a short review that we conducted, the importance of prebiotics, probiotics and synbiotics was expressed to be important across human lifespan from childhood to adulthood and the elderly [6].

2. The significance of prebiotics and probiotics

Probiotics in the presence of prebiotics undergo different biochemical pathways/messenger systems to inhibit pathogens and boost the immunity of the host, these includes

a. Presence of probiotics in the gut leads to competition for nutrients with pathogens which can then lead to starvation and reduction of these unwanted bacteria.

IntechOpen

b. Probiotics tend to compete for space via the adhesion effect to the mucosal lining by directly decreasing the adhesion of the pathogens and their toxins; this has been confirmed by in vitro studies demonstrating that probiotics possess lectin-like adhesion properties capable of binding carbohydrates from the receptors of glycoconjugate of epithelial cell surface [7] which blocks pathogen binding to the epithelial cell surface. Some probiotic strains of the *Lactobacillus* genus have shown some features and ability to bind to the enterocyte surface in vitro [8].

c. Probiotics are responsible for the synthesis of bacteriocins such as lantibiotics (class I) and class II bacteriocins by the probiotics, and this mainly by lactic acid bacteria (LAB) can help prevent the growth, colonization, and establishment of pathogens in the gut environments. These bacteriocins present a better activity on the pathogens than antibiotics due to their narrow-spectrum activity on foreign unwanted bacteria. Bacteriocins from Gram-positive bacteria are composed of membrane peptides capable of targeting and causing apoptosis of the cell membrane; however, most antibiotics inhibit enzymes and biosynthesis pathway in cells such as DNA, RNA, protein and cell-wall synthesis [9].

Probiotic microorganisms may also be able to produce enzymes, such as lipase, esterase, and co-enzymes A, Q, NAD, and NADP [10]. Likewise, some of the by-products of probiotics' metabolism may exhibit antibiotic properties and these include bacitracin, lactacin and acidophiline [11].

d. The bio-metabolization of prebiotics into lactate and short chain fatty acids (SCFAs) such as acetate, mainly produced by *Bifidobacteria*, *Lactobacilli* and *Akkermansia muciniphilia* through fermentation by probiotics has significant beneficial role to the health. Acetate is the most abundant in the human colon. Butyrate is produced by *Faecalibacterium prausnitzii*, *Eubacterium rectale* and *Roseburia* spp. and mainly by *Lachnospiraceae* and *Ruminococcaceae* and propionate which is produced by *Propionibacteria*,, *Firmicutes, Lachnospiraceae* and *Bacteroidetes* [12]. The release of these SCFAs by the prebiotic fermentation reduces the intestinal pH level and also reduces the production of putrefactive compounds such as ammonia, phenol, as well as indole and branched-chain fatty acids (BCFAs) [13]. SCFA synthesis are mainly by anaerobic saccharolytic fermentation of carbohydrates that have not been digested or absorbed in the small intestine. Acetate is metabolized in the muscles, kidney, brain and heart, butyrate acts mainly in the colon while propionate and butyrate are cleared by the liver. SCFAs may also regulate fat and glucose metabolism as reported in rat adipocytes [14]. In chronic inflammatory diseases such as IBD, it has been shown that fecal butyrate levels are significantly reduced while high levels of lactic acid are observed [15].

The production of butyrate is mainly from complex carbohydrates through the pyruvate and acetyl-coenzyme A (CoA) pathway; however, it can also be produced from amino acids via the glutarate, 4-aminobutyrate and lysine pathways in the gut [13]. Butyrate acts epigenetically as histone deacetylase (HDAC) inhibitors and the research into HDAC may be capable of providing cancer chemoprevention and therapies [16]. There are different functions of butyrate in the colon; it is the main source of energy for colonocytes. Furthermore, butyrate has been documented to inhibit proinflammatory cytokines such as tumor necrosis α (TNF-α) in monocytes [17], interferon-α (IFN-α) and IL-2 in rat mesenteric lymph nodes [18], chemokine CXCL-8 (IL-8) in Caco-2 cells [19].

e. Intake of prebiotics and probiotics has been linked to the development of immunomodulatory capacity by decreasing inflammation, antibody response and phagocytosis. Probiotics may be involved in the prevention of cytokine-induced epithelial damage. *Lactobacillus rhamnosus* GG (LGG) promoted the survival and enrichment of epithelial cells by the activation of antiapoptotic and inhibition of proapoptopic pathways [20].

f. Probiotic and prebiotic intake results in the improvement of the epithelial barrier integrity by the secretion of mucin [21] and defensins [22] including antimicrobial proteins (AMPs). Probiotics enhance the mucosal integrity also by inducing cytoprotective substance production by enterocytes such as heat shock proteins [23]. In an in vitro study, *Bifidobacterium infantis* enhanced the intestinal mucosal barrier (T84 human epithelial cells) [24]. Similarly, *Lactobacillus plantarum* is responsible for acting on the tight junctions via increasing the expression of occludins and *zonula occludens* proteins [25].

g. Prebiotics and probiotics are capable of the stimulation and production of antioxidant-related enzymes, systemic hormones, and neurochemicals such as serotonin, gamma-aminobutyric acid (GABA) and cortisol, as well as production of bile salt hydrolase. Consumption of probiotics and prebiotics has also been reported to be able to reduce cholesterol levels. Prebiotic fibers increased levels of satiety hormones (glucagon-like peptide-1, proglucagon and peptide YY mRNA) and decreased levels of ghrelin O-acyltransferase mRNA in rats [26]. Furthermore, prebiotic fermentation in the gut likewise improved satietogenic and incretin gut peptide production, thereby increasing the plasma glucagon-like peptide 1 and peptide YY concentrations in humans [27].

h. Prebiotics and probiotics are responsible for the synthesis of antigens via production of anti-inflammatory cytokine such as IL-10 which inhibits the T-helper cells (1, 2, 7 and 17) and transforming growth factor-β responsible for the production of immunoglobulin A [28].

The concept and use of prebiotics has been argued to be more important when compared to probiotics due to the vulnerability and susceptibility of probiotics to environmental stresses, manufacturing process (such as heat) and endangered conditions during storage [29].

3. Prebiotics and human health

Glenn Gibson and Marcel Roberfroid launched the prebiotic concept in 1995 as 'a nondigestible food ingredient that beneficially affects the host by selectively stimulating the growth and/or activity of one or a limited number of bacteria in the colon, and thus improves host health' [30]. This definition has however been modified several times, but the initial main features have been retained. Prebiotics tend to stimulate the growth of the gut bacteria endogenously. The pH of the gut environment plays a major role in determining bacterial interspecies competition outcome.

Food sources of prebiotics consist of edible plants such as fruits, vegetables, cereal component which provides the body with carbohydrate. Specific potential sources are artichokes, tomatoes, bananas, asparagus, garlic, berries, kiwi fruit, onions, chicory, green leafy vegetables, legumes as well as linseed, barley, oats, and wheat.

Even though various molecules can be prebiotics, the great majority are dietary fibers which are oligosaccharides such as inulin (mainly from chicory), GOS (obtained from lactose using β-galactosidase), Fructooligosaccharides (FOS) (from chicory by partial enzymatic hydrolysis), soybean oligosaccharides (SOS), and xylooligosaccharides (XOS). Inulin, GOS and FOS have been widely studied. The list of prebiotics also includes compounds such as resistant starches, arabinoxylan, pectin, whole grains as well as non-carbohydrate complex such as polyphenols [13]. Absence of dietary fiber in the colon causes anaerobic bacteria to obtain their energy from protein fermentation, and this metabolism leads to the production of potentially toxic and carcinogenic compounds such as ammoniac and phenolic compounds [31]. In contrast, carbohydrate fermentation (for example dietary fiber) will produce non-toxic SCFAs which can serve as fuel for the epithelial cells. The production of volatile fatty acids, including, SCFAs and BCFAs, play a role in energy homeostasis maintenance as well as in the regulation of functionality in peripheral tissues [32]. Prebiotics are also mainly active in the large intestine/colon.

Different strains of bacterial genus or species would prefer different substrates for fermentation in the colon. Generally, the strains of *Bifidobacterium* and *Lactobacillus* genera have been reported to prefer fructans as substrate, as opposed to glucose while other bacteria such as *Clostridia* and *Bacteroides* have been reported to thrive on fructans [33, 34].

The use of prebiotics has been shown to be efficient and effective against a few human health disorders such as Type 2 diabetes mellitus and inflammatory bowel diseases which has been termed the "Western" chronic diseases and colorectal cancer. This is accomplished by the modulation of the intestinal gut microbiota which confer a protective, metabolic, and trophic benefits to the host [13].

4. Probiotics and human health

The history of probiotics spans back to the 20th century when Mechnicoff (1907) revealed the virtues associated with the consumption of fermented dairy products, he hypothesized that the aging process resulted from the putrefaction of the large intestine. Almost simultaneously, another scientist Tissier indicated that the main component of the gut flora of breast-fed infants were bifidobacterial [35]. Even earlier, biblical recommendations have pointed out yoghurt as important/significant for the treatment of some ailments [36]. Furthermore, the indication has been that probiotics is more beneficial when consumed with food as opposed to supplement due to the available nutrient and energy sources. Probiotics are mainly active in the small and large intestine.

Organizations such as FAO, WHO and the European Food Safety Authority have indicated probiotic strains must meet both safety and effectiveness criteria for their selection process. The regulations require that safety and absence of risks is paramount for human and animal health. The human probiotic products usually belong to the *Lactobacillus*, *Bifidobacterium*, *Lactococus*, *Streptococcus* and *Enterococcus* genus. In addition, there are some Gram-positive bacteria of genus Bacillus and some yeast of Saccharomyces genus which are also used as probiotics.

Probiotic use has been postulated to be potent against human disorders such as inflammatory enteral diseases such as Crohn's disease, colitis, and non-specific ileitis. Intake of probiotics has also been assessed by various studies as capable of treating lactose intolerance, irritable bowel syndrome [37] and in the prevention of peptic ulcers and colorectal cancer [38]. Beneficial effects of probiotics have been observed in the process of digestion, food allergies treatment [39], dental caries [40], and candidoses [41]. The beneficial effects of probiotics observed by the host through augmentation of the epithelial wall, intestinal mucosal and competitive elimination of pathogens has been reported to aid inflammatory bowel disease (determined by cytokine-induced harm to the epithelial cell walls). Probiotics is capable of repressing gut inflammation via the downregulation of Toll-like Receptors' expression, the prevention of TNF-α entrance into the mononuclear cell in blood and the suppression of enterocyte's NF-kB (Nuclear Factor kappa-light-chain-enhancer of activated B cells) signaling pathway [42].

5. Synbiotics and human health

Synbiotics are a combination of prebiotics and probiotics. The consumption and intake of the combination of prebiotics and probiotics has been reported to stimulate, modulate, and alter the gut microbiota by lowering the colonic secretion of pro-inflammatory and immunoregulatory cytokines such as TNF-α, IL-1β and IL-6. Synbiotics can be used to help improve the beneficial microbes as well as increase the number of specific beneficial strains in the gastrointestinal tract [11].

Immunomodulatory effects of prebiotics and probiotics on human health.

One the putative ways by which prebiotics and probiotics affect the health is altering the immune system. There are two categories of the immune system: either the innate immunity or the adaptive immune system. The immune system is responsible for protecting the host against pathogens. The type of effective immune response which recognizes and mounts reactions to eliminate the pathogen is determined by the site and type of pathogen present. Prebiotics and probiotics modulate the gut immune system thereby also having effects on bone health.

Further studies are needed to investigate the benefits of synbiotics on bone health both in human and animal model.

6. Probiotics and bone health

Bone loss/osteoporosis is a major health problem that is associated with the imbalance between bone formation and bone resorption; often resulting in osteoporotic fractures. In addition, the estimation is that one in two women and one in four men over the age of 50 years will break a bone due to osteoporosis in their life time [43]. Postmenopausal osteoporosis is largely attributed to estrogen deficiency in women age 50 years and above due to ablation of the ovarian function which stimulates bone resorption resulting in bone loss. Risk factors leading to bone diseases include internal (genetic and aging) and external modifiable factors (e.g., diet, exercise, environment, medication etc). In osteoporosis treatment, different approaches have been used but lately due to the safety, low adverse effect and lack of major side effects, probiotics and prebiotics have been introduced. Treatment of bone diseases including osteoporosis and fracture has been mainly through hormone replacement therapy (HRT) as well as others such as bisphosphonates and more recently low-dose parathyroid hormone. However, there are side effects reported with this such as tumorigenesis, mood swings, fluid retention and bleeding as well as low compliance of daily injections [44].

7. The role probiotics in inflammatory homeostasis

Probiotics may aid the modulation of the hosts' inflammatory status by reducing the cytokine secretion levels. The downregulation of proinflammatory cytokines such as IL-6 [45] and TNF-α [46, 47] by probiotics has been reported on several occasions. Studies have shown that some peptides such as p40 and p75 secreted by *Lactobaccillus rhamnosus GG* (LGG) may prevent cytokine-induced apoptosis, increase heat-shock proteins, and could lead to the activation of mitogen-activated protein kinase (MAPK) [48]. Furthermore, TNF (as well as IL-1 and RANKL) has been described as the major physiological inducer of NF-kappa B, one of the transcription factors responsible for the regulation of normal cell functions and the development of inflammatory osteolysis [49].

The role of the intestinal microbiota has been implicated in influencing bone health. A way by which the intestinal tract aids bone is by the regulation of the absorption of minerals such as calcium, phosphorus, and magnesium. This can also be accomplished by endocrine and gut-derived factors such as incretins and serotonins which may influence bone remodeling. Evidence from using germ-free mice indicated the effect of the intestinal microbiome on bone physiology. These studies observed higher bone mass in germ-free mice as compared to the conventional mice. In addition, a decrease in the number of osteoclasts per bone surface and a reduction in CD4+ T cells and osteoclasts precursors were observed in the bone marrow of the mice [50].

The RANKL/RANK/OPG pathway is one of the mechanisms that influence bone turnover/remodeling. Osteoclast's formation and activities are controlled by the RANKL/RANK pathway. They are also an essential pathological process of the bone remodeling. Concomitantly, OPG (decoy receptor of RANKL) acts as a bone protector by binding to RANKL and preventing further resorption [42]. Probiotics (beneficial microbes) have been postulated to reduce inflammation [51] and increase OPG expression in bone [52].

8. Studies emphasizing the importance of probiotics for bone health

8.1 Animal studies

Studies have shown that various strains of *Lactobacillus* [52–54] and *Bifidobacterium* [55, 56] possess the ability to prevent and restore estrogen deficiency-related bone loss in animal models. However, not many studies have been conducted in humans. The study by Ohlsson et al. showed that C-terminal telopeptides (resorption markers) levels were not increased in probiotic treated mice as compared to the vehicle treated mice. Furthermore, there was a reduction in expression of two proinflammatory cytokines (TNF-α and IL-1β), and an increase in the expression of OPG in the cortical bone of ovariectomised mice [52].

Lactobacillus reuteri ATCC PTA 6475 has been used in two animal studies to modulate bone outcomes. Findings from the first study showed increase in femoral trabecular BV/TV, BMD, BMC, trabecular number, spacing, and thickness as well as suppression of the basal TNF-α mRNA expression in the ileum and jejunum in 14-week-old C57Bl/6 J male mice [51]. Meanwhile, the second study showed similar positive bone effects in Ovx Balb/c mice when treated with *Lactobacillus reuteri* for four weeks and changes in the gut microbiota composition was observed revealing an increase in *Clostridiales* and a decrease in *Bacteroidales* in the ileum and jejunum [57]. Furthermore, a study by Collins et al. showed that supplementation with *Lactobaccillus reuteri* 6475 could influence inflammatory status and bone formation after the inflammatory state of female mice were mildly induced. This was achieved via a dorsal surgical incision (DSI) and then administration of the probiotic. The findings indicated that the probiotic supplementation increased bone density, the DSI-treated female mice showed higher trabecular number and mineral apposition rate when compared to the non-treated mice. Although *L. reuteri* treatment had no effect on $CD4^+$ T cell numbers, it led to a decrease in IL-1β and TGFβ expression in the non-surgery cohort [58].

Probiotics are known to aid mineral absorption for the purpose of bone health maintenance. A study showed that supplementation of growing rats with *L. rhamnosus* HN001 enhanced calcium and magnesium absorption [59]. In addition, rats treated with yoghurt with a mix of *Lactobacillus casei*, *L. reuteri* and *L. gasseri* presented higher calcium absorption which resulted in an increased BMC in comparison to the control as well as production of SCFAs [60].

Narva et al. demonstrated the effect a bioactive peptide (valylprolyl-proline) and *Lactobacillus helveticus* LBK-16H fermented milk on bone loss in ovariectomized rats. Their findings showed that *L. helveticus* fermented milk decreased bone turnover and increased BMD in growing rats [61], ovariectomised rats [62] and increased serum calcium while reduced serum PTH was observed in postmenopausal women [63].

Studies have also shown that supplementation with *Bifidobacterium longum*-fermented broccoli suppressed TRAP-positive osteoclast differentiation on the alveolar bone surface in rats [64]. Similarly, administration of yacon flour as prebiotics with *B. longum* as probiotics resulted in significant retention of minerals (such as Ca, Mg and P) in bones of Wistar rats [56]. *B. longum* also increased the BMD of ovariectomised rats by increasing the expression of Sparc and Bmp-2 genes [55].

In a study, male senescence-accelerated mice prone to developing osteoporosis with aging were orally administered heat-killed and living (viable) *Lactococcus lactis* subsp. *cremoris* H61 (strain H61). The protective effect of the heat-killed bacterium included reduction in loss of bone density, reduction in incidence of skin ulcer and reduction in hair loss of the aged SAMP6 [65]. On the other hand, reduction of bone density loss was not observed for the administration of the viable bacterium which may suggest the role of membrane-bound protein, inactivated microbial cells or cell fractions from the cellular death, that is, paraprobiotic and/or postbiotic effect.

The growth of bone as an extra-intestinal organ is suppressed by undernutrition in children. The study by Schwarzer et al. indicated that *L. plantarum* promoted juvenile growth in a strain-dependent manner using mono-colonized mouse model [66]. Supplementation with the bacterium increased the levels of insulin growth factor (IGF-1) and IGF-1 binding protein-3 (IGFBP- 3), the endocrine determinants of somatic growth to wild type levels [66].

Furthermore, the effects of probiotics have also been reported in dysbiosis-induced bone loss observed in the periodontal model [67, 68], Type-1 diabetes-induced bone loss [69] and IBD-induced bone loss [70, 71].

8.2 Human studies

A human study conducted in Denmark evaluated the combined effects of bioavailable isoflavones and probiotics on bone health and estrogen metabolism using a randomized controlled trial in postmenopausal women. Their findings showed that administration red clover extract (isoflavones) and probiotic attenuated BMD at the lumbar spine and femoral neck, reduced plasma concentrations of C-terminal telopeptide of type I collagen (CTX-1) as well as increased the urinary 2-hydroxyestrone (2-OH) to 16α-hydroxyestrone (16α-OH) ratio (the equol producer status) [72].

The use of probiotics however needs to be administered with caution since although the potential beneficial effect in the treatment of inflammatory and auto-immune gastrointestinal diseases for the modulation of immune response is well recognized, individuals with weaker immune systems may still be at risk of viable bacterial cells; in which case the administration the use of killed/inactivated bacteria might be more beneficial [73].

9. Prebiotics and bone health

Prebiotics are non-digestible short-chain carbohydrates also known as oligosaccharides (and maybe polysaccharides) which selectively improves the function and activities of specific types of beneficial microbes. The chemical compounds are neither hydrolyzed by the human digestive system nor absorbed in the upper gastrointestinal tract. Prebiotics have been termed 'colonic foods' due to the ability of these types of foods to move through the colon serving as a substrate to endogenous bacteria while benefitting the host by providing energy and essential nutrients [74].

9.1 Animal studies

Some varieties of benefits have been attributed to the consumption of prebiotics. These include the ability of prebiotics to increase the absorption of minerals such as calcium, magnesium, and phosphorus [75–78] as well as iron [79] as reported quite recently. The absorption of these minerals has consequently been observed to improve bone mineralization and density [80], trabecular structure and increase equol production [81] which is known to reduce bone loss.

9.2 Human studies

FOS supplementation has been administered to both Korean [82] and Chinese [83] postmenopausal women to investigate its effect in the prevention of osteoporosis, modulation of bone biomarkers and mineral absorption. Their findings indicate that there is potential for prebiotics to play a pivotal role in the above mentioned. The study by van den Heuvel et al. reported the benefit of intake of both GOS and inulin in increasing calcium absorption in postmenopausal women [84] and oligofructose stimulating calcium absorption in adolescents [85]. Intake of oligofructose-enriched inulin resulted in improved mineral absorption and impacted the bone turnover markers in postmenopausal women [86]. Other studies also looked into the effect of prebiotics in infants as was recorded with GOS, polydextrose [87] and inulin [88]. Some of these studies have also been conducted in animal models as has been shown in a recent review [89].

10. Other clinical benefits of prebiotics

Due to the effect of the change in metabolism from protein fermentation causing the release of ammonia that leads to an increase in pH to more carbohydrate fermentation resulting in the release of acids, a reduction in the intestinal pH is observed. Low intestinal pH tends to increase bowel movement while protecting against pathogens. Diseases such as inflammatory bowel disease (IBD), irritable bowel syndrome (IBS) and Crohn's diseases are characterized by high pH levels [90]. Prebiotics are therefore able to reduce the symptoms and severity of these diseases. In addition, they are able to restore intestinal bacterial imbalance created by antibiotics, diarrhea, stress and sometimes medication and drugs intake [74].

Prebiotics are also known to help relief constipation. Most carbohydrates are able to increase water retention of the intestine and the acids' production thereby increasing intestinal motility [91]. Furthermore, prebiotics have been used as bioactive functional foods to modulate blood lipid levels [92] and it also been effective in weight loss and metabolic syndrome [93]. The anti-carcinogenic effects of both prebiotics and probiotics have been reported in the inhibition of aberrant crypt foci (ACF) which is a biomarker of colon cancer [94–96].

Recently, prebiotic food and Bidobacterium spp. have been reported to improve bone resorption and reduce serum TRACP-5b levels of Japanese female athletes [97]. Application of the combination of probiotic and prebiotic has been reported to confer a synergistical effect on the host due to the combined benefits of the two. This has been backed with the study by Scholz-Ahrens et al. which showed that probiotics supports the growth of other habitual microbiota strains and prebiotics chain length impacts the composition colonic, caecal, and fecal microflora. The combined administration of oligofructose and *Lactobacillus acidophilus* reduced the pH in the intestinal segments including the caecum, stimulated the colonic absorption as is indicated by increase in the colon weight [98].

11. Conclusion

The study of the effect of synbiotics on gut microbiota and bone health profile is now growing rapidly. Probiotic strains have differing genotype and phenotype and may therefore show different metabolic and immunological functions. The mechanisms however still need further investigation to look into the effect of synbiotics on the gut for the regulation of bone metabolism via the process of mineral absorption, the immune, endocrine system. Further studies are needed to elucidate the importance and mechanisms by which prebiotics and probiotics modulates the microbiota-gut-bone axis in order to get the full benefit of the long-term safety and efficacy of consumption of these functional bioactive products.

Author details

Bolaji Lilian Ilesanmi-Oyelere[1*] and Marlena Cathorina Kruger[1,2]

1 School of Health Sciences, College of Health, Massey University, New Zealand

2 Riddet Institute, Massey University, New Zealand

*Address all correspondence to: b.ilesanmi-oyelere@massey.ac.nz

References

[1] Klaenhammer, T.R., et al., *The impact of probiotics and prebiotics on the immune system.* Nature Reviews Immunology, 2012. **12**(10): p. 728-734.

[2] Dong, Y., et al., *Probiotic foods and supplements interventions for metabolic syndromes: a systematic review and meta-analysis of recent clinical trials.* Annals of Nutrition and Metabolism, 2019. **74**(3): p. 224-241.

[3] Lye, H.-S., et al., *The improvement of hypertension by probiotics: effects on cholesterol, diabetes, renin, and phytoestrogens.* International journal of molecular sciences, 2009.**10**(9): p. 3755-3775.

[4] Górska, A., et al., *Probiotic bacteria: a promising tool in cancer prevention and therapy.* Current microbiology, 2019.**76**(8): p. 939-949.

[5] Upadrasta, A. and R.S. Madempudi, *Probiotics and blood pressure: current insights.* Integrated blood pressure control, 2016.**9**: p. 33.

[6] Ilesanmi-Oyelere, B.L. and M.C. Kruger, *The Role of Milk Components, Pro-, Pre-, and Synbiotic Foods in Calcium Absorption and Bone Health Maintenance.* Frontiers in Nutrition, 2020.**7**: p. 182.

[7] Mukai, T., et al., *Binding of Bifidobacterium bifidum and L. reuteri to the carbohydrate moieties of intestinal glycolipids recognized by peanut agglutinin.* International journal of food microbiology, 2004.**90**(3): p. 357-362.

[8] Schiffrin, E.J., et al., *Immune modulation of blood leukocytes in humans by lactic acid bacteria: criteria for strain selection.* The American journal of clinical nutrition, 1997.**66**(2): p. 515S–520S.

[9] Umu, Ö.C., K. Rudi, and D.B. Diep, *Modulation of the gut microbiota by prebiotic fibers and bacteriocins.* Microbial ecology in health and disease, 2017.**28**(1): p. 1348886.

[10] Arevalo-Villena, M., et al., *Biotechnological application of yeasts in food science: starter cultures, probiotics and enzyme production.* Journal of applied microbiology, 2017.**123**(6): p. 1360-1372.

[11] Markowiak, P. and K. Śliżewska, *Effects of probiotics, prebiotics, and synbiotics on human health.* Nutrients, 2017.**9**(9): p. 1021.

[12] Yang, J., et al., *In vitro characterization of the impact of selected dietary fibers on fecal microbiota composition and short chain fatty acid production.* Anaerobe, 2013.**23**: p. 74-81.

[13] Valcheva, R. and L.A. Dieleman, *Prebiotics: Definition and protective mechanisms.* Best Practice and Research Clinical Gastroenterology, 2016.**30**(1): p. 27-37.

[14] Heimann, E., M. Nyman, and E. Degerman, *Propionic acid and butyric acid inhibit lipolysis and de novo lipogenesis and increase insulin-stimulated glucose uptake in primary rat adipocytes.* Adipocyte, 2015.**4**(2): p. 81-88.

[15] Machiels, K., et al., *A decrease of the butyrate-producing species Roseburia hominis and F. prausnitzii defines dysbiosis in patients with ulcerative colitis.* Gut, 2014.**63**(8): p. 1275-1283.

[16] Canani, R.B., M. Di Costanzo, and L. Leone, *The epigenetic effects of butyrate: potential therapeutic implications for clinical practice.* Clinical epigenetics, 2012.**4**(1): p. 1-7.

[17] Rodrıguez-Cabezas, M., et al., *Intestinal anti-inflammatory activity of dietary fiber (Plantago ovata seeds) in HLA-B27 transgenic rats.* Clinical nutrition, 2003.**22**(5): p. 463-471.

[18] Tedelind, S., et al., *Anti-inflammatory properties of the short-chain fatty acids acetate and propionate: a study with relevance to inflammatory bowel disease.* World journal of gastroenterology: WJG, 2007.**13** (20): p. 2826.

[19] Weng, M., W.A. Walker, and I.R. Sanderson, *Butyrate regulates the expression of pathogen-triggered IL-8 in intestinal epithelia.* Pediatric research, 2007.**62**(5): p. 542-546.

[20] Yan, F. and D.B. Polk, *Probiotic bacterium prevents cytokine-induced apoptosis in intestinal epithelial cells.* Journal of biological chemistry, 2002. **277** (52): p. 50959-50965.

[21] Mack, D.R., et al., *Extracellular MUC3 mucin secretion follows adherence of Lactobacillus strains to intestinal epithelial cells in vitro.* Gut, 2003. **52**(6): p. 827-833.

[22] Salzman, N.H., et al., *Enteric defensins are essential regulators of intestinal microbial ecology.* Nature immunology, 2010. **11**(1): p. 76-82.

[23] Tao, Y., et al., *Soluble factors from Lactobacillus GG activate MAPKs and induce cytoprotective heat shock proteins in intestinal epithelial cells.* American Journal of Physiology-Cell Physiology, 2006. **290**(4): p. C1018-C1030.

[24] Ewaschuk, J.B., et al., *Secreted bioactive factors from B. infantis enhance epithelial cell barrier function.* American journal of physiology-gastrointestinal and liver physiology, 2008. **295**(5): p. G1025-G1034.

[25] Buckley, A. and J.R. Turner, *Cell biology of tight junction barrier regulation and mucosal disease.* Cold Spring Harbor perspectives in biology, 2018. **10**(1): p. a029314.

[26] Parnell, J.A. and R.A. Reimer, *Prebiotic fibers dose-dependently increase satiety hormones and alter Bacteroidetes and Firmicutes in lean and obese JCR: LA-cp rats.* British Journal of Nutrition, 2012. **107**(4): p. 601-613.

[27] Cani, P.D., et al., *Gut microbiota fermentation of prebiotics increases satietogenic and incretin gut peptide production with consequences for appetite sensation and glucose response after a meal.* The American journal of clinical nutrition, 2009. **90**(5): p. 1236-1243.

[28] Ashaolu, T.J., *Immune boosting functional foods and their mechanisms: A critical evaluation of probiotics and prebiotics.* Biomedicine & Pharmacotherapy, 2020. **130**: p. 110625.

[29] Rad, A.H., F. Akbarzadeh, and E.V. Mehrabany, *Which are more important: Prebiotics or probiotics?* Nutrition, 2012. **28**(11/12): p. 1196.

[30] Gibson, G.R. and M.B. Roberfroid, *Dietary modulation of the human colonic microbiota: introducing the concept of prebiotics.* The Journal of nutrition, 1995. **125**(6): p. 1401-1412.

[31] Manning, T. and G. Gibson, *Microbial-gut interactions in health and disease.* Prebiotics. Best Pract. Res. Clin. Gastroenterol, 2004. **18**(2): p. 287-298.

[32] Plaza-Diaz, J., et al., *Mechanisms of action of probiotics.* Advances in Nutrition, 2019. **10**(suppl_1): p. S49-S66.

[33] Gibson, G.R. and X. Wang, *Enrichment of bifidobacteria from human gut contents by oligofructose using continuous culture.* FEMS microbiology letters, 1994. **118**(1-2): p. 121-127.

[34] Van der Meulen, R., et al., *In vitro kinetic analysis of oligofructose consumption by Bacteroides and Bifidobacterium spp. indicates different degradation mechanisms.* Applied and environmental microbiology, 2006. **72**(2): p. 1006-1012.

[35] Rad, A.H., et al., *Do probiotics act more efficiently in foods than in supplements?* Nutrition, 2012. **28**(7/8): p. 733.

[36] Lourens-Hattingh, A. and B.C. Viljoen, *Yoghurt as probiotic carrier food.* International dairy journal, 2001. **11**(1-2): p. 1-17.

[37] Guandalini, S., E. Cernat, and D. Moscoso, *Prebiotics and probiotics in irritable bowel syndrome and inflammatory bowel disease in children.* Beneficial microbes, 2015. **6**(2): p. 209-217.

[38] Hibberd, A.A., et al., *Intestinal microbiota is altered in patients with colon cancer and modified by probiotic intervention.* BMJ open gastroenterology, 2017. **4**(1): p. e000145.

[39] Tan-Lim, C.S.C. and N.A.R. Esteban-Ipac, *Probiotics as treatment for food allergies among pediatric patients: a meta-analysis.* World Allergy Organization Journal, 2018. **11**(1): p. 1-13.

[40] Hasslöf, P. and C. Stecksén-Blicks, *Probiotic bacteria and dental caries.* The Impact of Nutrition and Diet on Oral Health, 2020. **28**: p. 99-107.

[41] Kraft-Bodi, E., et al., *Effect of probiotic bacteria on oral Candida in frail elderly.* Journal of dental research, 2015. **94**(9_suppl): p. 181S–186S.

[42] Amin, N., et al., *Probiotics and bone disorders: the role of RANKL/RANK/OPG pathway.* Aging clinical and experimental research, 2020. **32**(3): p. 363-371.

[43] International Osteoporosis Foundation. *Osteoporosis - Incidence and burden*. 2017; Available from: https://www.iofbonehealth.org/facts-statistics.

[44] Montazeri-Najafabady, N., et al., *Supportive role of probiotic strains in protecting rats from ovariectomy-induced cortical bone loss.* Probiotics and antimicrobial proteins, 2019. **11**(4): p. 1145-1154.

[45] Matsumoto, S., et al., *Probiotic Lactobacillus-induced improvement in murine chronic inflammatory bowel disease is associated with the down-regulation of pro-inflammatory cytokines in lamina propria mononuclear cells.* Clinical & Experimental Immunology, 2005. **140**(3): p. 417-426.

[46] Vincenzi, A., M.I. Goettert, and C.F.V. de Souza, *An evaluation of the effects of probiotics on tumoral necrosis factor (TNF-α) signaling and gene expression.* Cytokine & Growth Factor Reviews, 2020.

[47] Lin, Y.P., et al., *Probiotic L. reuteri suppress proinflammatory cytokines via c-Jun.* Inflammatory bowel diseases, 2008. **14**(8): p. 1068-1083.

[48] Bermudez-Brito, M., et al., *Probiotic mechanisms of action.* Annals of Nutrition and Metabolism, 2012. **61**(2): p. 160-174.

[49] Abu-Amer, Y., *NF-κB signaling and bone resorption.* Osteoporosis International, 2013. **24**(9): p. 2377-2386.

[50] Sjögren, K., et al., *The gut microbiota regulates bone mass in mice.* Journal of bone and mineral research, 2012. **27**(6): p. 1357-1367.

[51] McCabe, L.R., et al., *Probiotic use decreases intestinal inflammation and increases bone density in healthy male but not female mice.* Journal of cellular physiology, 2013. **228**(8): p. 1793-1798.

[52] Ohlsson, C., et al., *Probiotics protect mice from ovariectomy-induced cortical bone loss.* PLoS One, 2014. **9**(3): p. e92368.

[53] Parvaneh, M., et al., *L. helveticus (ATCC 27558) upregulates Runx2 and*

Bmp2 and modulates bone mineral density in ovariectomy-induced bone loss rats. Clinical interventions in aging, 2018. **13**: p. 1555.

[54] Kim, J.G., et al., *Effects of a L. casei 393 fermented milk product on bone metabolism in ovariectomised rats.* International Dairy Journal, 2009. **19**(11): p. 690-695.

[55] Parvaneh, K., et al., *Probiotics (B. longum) increase bone mass density and upregulate Sparc and Bmp-2 genes in rats with bone loss resulting from ovariectomy.* BioMed research international, 2015. **2015**.

[56] Rodrigues, F.C., et al., *Yacon flour and B. longum modulate bone health in rats.* Journal of medicinal food, 2012. **15**(7): p. 664-670.

[57] Britton, R.A., et al., *Probiotic L. reuteri treatment prevents bone loss in a menopausal ovariectomized mouse model.* Journal of cellular physiology, 2014. **229**(11): p. 1822-1830.

[58] Collins, F.L., et al., *L. reuteri 6475 increases bone density in intact females only under an inflammatory setting.* PloS one, 2016. **11**(4): p. e0153180.

[59] Kruger, M.C., et al., *The effect of L. rhamnosus HN001 on mineral absorption and bone health in growing male and ovariectomised female rats.* Dairy Science and Technology, 2009. **89**(3-4): p. 219-231.

[60] Ghanem, K., I. Badawy, and A. Abdel-Salam, *Influence of yoghurt and probiotic yoghurt on the absorption of calcium, magnesium, iron and bone mineralization in rats.* Milchwissenschaft, 2004. **59**(9-10): p. 472-475.

[61] Narva, M., et al., *Effects of long-term intervention with L. helveticus-fermented milk on bone mineral density and bone mineral content in growing rats.* Annals of nutrition and metabolism, 2004. **48**(4): p. 228-234.

[62] Narva, M., et al., *Effects of bioactive peptide, valyl-prolyl-proline (VPP), and L. helveticus fermented milk containing VPP on bone loss in ovariectomized rats.* Annals of Nutrition and Metabolism, 2007. **51**(1): p. 65-74.

[63] Narva, M., et al., *The effect of L. helveticus fermented milk on acute changes in calcium metabolism in postmenopausal women.* European Journal of Nutrition, 2004. **43**(2): p. 61-68.

[64] Tomofuji, T., et al., *Supplementation of broccoli or B. longum–fermented broccoli suppresses serum lipid peroxidation and osteoclast differentiation on alveolar bone surface in rats fed a high-cholesterol diet.* Nutrition Research, 2012. **32**(4): p. 301-307.

[65] Kimoto-Nira, H., et al., *Anti-aging effect of a lactococcal strain: analysis using senescence-accelerated mice.* British Journal of Nutrition, 2007. **98**(6): p. 1178-1186.

[66] Schwarzer, M., et al., *L. plantarum strain maintains growth of infant mice during chronic undernutrition.* Science, 2016. **351**(6275): p. 854-857.

[67] Garcia, V., et al., *Effect of the probiotic Saccharomyces cerevisiae on ligature-induced periodontitis in rats.* Journal of periodontal research, 2016. **51**(1): p. 26-37.

[68] Messora, M.R., et al., *Probiotic therapy reduces periodontal tissue destruction and improves the intestinal morphology in rats with ligature-induced periodontitis.* Journal of periodontology, 2013.**84** (12): p. 1818-1826.

[69] Zhang, J., et al., *Loss of bone and Wnt10b expression in male type 1 diabetic mice is blocked by the probiotic L. reuteri.* Endocrinology, 2015. **156**(9): p. 3169-3182.

[70] Madsen, K.L., et al., *Lactobacillus species prevents colitis in interleukin 10 gene–deficient mice.* Gastroenterology, 1999. **116**(5): p. 1107-1114.

[71] Srutkova, D., et al., *B. longum CCM 7952 promotes epithelial barrier function and prevents acute DSS-induced colitis in strictly strain-specific manner.* PloS one, 2015. **10**(7): p. e0134050.

[72] Lambert, M.N.T., et al., *Combined bioavailable isoflavones and probiotics improve bone status and estrogen metabolism in postmenopausal osteopenic women: a randomized controlled trial.* The American journal of clinical nutrition, 2017. **106**(3): p. 909-920.

[73] Taverniti, V. and S. Guglielmetti, *The immunomodulatory properties of probiotic microorganisms beyond their viability (ghost probiotics: proposal of paraprobiotic concept).* Genes & nutrition, 2011. **6**(3): p. 261-274.

[74] Ashwini, A., et al., *Reactive mechanism and the applications of bioactive prebiotics for human health.* Journal of microbiological methods, 2019. **159**: p. 128-137.

[75] Coudray, C., et al., *Effects of inulin-type fructans of different chain length and type of branching on intestinal absorption and balance of calcium and magnesium in rats.* European journal of nutrition, 2003. **42**(2): p. 91-98.

[76] Coudray, C., et al., *Dietary inulin intake and age can significantly affect intestinal absorption of calcium and magnesium in rats: a stable isotope approach.* Nutrition Journal, 2005. **4**(1): p. 1-8.

[77] Scholz-Ahrens, K.E., Y. Açil, and J. Schrezenmeir, *Effect of oligofructose or dietary calcium on repeated calcium and phosphorus balances, bone mineralization and trabecular structure in ovariectomized rats.* British Journal of Nutrition, 2002. **88**(4): p. 365-377.

[78] Tahiri, M., et al., *Five-week intake of short-chain fructo-oligosaccharides increases intestinal absorption and status of magnesium in postmenopausal women.* Journal of Bone and Mineral Research, 2001. **16**(11): p. 2152-2160.

[79] Zhang, F., K.K. Yung, and C. KongYeung, *Effects of common prebiotics on iron status and production of colonic short-chain fatty acids in anemic rats.* Food Science and Human Wellness, 2021. **10**(3): p. 327-334.

[80] Takahara, S., et al., *Fructooligosaccharide consumption enhances femoral bone volume and mineral concentrations in rats.* The Journal of nutrition, 2000. **130**(7): p. 1792-1795.

[81] Ohta, A., et al., *A combination of dietary fructooligosaccharides and isoflavone conjugates increases femoral bone mineral density and equol production in ovariectomized mice.* The Journal of nutrition, 2002. **132**(7): p. 2048-2054.

[82] Kim, Y.-Y., et al., *The effect of chicory fructan fiber on calcium absorption and bone metabolism in Korean postmenopausal women.* Nutritional sciences, 2004.

[83] Kruger, M.C., et al., *Differential effects of calcium-and vitamin D-fortified milk with FOS-inulin compared to regular milk, on bone biomarkers in Chinese pre-and postmenopausal women.* European journal of nutrition, 2016. **55**(5): p. 1911-1921.

[84] van den Heuvel, E.G., M.H. Schoterman, and T. Muijs, *Transgalactooligosaccharides stimulate calcium absorption in postmenopausal women.* The Journal of nutrition, 2000. **130**(12): p. 2938-2942.

[85] van den Heuvel, E.G., et al., *Oligofructose stimulates calcium absorption in adolescents.* The American journal of clinical nutrition, 1999. **69**(3): p. 544-548.

[86] Holloway, L., et al., *Effects of oligofructose-enriched inulin on intestinal absorption of calcium and magnesium and bone turnover markers in postmenopausal women.* British Journal of Nutrition, 2007. **97**(02): p. 365-372.

[87] Hicks, P.D., et al., *Total calcium absorption is similar from infant formulas with and without prebiotics and exceeds that in human milk-fed infants.* BMC pediatrics, 2012. **12**(1): p. 1-6.

[88] Yap, K., et al., *Dose–response effects of inulin on the fecal short-chain fatty acids content and mineral absorption of formula-fed infants.* Nutrition & Food Science, 2005.

[89] Bakirhan, H. and E. Karabudak, *Effects of inulin on calcium metabolism and bone health.* International Journal for Vitamin and Nutrition Research, 2021.

[90] Hemarajata, P. and J. Versalovic, *Effects of probiotics on gut microbiota: mechanisms of intestinal immunomodulation and neuromodulation.* Therapeutic advances in gastroenterology, 2013. **6**(1): p. 39-51.

[91] Den Hond, E., B. Geypens, and Y. Ghoos, *Effect of high performance chicory inulin on constipation.* Nutrition Research, 2000. **20**(5): p. 731-736.

[92] Sharma, S. and S. Puri, *Prebiotics and lipid metabolism: a review.* Altern Ther Health Med, 2015. **21**(suppl 3): p. 34-42.

[93] Ferrarese, R., et al., *Probiotics, prebiotics and synbiotics for weight loss and metabolic syndrome in the microbiome era.* Eur Rev. Med Pharmacol Sci, 2018. **22**(21): p. 7588-7605.

[94] Bolognani, F., et al., *Effect of lactobacilli, bifidobacteria and inulin on the formation of aberrant crypt foci in rats.* European journal of nutrition, 2001. **40**(6): p. 293-300.

[95] Reddy, B.S., R. Hamid, and C. Rao, *Effect of dietary oligofructose and inulin on colonic preneoplastic aberrant crypt foci inhibition.* Carcinogenesis, 1997. **18**(7): p. 1371-1374.

[96] Reddy, B.S., *Prevention of colon cancer by pre-and probiotics: evidence from laboratory studies.* British Journal of Nutrition, 1998. **80**(S2): p. S219-S223.

[97] Ishizu, T., et al., *Prebiotic Food Intake May Improve Bone Resorption in Japanese Female Athletes: A Pilot Study.* Sports, 2021. **9**(6): p. 82.

[98] Scholz-Ahrens, K.E., et al., *Effects of probiotics, prebiotics, and synbiotics on mineral metabolism in ovariectomized rats—impact of bacterial mass, intestinal absorptive area and reduction of bone turn-over.* Nfs Journal, 2016. **3**: p. 41-50.

Chapter 12

The Domino Effects of Synbiotic: From Feed to Health

Flávia Pelá

Abstract

Around of 60,000 tons per year of antibiotics are consumed to produce our food through subtherapeutic dosage usage which aim is improve healthy and performance of animal in intensive system production. If the use of antibiotics allowed greater access to food, on the other hand, it allowed a selective pressure of antimicrobial resistant strains, the superbugs. Considered a worldwide public health problem, this ultimately led to the prohibition of antibiotics as growth enhancers in animal production and the synbiotic, prebiotic and probiotic, is claimed to be effective alternative to withdraw of antibiotics in poultry farm. Hence, in this chapter, an antimicrobial resistance, animal health regulatory affairs and synbiotic influences will be summarized. The results of scientific assays and field trials from our synbiotics commercial formulations will be described to concerning the effect of zootechnical performance and sanitary control in the poultry production.

Keywords: synbiotics additive, antimicrobial resistance, poultry production, quality food, human health

1. Introduction

The human health is intrinsically associated from health and nutrition to animal and plants. This direct proportionality stems from the fact of that animals and plant, as food, can be by a direct source of contamination by pathogens, is been a common strain or an antimicrobial resistance strain [1].

The constant growth of human population rise the food demand which imply in a better intensive animal productivity. The intensive system has several challenges to produce eggs, meat, milk, fish and others, with high productivity, low costs and a quality and safety standard conditions. One of the most practices to improve the animal production is a use of subtherapeutic dosages of antibiotics for animal growth performance and sanitary control [1].

However, since 1970, the international agencies like as World Health Organization (WHO), Food and Agriculture Organization of the United Nations (FAO), U.S. Food and Drug Administration (FDA), World Organization for Animal Health (OIE) are doing severe appointments through by global public campaign for limit and/or ban the use of antibiotics as feed additive, because, this subtherapeutic practical for growth performance is one of the causes that triggers antimicrobial resistance from the selective pressure carried out by antibiotics [2–4].

Antimicrobial resistance, nowadays, is one of public health problem in the world. Each year it causes the death of more than 700,000 people worldwide, which the most common serotypes of infections are being Salmonella ssp., followed by

Escherichia coli and *Staphylococcus aureus*. Spending on patient care is high, reaching costs of around $29,000 per patient in the United States.

Efforts to substitute the antibiotics are occurring and the synbiotics additive has been one of potential alternative feed additives for the banned antibiotic-based stimulators [2–4].

Synbiotic is described by "a mixture comprising live microorganisms and substrate(s) selectively utilized by host microorganisms that confers a health benefit on the host" [5]. Refers to nutritional supplements combining prebiotic and probiotic in complementary or synergism form which will beneficially affect the host by improving the implantation of live microbial dietary supplements in gastrointestinal (TGI) tract by selectively stimulating the growth and/or by activating the metabolism of one on limited number of health promoting bacteria [6, 7].

The mechanisms of synbiotic influence the host is the prebiotic stimulates growth of probiotic bacteria or the prebiotic and probiotic act independently in the GIT tract, both stimulating the intestinal microbiota. Non-digestible elements (prebiotics) are fermented in the GIT, while beneficial live microorganisms (probiotics) colonize it [5].

In this chapter, an antimicrobial resistance, animal health regulatory affairs and synbiotic influences will be summarized. The results of scientific assays and field trials from our synbiotics commercial formulations will be described to concerning the effect of zootechnical performance and sanitary control in the poultry production.

2. The domino effect

2.1 Antibiotic resistance

Antibiotics are in fact one of the best drugs developed. Initially applied for the treatment of infections, these drugs revolutionized modern medicine and changed the therapeutic paradigms [8]. Discovered in 1928 by Alexandre Fleming with penicillin, successive antimicrobials were developed and applied in the period between 1930 and 1960, the golden age [9–11]. However, concurrently with the findings, resistance to antibiotics has been identified, with the marked increase in patients relapsing to the infection of common bacterial pathogens. The truth is that every molecule used in the treatment of bacteria, fungi, parasites, viruses and, still, chronic diseases, by biochemical and physiological mechanisms favor the potential development of tolerance or resistance to the compound since the first use [10, 11]. This resistance associated with factors such as: overpopulation, improved global migration, indiscriminate use of antibiotics, as well as, the incorrect use neglecting the prescribed treatment, the intensification of animal production and the underdosing used as a zootechnical additive, selective pressure and basic sanitation precarious conditions have accentuated antibiotic resistance by living beings, making it one of the most important threats to public health in the 21st century, according to the WHO [2, 8, 12].

Results of genomic studies indicate the existence of more than 20,000 potential resistance genes (r genes) with about 400 different types [10], which mutation, horizontal gene transfer, conjugation and transduction are key hypothesis of the selective pressure that contributes to the distribution and co-selection of resistance and virulence genes. The impact of this selective pressure is reflected in the mechanisms of action of pathogenic strains that, in general, can modify the target site of antibiotics on the chromosome, promote the efflux of the molecule and degrade or modify the conformation of the compounds through enzymatic actions, thus favoring colonization and invasion of pathogens and, consequently, causing damage to the host by expressing clinical picture of infection [9, 12–14].

Li *et al*. in a metagenomic assay identified profiles of a wide spectrum of multiresistance genes from different environments. These profiles were correlated and grouped according to incidence, and the results showed a higher prevalence of multiresistance genes in animal feces and in residual water from farms, followed by sewage and human feces, STP effluents, STP ADS and STP AS & BF and, finally, in drinking water, rivers, soils and sediments [15].

The result by Li *et al*. corroborates with the identification of multiresistance genes in animal production environments systems from the practice of indicating subtherapeutic amounts of antibiotics to animals for the purpose of improving performance [8, 9, 15]. In addition to the zootechnical performance, the increase in the intensive practice of animal husbandry, with overcrowding of the sheds, absent or precarious hygiene and disinfection practices, increased the prophylactic use of antibiotics. [8]. It is estimated that 60,000 ton per year are consumed on agricultural farms, and 80% of antibiotics consumed in the USA are used in livestock, with around 27 different antimicrobial classes being used in animals [9–11]. Antibiotics depending on the drug and the species treated will have an absorption or metabolization range between 10–80%, with the remainder being excreted as active compounds in the urine and feces to the environment. Thus, soils, water, effluents are contaminated and the selective pressure on the microbiota of these environments is selected, increasing the resistance to antibiotics [9–11]. In the holistic analysis of the ecosystem, each environment and living being serves as a regulator or regulated agent of selective pressure to multiresistance genes, serving an evolutionary cycle.

Unfortunately, global resistance to antibiotics has no tendency to decline. Data show that around 700,000 deaths per year worldwide are due to antimicrobial resistance. In Europe this number is 33,000 and the estimative of resistance to antibiotics represents a costs of €1.5 billion per year with healthcare expenses and productivity losses. In the US, the of deaths is 99,000, estimated cost with patients treatment is about $20 billion and the social costs reach $35 billion. In the Americas, about 77 million people per year fall ill after consuming contaminated food. Out of these, nine thousand die. In Brazil, from 2007 to 2016, 90.5% of the cases of foodborne diseases were caused by bacteria, mostly *Salmonella spp* (7.5%), followed by *Escherichia coli* (7, 2%) and *Staphylococcus aureus* (5.8%). Therefore, coordinated efforts to implement new policies to regulate the use of antibiotics, stimulate the research efforts and seek measures to manage the crisis are necessary to maintain intensive livestock productivity, animal and human health, and the ecosystem balance [2–4].

2.2 Animal health regulatory affairs

As an effort to reduce the antimicrobial resistance promoted by antibiotics used asr growth promoter, international agencies are searching to regulate a tolerance levels to antibiotics used for animals. The problem has been obtain similar commitments by the WHO, FAO and OIE in which measures of banned or establishment of minimum tolerance level of the drug shall be evaluated for mitigated noise and, consequently, avoid opportunities to inappropriate use of antimicrobial [16].

Despite the divergences, countries have been establishing regulatory measures regarding the use of antibiotics as growth promoters. The Europe (EU), in 2006, finished the progressive elimination of antibiotics program, used as growth promoters, banning sodium monensin, sodium salinomycin, avilamycin and flavophospholipol. These final measures aim to combat the emergence of superbugs, due to antibiotics overexploitation or misuse [17–19]. In 2017, the European

Commission adopted a "EU AMR Action Plan" which the key objectives are to make EU an example practice region; improve the research, development and innovation; and, shape the global agenda. Nowadays, since the plan implementation, updates have been made in order to further strengthen EU's response to AMR, such as, Pharmaceutical Strategy for Europe, creation of a new EU authority named Health Emergency Response Authority (HERA), creation of Commission Implementing Decision (EU) 2020/1729 for monitor and report antimicrobial resistance; adoption a tool Farm to Fork Strategy for sustainable food systems, implementation of Regulation (EU) 2019/6 on Veterinary Medicinal Products (VMP Regulation) and Regulation (EU) 2019/4 on Medicated Feed (MF), an implementation of better animal welfare, and others [20, 21].

In United States (USA), the antibiotic reforms were difficult, marked by constant clashes with the industries. Only from 2000, some formal procedures were started to withdrawal the antibiotics in animals for growth promoters. In 2013, FDA published a guidance for industry to phase out antibiotic growth promotion via label changes [22, 23]. In 2017, the completed implementation of guidance represented a changed of antimicrobial drugs used in the feed animal production. Of the 292 animal drug applications, 84 were banned and 208 remaining applications were converted from over the counter to prescription status or to veterinary feed directive status [23].

In Brazil, the Ministry of Agriculture, Livestock and Supply, through Normative Instruction N° 45, of November 22, 2016, prohibited the import and manufacture of the antimicrobial substance colistin sulfate with a performance-enhancing zootechnical additive throughout the territory in animal feeding [24]. Ordinance N°·195, of July 4, 2018 establishes good management practices in commercial farms, in order to obtain sustainable production, preserving health and well-being [25]. Furthermore, Ordinance N° 171, of December 13, 2018, informed that the use of the antimicrobials tylosin, lincomycin, bacitracin and tiamulin is prohibited for the purpose of performance-enhancing additives in farm animals [26].

Despite the alarming situation that resistance to antimicrobials has triggered in public health worldwide and the repeated appeals to reduce the inclusion of antibiotics in animal production by internationals agencies, many low- and middle-income countries do not include these recommendations in their national commitments. China is a country example: considered one of the largest consumers of antibiotics in livestock animals, elaborated a National Action Plan to Combat Antimicrobial Resistance from Animal Resources which regulates the withdraw all antibiotics used as feed additive; revised indicative use that antimicrobials are used only for prevention or treatment and stablished that new approvals of antimicrobials are only indicate for veterinary medicine [27]. South Africa, in 2018, by Africa Centers for Disease Control and Prevention (Africa CDC) has also developed a national framework plan which aimed detect to respond the infectious diseases in country [28].

In summary, the overview commitments of the recommendations are: i) implement a global public campaign to awareness about the importance to reduce antimicrobial used; ii) improve practical of hygiene and disinfections in daily routine either for human health or for animal management; iii) reduce the indiscriminate use of antimicrobials; iv) develop new diagnostics tools for rapid and reliable assay, including for accuracy monitoring antimicrobial development; v) improve management procedures for disease prevention and control; vi) develop sustainable and effective substitutes for antibiotics in animal production system [29].

During recent years, efforts focused to develop and work on providing novel and alternative supplements for growth performance and therapeutics to prevent diseases and enhance animal immunity. One of the potential substitutes evaluate is the synbiotic additive.

2.3 Synbiotic mode of action: an overview

The synbiotic concept is "a mixture comprising live microorganisms and substrate(s) selectively utilized by host microorganisms that confers a health benefit on the host". The symbiotic term is a Greek word compound of prefix 'syn', meaning 'together' and the suffix 'biotic', meaning 'pertaining to life' [5]. The prebiotic and probiotic combination product might not have any co- dependent function, acting trough by complementary and synergistic mechanisms. Both, independently promote an eubiosis, a maintain physiology homeostasis, modulating the digestive and immune system, and others functions in the host. The synbiotic product can be applied to intestinal or extra-intestinal microbial ecosystems in human, animals and agricultural species by regulatory categories, such as, feed additive, foods, non-foods, nutritional supplements or drugs [5].

The symbiotic formulation performs its function in a gastrointestinal tract, where more than 100 trillion (10^{14}) microorganisms inhabit. The resident microbial groups are affected by endogenous factors, such as, temperature, pH, oxygen concentration, diet, secretions, and others. Particularly, diets rich in non-digestible ingredient can highly modify the composition and function of gut microbiota by selectively influence [5, 30].

These non-digestible food ingredient as named prebiotics was described as "a non-digestible components of food, fiber or non-carbohydrate digestible, that beneficially affects the host by selectively stimulating the growth and/or activity of one or a limited number of bacteria in the colon, and thus improves host health" [5, 30–32]. The criteria for prebiotic classification are: i) resist acidic pH, digestion action and adsorption by their host; ii) should be metabolized or fermented by microorganism residing in the TGI tract; iii) should promote a microbiota selectively stimulation, conferring beneficial physiological effect on the host; iv), not to all or poorly metabolized by pathogenic organism in gut bowel [5, 30, 31]. Most commonly known and characterized prebiotics include inulin, fructooligosaccharide (FOS), glucooligosaccharide (GOS), mannanoligosaccharide (MOS) [5, 30–33].

Prebiotics are considered a specific fuel that indigenous probiotic bacteria can utilize to grow. The selective fermentation of prebiotic occurs through correlation between chemical oligosaccharide structure and biochemicals metabolites of gut microbiota. The presence of carbon anomeric, the molecular weight and the number of branching present in prebiotic structure select microbiome preferences. For example, *Bifidobacterium sp* prefer to ferment low weight molecular of trisaccharides and tetrasachhrides in a series of oligosaccharides with reduced number of branching [30]. Beside this, the prebiotic metabolization by gut microbiome are influenced by secretion of a wide range of specific enzymes such as polysaccharidases, aminopeptidases, proteases, glycosidases, glycanases and others that will digest the prebiotics in a monomeric constituent. These parameters influence results the microbiome selective fermentation and explain the a non-digestion of prebiotic by host enzymes and the non-metabolization of them by pathogens strains, such as, *Salmonella spp.*, *E. coli*, and *Clostridial* population [30, 32].

Furthermore, the metabolic fermentation results in a lactic acid, short-chain fatty acid (SCFA), or some antibacterial substances, such as bacteriocins, leading to a reduction of the metabolic activity of potentially harmful bacteria [30–34]. In general, the SCFA acts acidifying the luminal pH which suppresses the growth of pathogens, influence intestinal motility and acts stimulating enterocytes proliferation and mucin secretion. The rapidly absorption of SCFA by the enteric mucosa contributes to the quickly supply of host's energy requirements. Furthermore, they can be recognized by protein coupled receptors (GPR) expressed on polymorphonuclear immune cells, enterocytes and enteroendocrine cells stimulating the chemokine and cytokines expression, such as, pro-inflammatory IL-2 and interferon (IFN)-γ and immuno-regulatory IL-10 production [30, 32, 33].

In addition, to modulating the immune system by SCFA, prebiotics can be direct recognized by toll-like receptors (TLRs) and NOD-like receptors (NLRs), both a pattern recognition receptor (PRR) present in immune membrane cells. This recognition will modulate the innate immune response inducing an overexpression of innate immune cells such as epithelial cells, macrophages, mast and dendritic cells. Another way of prebiotic action in immune systems is promoting the recognition of PAMPs signs by PRR, activating innate immune cells and the production of cytokines [30, 32, 33].

Finally, new scientific results correlate show that prebiotics also accelerate uptake of various micronutrients like iron, zinc, and calcium and significantly reduces or prevent the chances of colon-associated cancers, cholesterol, and elevated levels of triacylglycerols [30, 32, 33].

For establishment of health microbiota in host, probiotics play an important role enhancing the gut balance. Several studies revealed that supplementation of probiotics has positive impacts on TGI tract development and on the immune system modulation, consequently, improving the feed efficiency ratio, nutrient absorption, growth performance and the animal productivity. Probiotics are defined as "Live microorganisms which when administered in adequate amounts confer a health benefit on the host" [35].

There are several species with probiotics abilities such as live bacteria, *Bacillus sp., Lactobacillus sp, Bifidobacterium sp,* yeast, *Saccharomyces cerevisiae* and *Saccharomyces boulardii*, fungi, *Aspegillus*, which are isolated from fermented products and human and animal body like as gut, breast milk, feces and other [36]. A good probiotic should have the following characteristics: i) the fermentation process should result in a minimum $1x10^9$ CFU culture; ii) the stain should be specie specify with high ability to survive and multiply fast in TGI tract host; iii) should be stable and safe to the host, GRAS 0, resisting an acid and bile action; iv) should have an ability in maintaining the normal physiology of host animals by strong adhesive capability in TGI tract, an effective competitive exclusion to reduce pathogenic microorganisms, and others; v) should have a durable shelf-life of commercial manufacturing, processing and distribution [36, 37].

The mode of action of probiotics in animal includes: i) maintaining normal intestinal microflora by competitive exclusion and antagonism; ii) altering metabolism by increasing digestive enzyme activity and decreasing bacterial enzyme activity and ammonia production; iii) improving feed intake and digestion; iv) and neutralizing enterotoxins and stimulating the immune system [38].

The main major mechanisms triggered by probiotics described are: i) modulation of the physical–chemical environment; ii) synthesis of biologically active molecules with antimicrobial properties; iii) and, modulation of the immune system.

The modulation of the physical–chemical environment of the enzymatic activities through the gastrointestinal tract and enzymatic activities catabolism stimulate the food's energy and protein digestibility which favors, the absorption of nutrients promoting the growth of the probiotic microbiota in detriment of the pathogenic one by the establishment of competition between them. This dynamic is called competitive exclusion. Concomitant to competitive exclusion, probiotics are also able to decrease the gut pH, though fermentation of carbohydrates providing an inhospitable environment for pathogenic bacteria, which are more susceptible to acidic pH. This is called growth modulation by pH. Still, the consumption of lactic acid by lactic bacteria and yeast strains can occur, which will result in the buffering of the TGI tract and the production of organic acids and vitamins [39–41].

Regarding the synthesis of biologically active molecules, the production of bacteriocins, antibiotics, free fatty acids, hydrogen peroxide is mentioned, among others, in particular, when there is the establishment of the probiotic microbiota to the gastrointestinal mucosa. These biologically active molecules control the proliferation and/or survival of the surrounding microorganisms. For example, bacteriocins are cited as peptides or proteins that kill related bacteria by permeabilizing their cell membranes or by interfering with the structure of their essential enzymes [42–44]. Another benefit comes from the increase in the concentration of propionate, succinate, valerate which, as precursors of gluconeogenesis, favor the availability of glucose to the animal, favoring the increase production, as well as its quality [45].

Concerning the intestinal homeostasis, there are literature describing the commensal intestinal microbiota as the main modulator of host physiology. The presence of probiotics adhered to the intestinal mucosa forms the so-called intestinal barrier capable of reducing the installation of pathogenic microorganisms, interfering with intestinal permeability, increasing the degradation of enteric antigens, as well as altering their immunogenicity. The repercussion of probiotic activity in the intestine implies an immunological homeostasis which in adverse contexts will favor immunological tolerance through the development of tolerogenic dendritic cells, regulatory T cells, Toll-Like Receptors (TLR), production of cytokines, according to immunological balance patterns [46–50].

In summary, the ability of synbiotics to do a protective effect on the intestinal microbiota may be dependent of multiple factors regulations such as formulation composition, indicative use dosage, host's genetic background, age and health status, hygiene and disinfections ambient conditions and treatment condition and duration.

2.4 From feed to health: the influence of Synbiotic commercial formulations in the poultry farm

In 2019, around of 100 thousand tons of poultry meat were produced in worldwide, being the U.S the world production leader followed by China and Brazil. The combined production of these countries represents half of the world poultry meat production [51]. In the exports, Brazil is a largest exporter with 4,200 ton shipped to more than 150 countries [52]. In 2020, this number increased on4% in production due to the national consumption increase and due to continuity of Chinese demand for animal protein. Also, the consumption of eggs increased as well [53].

This rising in the poultry production impacted in increase of 3.6% in feed production and, consequently, in a higher consumption of macronutrients and micronutrients that compose them. Around 16,494 tons of zootechnical additives were consumed in 2020, in which 10,144 tons were enzyme consumption, 4,947 tons were prebiotics and probiotics and 1403 tons were performance enhancers [53].

Through a comparative analysis of this data to the same parameters rescued from 2011, it is possible to of almost 50% in the consumption of performance enhancers and an increase of 1649% in the consumption of prebiotics and probiotics. In 2011, 5,628 tons of additives were consumed in poultry production, distributed in 2,434 tons of enzymes, 2895 tons of antibiotics growth promoter and 300 tons of prebiotics and probiotics [54].

The expressive increase of prebiotics and probiotics consumption is a consequence of the guidelines of the international agencies about antimicrobial resistance, the prohibition of the use of certain antibiotics as a growth promoter, the elaboration and execution of the National Action Plan on Antimicrobial Resistance in Agriculture and the adjustments in the production chain in order to comply with the requirements of the foreign market.

The significant changes in the growth of commercial poultry have focused on intestinal development from two related but different directions. The tremendous genetic progress for largely grown poultry at ever decreasing ages turn recognize the first week posthatch represent a significant period of avian development and have a critical influence for intestinal growth. Immediately posthatch, the small intestine has proportional weight as body weight and will increase around 30% at 3 days. The contents of the residual yolk nutrients can be transferred to blood and intestine up 72 h, it represents a faster fed in chicks supplying their energy demand. At 7 days-old, the intestine will be twice as heavier weight than at day 1. Significant differences in villus height and crypt depth at day 3 from hatch noted, emphasizing the importance of intestinal development related to supporting accelerated growth and the importance of the intestinal given by histological measurements. A critical point in posthatch is the logistics of the chicks to the farm. During this period the birds are not feed with specific food, so they are susceptible to the environmental microbiota and, as a consequence, to a pathogen colonization [55, 56].

In this scenario of posthatch, in our trial research to evaluation of a commercial probiotic product, dispersive powder, composed by $3.5x10^7$ CFU/g *Bifidobacterium bifidum*, $3.5x10^7$ CFU / g *Enterococcus faecium*, 3, $5x10^7$ CFU/g *Lactobacillus acidophilus*, $4x10^7$ CFU / g *Bacillus subtilis* and $4x10^7$ CFU/g *Bacillus licheniformis*, indicated for application via spray, in the hatchery, on the chicks at a final concentration of $1.23x10^7$ CFU/ml, was applied in commercial layers to evaluate the microbial profile also too the product efficacy reduce the vulnerability that can occur by pathogen colonization in the gastrointestinal tract. Swabs from intestinal fragment, jejunum and ileum junction, were realized at times zero (D0), 7 days (D7) and 32 days (D32) and analyzed by next-generation sequencing technique, for evaluated the dynamic microbiome during the development of the gastrointestinal tract, also too, the better eubiosis establishment when probiotic intake is provided to the hens in the first moment of life.

At D0, hours after supplied the hens with probiotic supplement, were identified 12 bacterial species in the samples of jejunum and ileum junction, which 3189 reads (121 reads in treated group - SG; 3068 reads in control group - CG). The bacteria species identified are *Aeromonas hydrophila* (10 reads SG; 0 read CG), *Bacillus foraminis* (9 reads SG; 0 read CG), *Bacillus persicus* (5 reads SG; 0 read CG), *Brevundimonas bullata* (0 read SG; 185 reads CG), *Deftia acidovorans* (5 reads SG; 0 read CG), *Enterococcus faecalis* (82 reads SG; 1959 reads CG), *Noviherbaspirilum canariense* (0 read SG; 137 reads CG), *Ochrobactrum anthropi* (5 reads SG; 0 read CG), *Pantoea agglomerans* (0 read SG; 288 reads CG), *Pseusomonas koreensis* (0 read SG; 275 reads CG), *Pseudomonas putida* (5 reads SG; 129 CG), *Stenotrophomonas maltophilia* (0 read SG; 95 reads CG). These microbial profiles had a statistically significant difference to the treatment variable ($f(1) = 4.56$; *p-value* = 0.0353), and to the microbial diversity variable ($f(11) = 2.04$; *p-value* = 0.0329); and statistical trend for the interaction between the variables treatment and microbial diversity (*p-value* = 0.0765).

In start of feed consumption, at the first day of the birds' life (D1), hens of treated group were supplied with commercial product composed by $5x10^7$ CFU/g *Bacillus coagulans*, $5x10^8$ CFU/g *Bacillus subtillis*, $5x10^8$ CFU / g *Bacillus licheniformis*, $5x10^7$ CFU/g *Lactobacillus acidophilus* and $2x10^7$ CFU/g of *Saccharomyces cerevisae* and 2 g/kg Mannan oligosaccharides (MOS) was insert into the extruded feed at a final concentration of $2.24x10^5$ CFU/g of feed, to continue the gastrointestinal and immune system modulation. The analysis of the microbiome profile, at D7, had have a quantification of 88989 reads (18360 reads SG; 70629 reads CG) with identification of 17 bacterial strains distributed in *Bacillus cereus* (5 reads SG; 0 read CG), *Butyticicoccus pullicaecorum* (0 read SG; 385 reads CG); *Clostridium beijerinckii* (9 reads SG; 0 read CG), *Clostridium difficile* (0 read SG; 25 reads CG), *Clostridium innocuum* (0 read SG; 26 reads CG), *Clostridium spiroforme* (0 read SG; 243 reads CG), *Enterococcus faecalis* (0 read SG; 157 reads CG), *Enterococcus gallinarum* (0 reads SG; 38 reads CG), *Erysipelatoclostridium ramosum* (0 reads SG; 135 reads CG), *Kurthia gibsonii* (0 reads SG; 27 reads CG), *Lactobacillus gasseri* (0 read SG; 7293 reads CG), *Lactobacillus helveticus* (13869 reads SG; 1526 reads CG), *Lactobacillus intestinalis* (0 reads SG; 2029 reads CG), *Lactobacillus johnsonii* (0 read SG; 36340 reads CG), *Lactobacillus reuteri* (2070 reads SG;4471 reads CG); *Lactobacillus vaginalis* (6 reads SG; 659 reads CG) and *Lactobacillus oris* (0 read SG; 1076 reads CG). These results in a statistical trend for the treatment variable (f(1) = 3.50; *p-value* = 0.0657) and a statistically significant difference for the microbial diversity variable (f(16) = 2.42; *p-value* = 0.0031), and to the interaction of these variables (*p-value* = 0.0071). In addition, at D7, greater intestinal length was observed in the hens of the treated group (X = 110.77 cm, Min = 100 cm, Max = 123 cm) compared to the control group (X = 103.5 cm, Min = 91 .5 cm, Max = 115.5 cm) resulting in a statistically significant difference, *p-value* = 0.0168.

At D32, end period of the microbial profile evaluation, there were a total quantification of 85069 reads (53042 reads SG; 32027 reads CG), with 37 bacterial strains identified distribute in *Acinetobacter junii* (0 read SG; 73 reads CG), *Acinetobacter ursingii* (0 reads SG; 106 reads CG), *Brachbacterium articum* (18 reads SG; 292 reads CG), *Brachbacterium faecium* (17 reads SG; 106 reads CG), *Brevibacterium epidermidis* (985 SG reads; 1557 CG reads), *Brevibacterium senegalense* (142 SG reads; 490 CG reads), *Brevundimonas diminuta* (0 SG reads; 283 CG reads), *Clostridium ruminantium* (18790 SG reads; 4844 CG reads), *Comamonas kerstersii* (121 SG reads; 0 CG reads), *Corynebacterium stationis* (1035 SG reads; 767 CG reads), *Corynebacterium casei* (997 SG reads; 915 CG reads), *Corynebacterium nuruki* (24 SG reads; 0 CG read), *Corynebacterium terpenotabidum* (0 SG reads); 75 reads CG), *Corynebacterium variabile* (227 reads SG; 382 reads CG), *Dietzia maris* (549 reads SG; 0 read CG), *Enterococcus cecorum* (506 reads SG; 290 reads CG), *Escherichia coli* (0 read SG; 10248 reads CG), *Facklamia tabacinalis* (148 reads SG; 0 read CG), *Fusobacterium mortiferum* (62 reads SG; 0 reads CG), *Fusobacterium necrogenes* (82 reads SG; 0 read CG), *Globicatella sanguinis* (35 reads SG; 0 reads CG), *Lactobacillus agiis* (0 read SG; 142 reads CG), *Lactobacillus aviarius* (611 reads SG; 0 read CG), *Lactobacillus helveticus* (21816 reads SG; 6348 reads CG), *Lactobacillus salivaris* (6061 reads SG; 1852 reads CG), *Ochrobactrum pseudogrignonense* (0 read SG; 47 reads CG), *Pantoea aeptica* (0 read SG; 121 reads CG), *Providencia rettgeri* (95 read SG; 0 read CG), *Pseudomonas veronii* (0 read SG; 41 read CG), *Staphylococcus gallinarum* (170 read SG; 178 read CG), *Staphylococcus lentus* (216 read SG; 0 read CG), *Staphylococcus saprophyticus* (229 read SG; 899 reads CG), *Staphylococcus sciuri* (18 reads SG; 0 read CG), *Streptococcus infantarius* (0 read SG; 192 reads CG), *Streptomyces rectiviolaceus* (17 reads SG; 0 reads CG), *Subdoligranulum variabile* (71 reads SG; 0 reads CG) and *Veillonela magna* (0 read SG; 1425 reads CG). There was no statistical difference for the treatment variable (f(1) = 0.81; *p-value* = 0.3692), there was statistical difference for microbial diversity variable (f(36) = 2.53; *p-value* < 0.0001), and no difference statistics for the interaction between variables (*p-value* = 0.4220).

As can be seen, immediately after posthatch, colonization of the gastrointestinal tract of the bird begins, whose quantitative and qualitative composition presents distinct microbial dynamics and profiles according to the influence of the zoogenic conditions of the environment, the components of the diet supplied to the animal, the interaction of microorganisms the physiology, metabolism and immunology of the host, and the dynamics of interaction between microorganisms to achieve the complex and dynamic establishment of the microbiota [57].

When analyzing the results of the microbial profile, at D0, the quantitative discrepancy of the microbial load present between the experimental groups is observed. Hypothetically, it is suggested that there was competitive exclusion between bacterial species: the environmental microbiota and the probiotic multi-strains supplied through the commercial product. This hypothesis is based on the analysis of the microbial distribution profile in the intestinal fragment in which an approximate percentage of pathogenic bacteria colonizing both experimental groups is observed, but with a lower microbial load in the treated group. As an example, there was a prevalence of colonization of *Enterococcus faecalis* strains (82 reads SG, 68%; 1959 reads CG, 61%; FC = 23.89) followed by *Pseudomonas putida* (5 reads SG, 4%; 129 reads CG, 4%; FC = 25.8) in both groups, however, in the control group the presence of 23.89 more *Enterococcus faecalis* and 25.8 more *Pseudomonas putida* is observed in relation to the treated group.

These same pathogenic strains prevalent at D0 are suppressed from the microbial profile at D7, at distribution of *Enterococcus spp* being 0.27% in the control group and 0% in the treated group. The genus *Pseudomonas spp* is absent in both experimental groups, which shows the occurrence of competitive exclusion in the colonization of the intestinal fragment. Still, at D7, when analyzing the microbial profile of the experimental groups, the control group showed the greatest diversity and quantity of bacterial strains colonizing the intestinal fragment, with a prevalence of 98.53% of lactic strains and the presence of pathogenic strains with 0.41% *Clostridium spp* and 0.27% *Enterococcus spp*. Meanwhile, the treated group had lower microbial diversity, but higher prevalence of lactic strains (99.92%).

This dynamic microbiota in the first life stage of chicken was also reported by Śliżewska *et al.* [58] since the posthatch, in which they observe a prevalence of coli, enterococcus and lactic bacteria genera present in the crop, duodenum and jejunum. In the first and second weeks of life, they described the prevalence of the Lactobacillus spp. genera in the composition of the gastrointestinal tract and, in the third week, the microbial constitution was distributed in *Lactobacillus spp.* (70%), *Clostridium spp.* (11%), *Streptococcus spp.* (6.5%), *Enterobacteriaceae* family bacteria (6.5%), *Enterococcus spp.* (6%), corroborating a distribution of a microbial profile close to that identified in our results. Another common correlation identified was the significant reduction of potential pathogenic bacteria such as *Escherichia coli* and *Clostridium spp* when adding the symbiotic in the feed. In summary, both results show the beneficial effects of the consumption of the synbiotic in favoring sanitary control by establishing the balance of the intestinal microbiota.

At D32, the period reported in the literature for the establishment of eubiosis, effective bacterial diversity is observed in both experimental groups, and in eubiosis the group treated with commercial synbiotic product had a higher and better microbial profile. It should be noted that the prevalence of probiotic strains in the treated group throughout the experiment, even with a smaller amount of reads identified at D0 and D7, favored the establishment of eubiosis with the proliferation of other lactic strains that benefited the development and maturation of the treatment. Gastrointestinal tract of birds. While the control group had 26% probiotic strains (*Lactobacillus agiis, Lactobacillus helveticus and Lactobacillus salivaris*), 32% *Escherichia coli*, 4% *Staphylococcus spp* and other environmental strains, the treated group had 54% probiotic strains (*Lactobacillus aviarius, Lactobacillus helveticus and Lactobacillus salivaris*), absence of *Escherichia coli*, 1% *Staphylococcus ssp* and other environmental strains, showing the impact of consumption of the synbiotic for the establishment of eubiosis with a better microbial profile in hens.

Adhikari [59] described the distribution of lactic strains along the gastrointestinal tract of birds correlated with what was identified in our results. This reports the identification of greater abundance of *Lactobacillus salivarius* and *Lactobacillus johnsonii* in all intestinal fragments analyzed: cecal lumen, cecal mucosa and ileum mucosa, with the highest concentration of lactic strains identified in the ileum mucosa and cecal lumen followed by the cecal mucosa. Similar colonization profiles of lactic strains were described by Ranjitkar *et al.* [60] and Wang et al. [61].

Dunislawska *et al.* [62] corroborate the benefits of consumption of synbiotics by describing effects of consumption of microflora-promoting bioactive compounds, even in a single dose of prebiotic or synbiotic *in ovo* and immediately posthatch, in interfering with the dynamics of microbiota colonization as well as across the entire spectrum of phenotypic characteristics in the broiler development stages, including zootechnical performance, development and modulation of the immune system, development and histological composition of the gastrointestinal tract, change in molecular expression in cecal tonsils, spleen and liver, change in the composition of meat quality.

The reflection of this dynamics of colonization of the gastrointestinal tract of birds has repercussions in various field scenarios in the results of zootechnical performance, in sanitary control and in the reduction of antimicrobial pulses administered to the birds. To report this scenario of the reality of the field, whose management variables are diverse and often distinct from each other, one of our field trials is presented. This assay was carried out on a commercial poultry farm producing broilers, which houses about 7,000,000 birds per month. Two farms, Farm 1 and Farm 2, composed of 15 and 16 sheds respectively, housed Ross lineage birds. Farm 1 had in its ambience a cepillo's bed, dating back to 1st and 2nd, conventional lighting, side plates and an oven per aviary. Farm 2 had a cepillo's bed, dating back to n°. 2, dark lighting, side and front plates and two ovens per aviary. As for the treatment, the commercial synbiotic product was composed of $5x10^7$ CFU/g *Bacillus coagulans*, $5x10^8$ CFU/g *Bacillus subtillis*, $5x10^8$ CFU/g *Bacillus licheniformis*, $5x10^7$ CFU/g *Lactobacillus acidophilus* and $2x10^7$ CFU/g of *Saccharomyces cerevisae* and 2 g/kg Mananooligosaccharide was administered on extruded feed mixture at a final concentration of 1.02x105 CFU/g feed at farm 1, while poultries from farm 2 received the probiotic product consisting of $1x10^8$ CFU CFU/g *Bifidobacterium animalis*, $6x10^8$ CFU CFU/g *Enterococcus faecium*, $2,5x10^7$ CFU/g *Lactobacillus reuteri*, $2,5x10^7$ CFU/g *Lactobacillus salivarius*, $2,5x10^8$ CFU/g CFU/g *Pediococcus acidilactici* added to the extruded feed with final concentration of $1.00x10^5$ UFC/g of feed. Farm 1 will be named as the treated group and farm 2 as the control group.

In terms of zootechnical performance, there were no statistical differences between both treatments, at the seventh day (D7), regarding weight gain, *p-value* = 0.966 (control group X = 183.2 g, Min = 159 g, Max = 203 g; treated group X = 185.4 g, Min = 167 g, Max = 228 g) and as for intestinal length, *p-value* = 0.977 (control group X = 106.2 cm, Min = 90 cm, Max = 122 cm; treated group X = 107.2 cm, Min = 94 cm, Max = 124 cm); at D14, as for weight gain, *p-value* = 0.6111 (control group X = 510.3 g, Min = 400 g, Max = 572 g; treated group X = 510.2 g, Min = 473 g, Max =542 g) and as for intestinal length, *p-value* = 0.114 (control group X = 137.9 cm, Min = 115 cm, Max = 166 cm; treated group X = 144.1 cm, Min = 125 cm, Max = 174 cm); at D21, as for weight gain, *p-value* = 0.368 (control group X = 1014 g, Min = 969 g, Max = 1118 g; treated group X = 1019 g, Min = 878 g, Max = 1145 g) and as for intestinal length, *p-value* = 0.160 (control group X = 164.2 cm, Min = 148 cm, Max = 178 cm; treated group X = 169.8 cm, Min = 153 cm, Max = 198 cm); at D28, as for weight gain, *p-value* = 0.989 (control group X = 1596 g, Min = 1435 g, Max = 1702 g; treated group X = 1600 g, Min = 1441 g, Max = 1763 g) and as for intestinal length, *p-value* = 0.808 (control group X = 187.6 cm, Min = 160 cm, Max = 220 cm; treated group X = 185.7 cm, Min = 166 cm, Max = 207 cm).

Despite the absence of significant statistics in the above results, at the end of the management, the treated group showed better performance in relation to the zootechnical results, as they had greater daily weight gain (control group = 68.82 g; treated group = 71.34 g), greater corrected slaughter weight (control group = 2573 g; treated group = 2853 g), better feed conversion (control group = 1.593; treated group = 1.571), consequently, better productivity factor (control group = 413.19; treated group = 430. 89). The only zootechnical results of the treated group with lower performance than the control group were the mortality parameter (control group = 4.27%; treated group = 5.17%) whose established hypothesis refers to the ambience, the presence of a single oven in the aviary, and the thermal challenges, variations from 8–25°C throughout the day, that the birds in the treated group went through in the first week of bird life.

As for sanitary control, it is routine in the management of farms to carry out at D21 the evaluation of the identification of the presence/absence of salmonella in the sheds using a drag swab, performing both polymerase chain reaction (PCR) methodology and the conventional method of microbial cultivation. The results for the PCR assay showed 4 positive samples for the control group and 2 positive samples for the treated group, while, for the conventional method of microbial cultivation, the control group showed 2 positive samples while the treated group did not show characteristic culture growth. These results show the best sanitary control of the synbiotic product to the sanitary control for salmonella. It is noteworthy that this drag swab is carried out in the bed of the sheds and does not necessarily reflect the presence of salmonella in the cecal content of the poultries. Further tests carried out in other poultry farms whose house received the treatment of the synbiotic product, despite showing identification of salmonella in the house and outside areas, did not show identification of salmonella in the cecal content of poultries.

As for the consumption of antibiotics, there was a significant reduction in the consumption of antibiotics in the treated group compared to the control group (FC = 0.37). The treated group consumed throughout the management three types of antibiotics which total of 33 administration pulses, while the control group consumed four types of antibiotics, totaling 89 administration pulses. The description of antibiotic consumption in the control group was, at D1, four aviaries received pulses of the antibiotic Cipronil for five days; at D7, seven farms received Trimoxil pulses for three days; at D9, 1 aviary also received Trimoxil for three days; at D13, 3 farms received Farmaxilin pulses for three days; at D20, three farms received Cipronil pulses for five days, two farms received Farmaxilin pulses for three days; and, at D28, one house received Farmaxilin pulses for three days and four houses received Amprol Base pulses for two days. While the birds in the treated group, distributed in 15 aviaries, at D7, three aviaries received Farmaxilin pulses for three days; at D18, two farms received three Farmaxilin pulses; at D26, two aviaries received three pulses of Amprol Base; at D29, one aviary received three pulses of Cipronil and three aviaries received three pulses of also Amprol Base.

There is an adversity in comparing the results of zootechnical performance obtained on the commercial farm with results published in the literature, as the indications for use of synbiotic products and the experimental environment variables are distinct and extrapolate the behavior of commercial products in the development of the gastrointestinal tract of birds. In short, when evaluating the results described by Syed *et al.* [63] whose treatment 4 (T4) used the same commercial synbiotic product present in the control group, but with an indication for use 5.00x10^5 CFU/g of feed, if the control group had a lower performance in body weight gain than reported by the authors, but with a performance similar to that observed by the treated group whose inclusion of synbiotic product was five times more lower (BWG = 2573 g CG, BWG = 2983.9 g T4 and BWG = 2853 g SG). The feed conversion rate also differs in the experimental and field settings, in this variable, the corrected feed conversion rate was better in the treated group, followed by the control group and treatment 4 (FCR = 1.57 SG, FCR = 1.59 CG and FCR = 1.87 T4). Finally, mortality, whose treatment 4 showed better results compared to the control group and the treated group (Mortality (%) = 1.11 T4, Mortality (%) = 4.27 CG and Mortality (%) = 5.17 SG). In conclusion, the treated group prevailed with better results in 2 of the 3 variables compared in zootechnical performance. The zootechnical results obtained in both experiments are a reflection of several variables such as management and ambience protocols, nutritional quality of the feed as well as the composition and indication of use of zootechnical additives, environment and sanitary challenges. And, these results are reproduced and can also be compared to the results described by Śliżewska *et al.* [58], Abdel-Wareth *et al.* [64] and others.

Synbiotic products in sanitary control promote resistance to infections by favoring morphological changes to the intestinal mucosa, developing longer villus, smaller crypts and better villus/crypt ratios, also by reducing the gastrointestinal pH due to higher lactic acids and by mitigating frequency and histopathological lesions [64]. Results described by Mora et al. [65] report the sanitary control of *Salmonella Typhimurium* and *Clostridium Perfringens* when birds are supplemented with symbiotics. Shanmugasundaram et al. [66], Markazi et al. [67], Luoma et al. [68], Asahara et al. [69], also report a reduction in salmonella proliferation in the cecum of birds.

It was not possible to carry out a comparative evaluation of the reduction in the consumption of antibiotics in therapeutic dosages, as a result of the use of synbiotics in the animals' diet and also of different compositions of synbiotics. The results presented are unprecedented and effectively report the benefits that the consumption of certain synbiotics influences on the modulation of animal health and reflects on the residual reduction of these antimicrobial agents in meat and the environment, as well as on the operational result of the creation.

It is in this dual scenario between science and the reality of the field that it is important to highlight the equalization between basic science and the application of development and innovation carried out in research centers, because although experimental tests are essential for the development and proof of new products, the reality of management on commercial farms presents adverse variables and challenges, often even unpredictable, that will compromise the zootechnical performance of the birds, the final quality of this food and, consequently, the operating result of the farm, on the health of the final consumer that consumes the food and in the environment that receives the residues from the handling operation.

The complexity of correlating the mode of action of synbiotic effects in poultry production demonstrates the wide spectrum of opportunities that science has to develop to understand all pathways influenced by prebiotics and probiotics in the TGI tract. Scientific results showed a specific interaction with the environment, the host and the synbiotic formulation. In addition, it demonstrated that the synbiotic participates in metabolic pathways little described in the scientific literature.

In summary, the results of scientific and field tests have shown a beneficial effect of all elaborated synbiotics on the balance of the intestinal microbiota, its metabolism and the performance of broiler chickens. Supports the ability of commercial synbiotic products to replace the use of antibiotics as a growth performance in order to mitigate rising antimicrobial resistance.

3. Conclusion

Synbiotic formulations are a potential choice to withdraw antibiotic as growth promoter. The complementary or synergic action of synbiotic improve the poultry production and control infections disease. Further studies should be developed to identify target microorganism's species according to farm management conditions. The hope is that, going forward, the prebiotic, probiotic or synbiotic will have greater representativeness among feed additive, reducing the use of antibiotics and the selective pressure of microorganism. Advances in symbiotic research will promote better understanding of interested parties, enabling better communication with consumers.

Acknowledgements

The author thanks Vanderson Camilo, João Ito, Marissol Cardoso, Kelly Pereira, Alisson Rotter and Filipe Ribeiro for their input and assistance in preparation of this review. This research was supported by PolySell Chemical Products LTDA.

Conflict of interest

The author declares no conflict of interest.

Author details

Flávia Pelá
Poly Sell Chemical Products LTDA, Brazil

*Address all correspondence to: flavia@polysell.com.br

References

[1] Markowiak P. & ŚliżewskaK. The role of probiotics, prebiotic and synbiotics in animal nutrition Gut Pathog.2018,10:21. DOI: https://doi.org/10.1186/s1

[2] Antimicrobial resistance and foods of plant origin [Internet]. Food and Agriculture Organization of United Nations, 2018. Available from: http://www.fao.org/3/BU657en/bu657en.pdf. Accessed on March 20, 2021.

[3] Bondad-Reantaso, MG., Lavilla-Pitogo CR., Karunasagar, I., Arthur, J.R., Hao, B., Irde, E., Garrido Gamarro, E. and Peñarubia, O.R. Outputs and activities of FAO Project FMM/RAS/298/MUL on antimicrobial resistance in fisheries and summary of FAO's recent work on antimicrobial resistance in aquaculture. FAO, 2020. Fisheries and Aquaculture Circular No. 1215. Rome, FAO.https://doi.org/10.4060/cb1209en

[4] Caruso G. Antibiotic Resistance in *Escherichia coli* from Farm Livestock and Related Analytical Methods: A Review. J AOAC Int. 2018; 1;101(4):916-922. DOI: 10.5740/jaoacint.17-0445.3099-018-0250-0

[5] Swanson KS., Gibson GR., Hutkins R., Reimer RA., Reid G., Verbeke K., Scott KP., Holscher HD., Azad MB., Delzenne NM., Sanders ME. The International Scientific Association for Probiotics and Prebiotics (ISAPP) consensus statement on the definition and scope of synbiotic. Nat Rev Gastroenterol Hepatol. 2020;17(11):687-701. DOI: 10.1038/s41575-020-0344-2.

[6] Hamasalim HJ. Synbiotic as feed additives relating to animal health and performance. Advances in Microbiology. 2016. 6, 288-302. http://dx.doi.org/10.4236/aim.2016.64028

[7] Sharma R., Sharma S., Shukla PC., Sharma V., Baghel RPS., Raikwar A., Pradhan S., Yadav V. The Pharma Innovation Journal 2018; 7(7): 62-68. DOI:

[8] Aminov RI. The role of antibiotics and antibiotic resistance in nature. Environ Microbiol. 2009; 11(12):2970-2988. DOI: 10.1111/j.1462-2920.2009.01972.x.

[9] Aslam B., Wang W., Arshad MI, Khurshid M., Muzammil S., Rasool MH., Nisar MA., Alvi RF., Aslam MA., Qamar MU., Salamat MKF., Baloch Z. Antibiotic resistance: a rundown of a global crisis. Infect Drug Resist. 2018; 11: 1645-1658. DOI: 10.2147/IDR.S173867.

[10] Davies J & Davies D. Origins and evolution of antibiotic resistance. Microbiol Mol Biol Ver 2010;74(3):417-433. DOI: 10.1128/MMBR.00016-10.

[11] Ventola CL. The Antibiotic Resistance Crisis. Part 1: Causes and Threats. P T. 2015; 40(4): 277-283. PMC4378521.

[12] Martinez JL. General principles of antibiotic resistance in bacteria. General principles of antibiotic resistance in bacteria. Drug Discovery Today: Technologies, 2014. 11, 33-39. DOI:10.1016/j.ddtec.2014.02.001.

[13] Munita J.M. & Arias C. A. Mechanisms of Antibiotic Resistance. Microbiol Spectr. 2016; 4(2):10.1128/microbiolspec. VMBF-0016-2015. DOI: 10.1128/microbiolspec. VMBF-0016-2015.

[14] Marshall BM., Levy SB. Food animals and antimicrobials: impacts on human health. Clin Microbiol Rev. 2011;24(4):718-733. DOI: 10.1128/CMR.00002-11.

[15] Li, B. et al. Metagenomic and network analysis reveal wide

distribution and co-occurrence of environmental antibiotic resistance genes. ISME J. 2015;9(11):2490-2502. DOI: 10.1038/ismej.2015.59.

[16] Innes GK., Randad PR., Korinek A., Davis MF, Price LB., So AD., Heaney CD. External Societal Costs of Antimicrobial Resistance in Humans Attributable to Antimicrobial Use in Livestock. Annu Rev Public Health. 2020; 41: 141-157. DOI:10.1146/annurev-publhealth-040218-043954.

[17] European Comission. Regulation 1831/2003/EC on additives for use in animal nutrition, replacing Directive 70/524/EEC on additives in feeding-stuffs. Downloaded from: https://eur-lex.europa.eu/legal-content/EN/TXT/?uri=CELEX%3A32003R1831. Accessed on March 20, 2021.

[18] Millet S & Maertens L. The European ban on antibiotic growth promoters in animal feed: from challenges to opportunities. Vet J. 2011;187(2):143-144. DOI: 10.1016/j.tvjl.2010.05.001.

[19] Castanon JIR. History of the use of antibiotic as growth promoters in European poultry feeds. Poult Sci. 2007;86(11):2466-2471. DOI: 10.3382/ps.2007-00249.

[20] European Comission. EU Action on Antimicrobial Resistance. Downloaded from: https://ec.europa.eu/health/antimicrobial-resistance/eu-action-on-antimicrobial-resistance_en. Accessed on March 20, 2021.

[21] European Comission. Farm to folk strategy. 2020. Downloaded from: https://ec.europa.eu/food/farm2fork_en. Accessed on March 20, 2021.

[22] Kirchhelle C. Pharming animals: a global history of antibiotics in food production (1935-2017). Palgrave Communications. 2018. Vol. 4, N°.96. DOI: 10.1057/s41599-018-0152-2.

[23] U.S. Food and Drug Administration (FDA). Timeline of FDA Action on Antimicrobial Resistance. Downloaded from: https://www.fda.gov/animal-veterinary/antimicrobial-resistance/timeline-fda-action-antimicrobial-resistance. Accessed on March 20, 2021.

[24] Ministry of Agriculture, Livestock and Supply (MAPA). Normative Instruction No 45, of November 22, 2016. Downloaded from: https://www.gov.br/agricultura/pt-br/assuntos/insumos-agropecuarios/insumos-pecuarios/alimentacao-animal/arquivos-alimentacao-animal/legislacao/instrucao-normativa-no-45-de-22-de-novembro-de-2016.pdf/view. Accessed on March 20, 2021.

[25] Ministry of Agriculture, Livestock and Supply (MAPA). Ordinance No.195, of July 4, 2018. Downloaded from: https://www.in.gov.br/materia/-/asset_publisher/Kujrw0TZC2Mb/content/id/29305677/do1-2018-07-10-portaria-n-195-de-4-de-julho-de-2018-29305658. Accessed on March 20, 2021.

[26] Ministry of Agriculture, Livestock and Supply (MAPA). Ordinance No 171, of December 13, 2018. Downloaded from: https://www.in.gov.br/materia/-/asset_publisher/Kujrw0TZC2Mb /content/id/55878469/do1-2018-12-19-portaria-n-171-de-13-de-dezembro-de-2018-55878239. Accessed on March 20, 2021.

[27] Hu YJ & Cowling BJ. Reducing antibiotic use in livestock, China. Downloaded from: https://www.who.int/bulletin/volumes/98/5/19-243501/en/. Accessed on March 20, 2021.

[28] Selaledi LA., Hassan ZM., Manyelo TG., Mabelebele M. The Current Status of the Alternative Use to Antibiotics in Poultry Production: An African Perspective. Antibiotics (Basel). 2020;11;9(9):594. DOI: 10.3390/antibiotics9090594.

[29] Marquardt RR., LI S. Antimicrobial resistance in livestock: advances and alternatives to antibiotics. Anim Front. 2018. 19;8(2):30-37. DOI: 10.1093/af/vfy001.

[30] Roberfroid M., Gibson GR, Hoyles L, McCartney AL., Rastall R., Rowland I., Wolvers D., Watzl B., Szajewska H., Stahl B., Guarner F., Respondek F., Whelan K., Coxam V., Davicco MJ, Léotoing L., Wittrant Y., Delzenne NM., Cani PD, Neyrinck AM, Meheust A. Prebiotic effects: metabolic and health benefits. Br J Nutr. 2010;104 Suppl 2:S1-63. DOI: 10.1017/S0007114510003363.

[31] Gibson GR. Dietary modulation of the human gut microflora using prebiotics. British Journal of Nutrition.1998; 80(S2), S209–S212. DOI:10.1017/S0007114500006048.

[32] Althubiani AS., Al-Ghamdi SB., Qais SFA., Khan MS., Ahmad I., Malak HA. Chapter 4 - Plant-Derived Prebiotics and Its Health Benefits. Advancements in Herbal Products as Novel Drug Leads. 2019, 63-88. DOI: https://doi.org/10.1016/B978-0-12-814619-4.00004-5

[33] Teng PY. & Kim WK. Review: Roles of Prebiotics in Intestinal Ecosystem of Broilers. Front. Vet. Sci. 5:245. DOI: 10.3389/fvets.2018.00245

[34] Davani-Davari D., Negahdaripour M., Karimzadeh I., Seifan M., Mohkam M., Masoumi SL., Berenjian A., Ghasemi Y. Prebiotics: Definition, Types, Sources, Mechanisms, and Clinical Applications. Foods. 2019; 8(3): 92. DOI: 10.3390/foods8030092.

[35] Food and Agriculture Organization of the United Nations (FAO). Probiotics in animal nutrition: production, impact and regulation. 2016. ISBN 978-92-5-109333-7

[36] Patterson JA. & Burkholder KM. Application of Prebiotics and Probiotics in Poultry Production. Poultry Science. 2003; 82:627-631. DOI: https://doi.org/10.1093/ps/82.4.627

[37] Khan RU, Naz S. The applications of probiotics in poultry production. World's Poultry Science Journal. 2013. 69(3), 621-632. DOI:10.1017/s0043933913000627

[38] Jin LZ., Ho YW, Abdullah N., Jalaludin S. Probiotics in poultry: modes of action. World's Poultry Science Journal. 1997. 53 (4) 351-368. DOI: https://doi.org/10.1079/WPS19970028

[39] Fong W., Li Q. & Yu J. Gut microbiota modulation: a novel strategy for prevention and treatment of colorectal cancer. Oncogene. 2020;39, 925-4943. DOI: https://doi.org/10.1038/s41388-020-1341-1

[40] Yirga, H. The use of probiotics in Animal Nutrition. Journal of Probiotics & Health. 2015. 3 (2) DOI: 10.4172/2329-8901.1000132

[41] Kim CH, Park J, Kim M. Gut microbiota-derived short-chain Fatty acids, T cells, and inflammation. Immune Netw. 2014; 14:277-288 DOI: 10.4110/in.2014.14.6.277

[42] Gillor O., Etzion A. & Riley MA. The dual role of bacteriocins as anti- and probiotics. Appl Microbiol Biotechnol. 2008 Dec; 81(4): 591-606. DOI: 10.1007/s00253-008-1726-5

[43] Dobson A, Cotter PA, Ross RP & Hill C. Bacteriocin Production: a Probiotic Trait? Appl Environ Microbiol. 2012 Jan; 78(1): 1-6. DOI: 10.1128/AEM.05576-11

[44] Vieco-Saiz N., Belguesmia Y., Raspoet R., Auclair, E., Gancel, F., Kempf, I., Drider, D. Benefits and Inputs From Lactic Acid Bacteria and Their Bacteriocins as Alternatives to

Antibiotic Growth Promoters During Food-Animal Production. Frontiers in Microbiology. 2019. 10(), 57–. DOI:10.3389/fmicb.2019.00057

[45] Engevik MA & Versalovic J. Biochemical features of beneficial microbes: foundations for therapeutic microbiology. Microbiol Spectr. 2017. 5(5) DOI: 10.1128/microbiolspec. BAD-0012-2016

[46] La Fata G, Weber P & Mohajeri M.H. Probiotics and the Gut Immune System: Indirect Regulation. Probiotics & Antimicro. Prot. 2018. 10:11-21. DOI: 10.1007/ s12602-017-9322-6.

[47] Ashraf R & Shah NP. Immune system stimulation by probiotic microorganisms, critical. Reviews in Food Science and Nutrition. 2014. 54:7, 938-956, DOI: 10.1080/10408398.2011.619671

[48] Belkaid Y. & Hand TW. Role of the microbiota in immunity and inflammation. Cell. 2014; 157(1): 121-141. DOI: 10.1016/j.cell.2014.03.011

[49] Hardy H., Harris J., Lyon E., Beal J, Foey AD. Probiotics, prebiotics and immunomodulation of gut mucosal defences: homeostasis and immunopathology. Nutrients. 2013; 5(6): 1869-1912. DOI: 10.3390/ nu5061869

[50] Calder PC. Feeding the immune system. Proc Nutr Soc. 2013;72(3):299-309. doi: 10.1017/S0029665113001286.

[51] Brazilian Agricultural Research Corporation (Embrapa). Poultry and swine intelligence center - Production performance statistics. 2021. Downloaded from: https://www. embrapa.br/suinos-e-aves/cias/ estatisticas. Accessed on March 21, 2021.

[52] Brazilian Agricultural Research Corporation (Embrapa). Poultry and swine intelligence center - Statistics | World | Broilers. 2021. Downloaded from: https://www.embrapa.br/suinos-e-aves/cias/estatisticas/frangos/mundo. Accessed on March 21, 2021.

[53] Sindirações. Boletim informativo do setor. 2021. Downloaded from https:// sindiracoes.org.br/produtos-e-servicos/ boletim-informativo-do-setor/. Accessed on March 21, 2021.

[54] Ministério do desenvolvimento, indústria e comércio exterior. Estudo de Viabilidade Técnica e Econômica destinado à implantação do Parque Produtivo Nacional de Aditivos da Indústria de Alimentação de Animais de Produção. 2012. Downloaded from: http://www.asbram.org.br/wp3/ wpcontent/uploads/2015/11/Estudo_ de_aditivos_da_industria_de_ alimentacao_de_anima is_de_producao. pdf Accessed on March 21, 2021.

[55] Lilburn MS. & Loeffler S. Early intestinal growth and development in poultry. Poultry Science. 2015. 94 (7) 1569-1576. DOI: 10.3382/ps/pev104

[56] Rubio LA. Possibilities of early life programming in broiler chickens via intestinal microbiota modulation. Poultry Science. 2019; 2(1) 695-706. DOI: https://doi.org/10.3382/ps/pey416

[57] Pan D & Yu Z. Intestinal microbiome of poultry and its interaction with host and diet. Gut Microbes. 2014; 5(1), 108-119. DOI: http://dx.doi.org/10.4161/gmic.26945

[58] Śliżewska K, Markowiak-Kopeć P, Żbikowski A & Szeleszczuk P. The effect of synbiotic preparations on the intestinal microbiota and her metabolism in broiler chickens. Scientific Reports. 2020; 10:4281 DOI: https://doi.org/10.1038/ s41598-020-61256-z

[59] Adhikari B. Investigation of Microbiota in Health and Disease of

Poultry. Theses and Dissertations. 2019, 3371. DOI: https://scholarworks.uark.edu/etd/3371

[60] Ranjitkar S, Lawley B, Tannock G & Engberg RM. Bacterial Succession in the Broiler Gastrointestinal Tract. Appl Environ Microbiol. 2016, 82(8): 2399-2410. DOI: 10.1128/AEM.02549-15.

[61] Wang Y, Sun J, Zhong H *et al*. Effect of probiotics on the meat flavour and gut microbiota of chicken. Scientific Reports. 2017, 7 6400. DOI:10.1038/s41598-017-06677-z.

[62] Dunislawska A, Slawinska A, Stadnicka K *et al*. Synbiotics for Broiler ChickensÐIn Vitro Design and Evaluation of the Influence on Host and Selected Microbiota Populations following In Ovo Delivery. PLoS ONE. 2016, 12(1): e0168587. DOI: 10.1371/journal.pone.0168587.

[63] Syed B, Wein S & Ruangapanit Y. The Efficacy of Synbiotic Application in Broiler Chicken Diets, Alone or in Combination with Antibiotic Growth Promoters on Zootechnical Parameters. J. World Poult. Res. 2020, 10(3): 469-479. DOI: https://dx.doi.org/10.36380/jwpr.2020.54

[64] Abdel-Wareth A. A.A, Hammad S, Khalaphallah, Rafat. et al. Synbiotic as eco-friendly feed additive in diets of chickens under hot climatic conditions. Poultry Science, 2019, 98, 4575-4583. DOI: 10.3382/ps/pez115.

[65] Mora ZV, Nuño K, Vázquez-Paulino O, *et al. Effect* of a synbiotic mix on intestinal structural changes, and *Salmonella typhimurium* and *Clostridium perfringens* colonization in broiler chickens. Animals. 2019, 9, 777.DOI:10.3390/ani9100777

[66] Shanmugasundaram R, Mortada M, Cosby DE *et al*. Synbiotic supplementation to decrease Salmonella colonization in the intestine and carcass contamination in broiler birds. PLoS ONE. 2019, 14(10): e0223577. DOI: https://doi.org/10.1371/journal.

[67] Markazi A, Luoma A, Shanmugasundaram, R. *et al.* Effects of drinking water synbiotic supplementation in laying hens challenged with Salmonella. Poultry Science, 2018, 97:3510-3518. DOI: http://dx.doi.org/10.3382/ps/pey234

[68] Luoma A, Markazi A, Shanmugasundaram, R. *et al.* Effect of synbiotic supplementation on layer production and cecal Salmonella load during a Salmonella challenge. Poultry Science. 2017, 0:1-9. DOI: http://dx.doi.org/10.3382/ps/pex251

[69] Asahara T, Nomoto K, Shimizu K. *et al.* Increased resistance of mice to *Salmonella enterica* serovar Typhimurium infection by synbiotic administration of Bifidobacteria and transgalactosylated oligosaccharides. Journal of Applied Microbiology. 2001, 91, 985±996. DOI: 10.1046/j.1365-2672.2001.01461.x

Chapter 13

Benefits of Probiotics on Aflatoxin Infected Birds

Muhammed Jimoh Ibrahim

Abstract

Aflatoxin are transferred from feed to animal products (Eggs, Meats and Milk). There is need to find alternative chemicals that is economically friendly to reduce the impact of aflatoxins. Probiotics additives especially Lactobacillus and Bacillus spp. biodegradation generally decreases aflatoxin residues in milk, egg and meat. They are low cost, economically friendly and accessible additives which could mitigate aflatoxin formation in feed and food. There is need for aggressive public health awareness on the implication of aflatoxin residues and as well as detoxification strategy that can reduce toxin absorption into animal feed.

Keywords: Probiotics, birds, aflatoxin, residues, implication

1. Introduction

Food safety is effectively achieved when the food pillars, such as; food availability, food access, food utilization, and food stability which permit individual at any time to have access to affordable, safe and healthy food to meet daily nutrient requirement [1]. Weakens of this four pillar pose a treat to food security. Human health and animal welfare are influenced by food insecurity and contaminant, which reflect on social and economic status of a society. Mycotoxin during pre, processing and post-harvest are driving factors of food insecurity since contamination occurs along the food value chain from farm to fork [2]. Poultry products are important international food commodity. Economic losses may occur due to the presence of natural feed contaminants, such as mycotoxins, which are secondary metabolites produced by certain toxigenic aflatoxins [3], poultry-derived products such as meat and eggs are carry-over of aflatoxin into the human food value chain which serve as potential threat to human health [4–7]. Contaminated food and feeds with aflatoxin prohibit trade of international concern [8]. The regulations on "acceptable health risk" usually depend on a country's level of economic development, extent of consumption of high-risk crops, and the susceptibility to contamination of crops to be regulated [9]. Safety limit of aflatoxin consumption for human ranges 4–30 mg/kg. European Union has set the strictest standards, which establishes that any product for direct human consumption cannot be marketed with a concentration of AF-B1 and total AFs greater than 2 mg/kg and 4 mg/kg, respectively [10–12]. Likewise, US regulations have specified the maximum acceptable limit for AFs at 20 mg/kg [13–16]. Worldwide European Union aflatoxin standard is adopted, meeting this standard Sub-Sahara Africa and Asia encounter both economic losses and financial costs. This situation requires alternative technologies at pre- and post-harvest levels aimed to minimize contamination of commercial foods and feeds, at least to ensure that AF levels remain below safe limits [15, 16].

Physical, chemical and biological approaches have been conducted to degrade mycotoxin. Most of these method are unsafe due to losses in the nutritional value, cost of equipment, and formation of intermediate metabolite [17]. Biological detoxification using microorganisms or enzymatic preparations is promising [18]. Probioitcs such as *Rhodococcus erythropolis*, *Armillariella tabescens*, and *Myxococcus fulvu, Rhizopus oryzaes, Pseudomonas sp* and *Bacillus subtilis*, have been reported to have different AF-degrading ability [19–21]. *Bacillus subtilis* applied directly on the feedstuffs degrade 81.5% AFB1 and 85% ZEA in naturally contaminated feed in vitro [22, 23]. *B. subtilis* had protective effects against aflatoxicosis in layers and broilers fed naturally AF-contaminated diets [24–26]. It is therefore, important to identify benefits of probiotics on aflatoxin contaminated poultry products to effectively monitor carry-over of residues to sustain healthy living and socioeconomic development.

1.1 Mycotoxin

Mycotoxin refers to harmful secondary metabolites produced by fungi in food and feed products that negatively impact animal and human health, by themselves or through synergistic interactions with each other [27]. Mycotoxins are structurally diverse low-molecular weight secondary metabolites produced by fungal growth [27]. Aspergillus, Penicillium, and Fusarium contaminate feed and food consumed by animals and humans. Globally, millions of dollars are losses annually on mycotoxins, on agricultural products, animal and human health [15].

1.2 Aflatoxins

Aflatoxins are polyketide secondary metabolites produced by toxigenic strains of *Aspergillus, Penicillium, Fusarium* and *Alternaria* fungi [28, 29]. They grow on a variety of nutritional substrates like cereals which is the main active ingredient of poultry and human food [30]. They are extremely harmful to the health of humans and animals, showing changes in biochemical and hematological indices effecting metabolism via alteration of enzymatic pathways of starch, proteins, lipids and nucleic acids. Hence, serum glutamate pyruvatate transaminase, serum gluatamate oxaloacetate tranferase and γ-glutamyl transferase activities are increased, inciting; hepatotoxic, carcinogenic, mutagenic, teratogenic, immunosuppressive actions and in severe intoxications may cause death [31–38]. Acute or chronic aflatoxicosis in poultry results in retarded growth, decreased production and egg quality, impaired immune response, increased mortality and liver and intestine damage [39, 40]. AF is also known to interfere with metabolism of vitamin D, iron and copper and can cause leg weakness. Aflatoxin has caused serious destructions in Africa, which has caused significant financial losses in agricultural commodities contaminated with toxins and consequently having effects on animal and human health point of view [41, 42]. Although most countries of the world has been affected by aflatoxin, it is sub-saharan Africa (SSA) that has suffered most [43]. Most of SSA agriculture occurs in impoverished rural areas and a lack of technical infrastructure in many African countries does not allow for routine quality control of even commercially produced commodities, never mind those produced by rural population for their own consumption [43]. Ultimately, the transmission of AF and its metabolites from feed to animal edible tissues and products, such as liver and eggs, becomes a potential hazard for human health.

1.2.1 Types of aflatoxins

Among the 18 different types of aflatoxins identified, the major members are aflatoxin B1 (AFB1), B2 (AFB2), G1 (AFG1) and G2 (AFG2), which are produced by *Aspergillus flavus* and *Aspergillus parasiticus A. nomius* [44]. M1 (AFM1) and M2 (AFM2) are metabolites of AFB1 and AFB2 in human and animal milk fed on contaminated food. Aflatoxin B1 (AFB1) being the most toxic among other species. Additionally other species which produce aflatoxin are *A. pseudotamarii, A. ochraceoroseus, A. rambellii, A. toxicarius* [45]. In addition other fungi of the genera *Aspergillus* (e.g. *A. ochraceus* and *A. carbonarius*) produces another important mycotoxin ochratoxin A (OTA) [38, 46]. *A. flavus* and *A. parasiticus* varies from highly toxigenic to non-toxigenic forms and are produced by AFB1 than AFG1. *A. parasiticus* are produce by AFB1 and varying amounts of AFB2, AFG1 and AFG2 with variable toxigenicity [47]. Aflatoxins B occur more frequently as contaminants, and are also believed to be more potent, than Aflatoxins G [48].

1.2.2 Chemical structure

Chemically aflatoxin B occur they are difuro-coumorins –cyclopentenone and difurocoumaro lactone series which are freely soluble in chloroform and methanol [49, 50], Other aflatoxins have different substitutes but share basic coumarine structure. The epoxidation of the 8, 9-double bond and cyclopentenone ring of B series is responsible for the order of acute and chronic toxicity as compared with the six-membered lactone ring of the G series AFB1 > AFG1 > AFB2 > AFG2 (**Figure 1**) [49].

1.2.3 Physical structure

Structurally they are dihydrofuran-coumorins moiety containing double bond which are freely soluble in chloroform and methanol. They are stable at high temperatures but unstable to UV light or polar solvents [49, 51]. Aflatoxins are toxic secondary metabolites upon exposure to fluorescence ultra violet (UV) light, aflatoxin B appear blue in color and G appear green in color (**Table 1**) [49, 52].

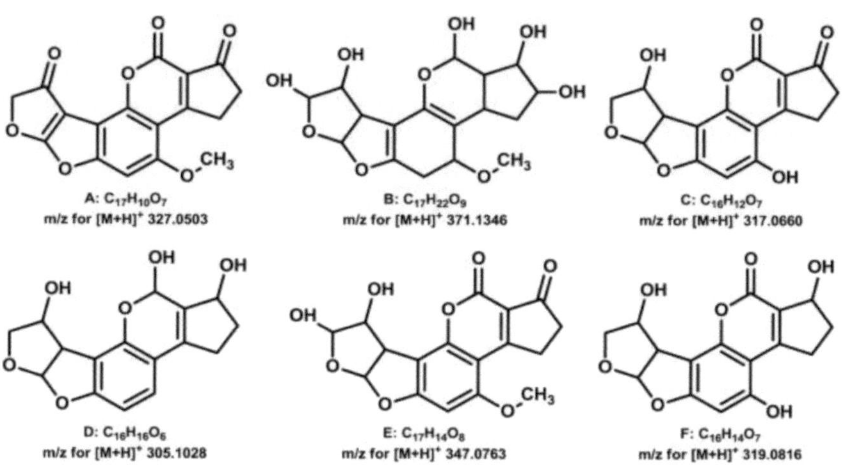

Figure 1.
Chemical properties of aflatoxin B and G (A–F). Source: Adapted from Agriopoulou et al. [38].

Aflatoxin	Molecular formular	Molecular weight	Melting point °C
B1	$C_{17}H_{12}O_6$	312	268–269
B2	$C_{17}H_{14}O_6$	314	286–289
G1	$C_{17}H_{12}O_7$	328	244–246
G2	$C_{17}H_{14}O_7$	330	237–240
M1	$C_{17}H_{12}O_7$	328	299
M2	$C_{17}H_{14}O_7$	330	293
B2A	$C_{17}H_{14}O_7$	330	240
G2A	$C_{17}H_{14}O_8$	346	190

Source: International Crop Research Institute for Semi-Arid Tropics.
Adapted from: Reddy et al. [49]

Table 1.
Physical properties of aflatoxins.

1.3 Occurrence of aflatoxin in food and feed

Eggs, milk and meat are sometimes contain residues of aflatoxins because of consumption of aflatoxin contaminated feed ingredients such as peanuts, cottonseed, nuts, almonds, figs, spices, soybean, rice and maize [53].

1.4 Mode of action

Cytochrome P450 enzymes (phase I metabolisation) convert aflatoxins to a reactive 8,9-epoxide form, which is essential for the toxicity. In mammals CYP1A2 and CYP3A4 are the enzymes responsible for conversion [54] in chicken and turkeys, the corresponding enzymes are CYP2A6 and to a lesser extent CYP1A1 orthologs [55, 56]. DNA and protein binds to guanine residues of nucleic acids to produced epoxide metabolite causing genotoxicity and cytotoxicity [57]. Aflatoxin B1-DNA adducts result in guanine-cytosine (GC) to thymine-adenine (TA) transversions [48], which leads to irreversible DNA damage, therefore results to hepatocellular carcinomas [58]. Gluthatione conjugation or hydrolysis detoxified the toxic epoxide metabolite and epoxide hydrolase to phase II metabolisation and AFB1–8,9-dihydrodiol (AFB1-dhd) respectively. AFBI Metabolisation to less toxic compounds such as aflatoxin M1 (AFM1) or Q1 (AFQ1) [54, 56]. AFM1 metabolite possesses carcinogenic properties which are 10 times lower than AFB1. These metabolites obtained from cattle milk. The maximum limits in milk permissible for human consumption have been established (0.05 μg/kg) [12, 59], 20 ppb in grain and 4 ppb in food and agricultural commodities [59].

1.4.1 Carcinogenesis

The International Agency for Research on Cancer [60] classify aflatoxin as class 1 carcinogen, transversion of G to T occur in guanine codon 249 of tumor suppressor gene p53 of DNA that induce mutagenesis by alkylation of nuclear DNA, leading to carcinogenesis and teratogenesis [61]. 8, 9,-epoxide is a potent carcinogen and induces chromosomal aberrations, mutation and cell toxicity [62].

1.4.2 Immunesuppression

Immunosuppressive effects on NK cell activity, humoral and cellular immune function are impair by aflatoxin through reducing the primary and secondary immune responses [63–66]. AFB1 induces; thymic aplasia, reduce T-lymphocyte function, lymphokines, suppress phagocytic and complement activity [67, 68]. Aflatoxin suppresses the levels of IL-1, IL-2, IL-6, IFN, TNF alpha, mRNA and proinflammatory cytokines [69, 70]. Embryonic chicks exposed to AFB1 showed a depressed graft-versus-host response, thymic bursal involution, delayed cutaneous hypersensitivity, macrophages function, reduced antibody titers to vaccines for Newcastle, Mareks and infectious bursal disease [32, 52, 71, 72].

1.4.3 Nutritional

In poultry a drop in feed conversion efficiency and decreased growth rate is observed following a chronic exposure to aflatoxin feed [73]. Aflatoxin modifies vitamin A nutrition in poultry halving the serum retinol and Plasma concentration of 25-hydroxyvitamin D and 1,25- dihydroxyvitamin D concentrations [48, 74]. Bennett and Klich [8], toxin has been a factor modulating the rate of recovery from protein malnutrition. Toxin contaminated diet affect zinc and selenium which are essential for healthy immune systems [75].

1.4.4 Aflatoxin control

Contamination of feed and food with aflatoxins occur during the preparation value chain. Several methods have been adopted in the prevention of aflatoxicosis in animal origin. Application of Good Agricultural Practices (GAP) are important strategy during pre-harvest. Appropriate GAP includes crop rotation, soil cultivation, irrigation and proper use of chemicals. Crop rotation is important and focuses on breaking the chain of infectious material, for example by maize/legume rotations. Any crop husbandry that includes destruction, removal or burial of the infected crop is seen as good soil cultivation. The deeper the soil is inverted (plowing), [76]. Reducing plant stress by irrigation is also valuable to prevent fungi infestation [77]. Damages caused by insects, birds and rodents increases susceptibility of aflatoxin invasion. Successive fungal infection must by controlled by appropriate use of critical pest management system and application of fungicides [77]. Climate change such as high temperature, relative humidity and drought influenced mold infection and mycotoxin production [17].

Mycotoxin are prevented during storage by improving the post-harvest storage conditions [78]. Jard et al. [79], reported storage of grain at less than 15% moisture, removal of infected grain by insect and visibly damaged this prevent favorable condition for mold growth, combination of multiple strategies to reduced moisture content of grain and prevent mold formations. Mycotoxin are destroyed, inactivated, or generate non-toxic products which do not altered the nutritional quality of the food or feed [79]. There are several decontamination processes which include radiation, oxidation, reduction, ammonization, alkalization, acidification and deamination [17]. These chemical methods are not allowed in the European Union [12] as chemical transformation might lead to toxic derivatives. In the United States, only ammonization is licensed for detoxifying aflatoxins.

1.4.5 Detoxifying

Detoxification of agricultural commodities through; radiation, oxidation, reduction, ammonization, alkalization, acidification and deamination is restricted due to problems associated with incomplete detoxification, cost implication and unavailability of equipment. Commonly used method to reduce mycotoxin exposure in the field is the inclusion of mycotoxin detoxifying agent in feed (mycotoxin detoxifiers) which decreases the bioavailability of the toxin [79, 80]. There are two different class of detoxifiers, namely mycotoxin binders and mycotoxin modifiers. The modes of action differs; mycotoxin binders adsorb the toxin in the gut, resulting in the excretion of toxin-binder complex in the feces, whereas mycotoxin modifiers transform the toxin into non-toxic metabolites [34]. Detoxifier are extensively use as feed additives for the reduction of contamination of feed by mycotoxin; which modify their mode of action, reduce absorption and secretion of metabolites [34]. Detoxifier does not mean that animal feed exceeding maximal regulatory limits used. Quality of feed can be improve by adding detoxifier making the product acceptable in market and providing safety for animal health [80].

1.4.6 Organic binder

Lactic acid bacteria (LAB), are divided into four genera: Lactococcus, Lactobacillus, Leuconostoc and Pediococcus. They are Gram-positive, catalase-negative, non-sporulating, usually non-motile rods, cocci, ferment carbohydrates, produced lactic acid [81]. Lactic acid bacteria are used in food processing industry for fermentation, preservation and mycotoxin binding abilities [82]. The mechanism of interaction involves the peptidoglycan structure (amino acid) which are common site for binding. However, different mycotoxin have different binding sites [82].

1.4.7 Probiotics

Application of biotechnological tools to reduced chemical residues and improved production efficiency that does not create any harm to poultry as well as consumers of the value chain [83]. Recent advancement in biotechnology on poultry feeds, banning of harmful growth promoters and antibiotics. Globally, probiotics is gaining acceptance in feed formulation [83]. Antimicrobial resistance is now a worldwide threat [84] with alteration of immune response due to feeding of antibiotic growth promoters, Probiotics are considered as an important tool as regard to antimicrobial resistance [85]. Chick gut are usually sterile immediately after hatch, colonization of microflora on the gut occur on the hatching tray, hatcher, feed and water intake. These Microorganisms in the gut could either be beneficial or harmful based on their response to the host immune system. The beneficial organisms maintain gut equilibrium, improve health and production of the birds. However, harmful bacteria like *E. coli*, *Salmonella*, *Coliform* and *Campylobacter* adjust the gut equilibrium to favor spread of infection. Probiotics supplementation mitigate the spread of infection on poultry. Commercial probiotics preparation can be administer as a single or multi-strain where they positively improved production and egg shell quality [86]. Probiotics depends on several factors for their survival on the host, this include; dose frequency, type of host animal, strain and stability of organism, genetic component of host, nutritional status of host age and physiological levels [87, 88]. Research findings showed that use of probiotics in layer diets enhanced egg production, improve body weight [89–92], reduced serum low density lipoprotein (LDL) cholesterol [93], decrease cholesterol and triglycerides in blood [94, 95]. Probiotics improved shell quality hardness and bone strength in laying hens [96]. Improvement in the production of darker yolk color Sobczak and Kozłowski [90].

1.4.8 Lactobacillus spp. *and* Bacillus spp.

Physical and chemical detoxification are associated with some disadvantages such as undesirable effects on products, loss of nutritional quality and altered organoleptic properties, high cost of production and time consumption [97].

Antibiotic are used in poultry to treat an infection, growth promoter and productivity thus causes antimicrobial resistance to the health of livestock and consumers of the bye products [98]. Multi-drug resistance genes (MDRG) occurs due to under administration, overdose, drug residues and extra label use of drugs which is emerging in both animal and human due to continuous use of antibiotic in the diet of poultry. However, biological methods based on competitive exclusion where probiotics colonized adhesive sites on the intestinal epithelium thereby, prevent colony formation of pathogenic bacteria, non-toxigenic fungal strains have been reported promising method for lessening the formation of mycotoxins and preventing their absorption animal to human [87, 99]. Lactobacillus, Bifidobacterium, Propionibacterium, and Lactococcus are found to be active in terms of binding AF-B1 and AF-M1 [97, 100, 101]. Probiotics are alternatives for growth promotion, food safety, enhanced nutrient assimilation, improve production and reducing harmful bacterial concentration of the gut [87, 102, 103]. Binding of aflatoxin depend on several factors such as temperature, incubation time, pH, matrix and strain of probiotics [104]. Probiotics act as antagonist against aflatoxin, by altering metabolism of gastrointestinal tract, production of volatile fatty acid, organic acid, antibacterial (lactocidin, acidophillin, bacteriocins and hydrogen peroxide), stimulation of essential nutrient for immune responses and inhibiting bacteria growth [105, 106]. Absorption of nutrient and digestive activity are increase with decreased in ammonia production and bacteria enzyme activity (glucoronidase, nitroreductase, azoreductase) produced by pathogenic bacteria. They stimulate immune system by higher production of immunoglobulins, macrophages, lymphocytes, γ-interferon increase villus height, goblet cells and crypt depth to create environment unfavorable to agent [107]. Strain composition and doses determines the potentiality of probiotics [86]. Single strain probiotics exact direct mechanism of action but for multi-strain, it exact synergistic synergistic action among different strains and in such condition, it is supposed that multi-strain probiotics have more adhesive power than single strain [108].

1.4.9 Intestine

Intestine and the intestinal epithelial cell layer are selective barrier between external and internal environment. The first barrier layer prevent exposure of high concentration of foreign antigens, natural toxins, pathogens and mycotoxin [109, 110]. Intestine are maintained by well-organized intercellular structures including tight junctions, adherence junctions and desmosomes surrounding the apical region of epithelial cells [111]. Physical and chemical factors can dynamically alter the structure and function of tight junctions. The trans-epithelial electrical resistance (TEER) of cell monolayers can be considered as a good indicator of the epithelial integrity and of the degree of organization of the tight junctions over the cell monolayer [112]. The primary function of intestinal cells are to act as a physical barrier, separating the contents of a harsh luminal environment from the layers of tissue comprising the internal milieu [113]. Intestinal epithelial cell studies performed on rats indicate that aflatoxin B1 decreases intestinal cell proliferation throughout the intestine [114]. The intestinal epithelial cells barrier function as both on innate and adaptive components of immunity [113].

1.5 Immune response

Various mycotoxins affect immune-related organs and cells, and influence host defenses against infectious agents and related microbial toxins [115]. Aflatoxins suppress immune functions, particularly cell-mediated immune responses [116].

For instance, high levels of aflatoxin B1 (AFB1)-albumin adducts change T-cell phenotypes and reduce the percentage of B cells in human immunodeficiency virus-positive individuals [117]. In addition to lymphocytes, embryonic exposure to AFB1 impairs the functions of phagocytes such as macrophages and neutrophils, via the depression of phagocytic potential, inhibition of antiviral activity, and reduction in chemotactic responses [118–120]. AFB1 also interferes with the innate immunity of macrophages by suppressing tumor necrosis factor-α (TNF- α), interleukin (IL)-1, and IL-6, resulting in the disruption of pulmonary and systemic host defenses [67, 121].

2. Conclusion

Probiotics significantly counteract the adverse effect of aflatoxins which effectively reduced accumulation of aflatoxin residues in milk, meat and eggs [122]. In conclusion, feed and food industry could benefit from the use of probiotics to mitigate aflatoxin residues in eggs, milk and meats. Hence, probiotics might be promising tools in decreasing economic and health damage caused by aflatoxin in poultry industry. The prevalence of aflatoxin residues in poultry products call for public health attention of food safety along the value chain, by creating awareness on the presence of aflatoxins on poultry products and health implication to both animal and human.

Author details

Muhammed Jimoh Ibrahim
Faculty of Veterinary Medicine, Department of Veterinary Public Health and Preventive Medicine, Ahmadu Bello University, Nigeria

*Address all correspondence to: muhammedibrahim407@gmail.com

References

[1] Food and Agriculture Organization of the United Nations (FAO). (1996). Rome declaration on world food security and world food summit plan of action. Rome, Italy: FAO.

[2] Udomkun, P., Wiredu, A.N., Nagle, M., Müller, J., Vanlauwe, J. and Bandyopadhyay, R. (2017). Innovative technologies to manage aflatoxins in foods and feeds and the profitability of application - A review. *Food Control,* 76: 127-138

[3] Ito, Y., Peterson, S.W., Wicklow, D.T. and Goto, T. (2001). A*spergillus pseudotamarii,* a new aflatoxin producing species in *Aspergillus* section *flavi*. *Mycology Research,* 105: 233-239.

[4] Aly, S.A. and Anwer, W. (2009). Effects of naturally contaminated feed with aflatoxins on performance of laying hens and the carryover of aflatoin B1 residues in table eggs. *Pakistan Journal of Nutrition*, 8: 181-186

[5] Herzallah, S.M. (2013). Aflatoxin B1 residues in eggs and flesh of laying hens fed aflatoxin B1 contaminated diet. *American Journal of Agriculture and Biological Sciences,* 8: 156-161.

[6] Iqbal, S.Z., Nisar, S., Asi, M.R. and Jinap, S. (2014). Natural incidence of aflatoxins, ochratoxin A and zearalenone in chicken meat and eggs. *Food Control,* 43: 98-103.

[7] Christofidou, M., Kafouris, D., Christodoulou, M., Stefani, D., Christoforou, E., Nafti, G., Christou, E., Aletrari, M. and Ioannou-Kakouri, E. (2015). Occurrence, surveillance, and control of mycotoxins in food in Cyprus for the years 2004-2013. *Food Agricultural and Immunology,* 26, 880-895.

[8] Juan, C., Ritieni, A. and Mańes, J. (2012). Determination of trichothecenes and zearalenones in grain cereal, flour and bread by liquid chromatography tandem mass spectroscopy. *Food Chemistry*, 134(4): 2389-2397.

[9] Kendra, D. F. and Dyer, R. B. (2007). Opportunities for biotechnology and policy regarding mycotoxin issues in international trade. *International Journal of Food Microbiology,* 119(1-2): 147-151.

[10] European Commission (2007). Commission Regulation (EC) No. 1126/2007 of 28 September 2007 amending Regulation (EC) No. 1881/2006 setting maximum levels for certain contaminants in foodstuffs as regards Fusarium toxins in maize and maize products. Official Journal of European Union. L 255/14.

[11] European Commission (2009). Commision Regulation 386/2009/EC of 12 May 2009 amending Regulation (EC) No 1831/2003 of the European Parliament and of the Council as regards the establishment of a new functional group of feed additives. Official Journal of the European Union L 118, 66.

[12] European Commission (2010). Commission Regulation (EU) No 165/2010 of 26 February 2010 amending Regulation (EC) No 1881/2006 setting maximum levels for certain contaminants in foodstuffs as regards aflatoxins. Official Journal of the European Union L 50, 8.

[13] Wu, J. N., Doan, H. and Cuenca, M. A. (2006). Investigation of gaseous ozone as an antifungal fumigant for stored wheat. *Journal of Chemical Technology and Biotechnology,* 81(7): 1288-1293

[14] Prietto, L., Moraes, P. S., Kraus, R. B., Meneghetti, V., Fagundes, C. A. A. and Furlong, E. B. (2015). Post-harvest operations and aflatoxin levels in rice (Oryza sativa). *Crop Protection,* 78: 172-177.

[15] Council for Agricultural Science and Technology (2003). Mycotoxins: risks in plant, animal, and human systems. Vol Task Force Report 138. Council for Agricultural Science and Technology, Ames, IA, USA, 199 pp.

[16] Council for Agricultural Science and Technology (2007). Probiotics: Their Potential to Impact Human Health. Issue paper 36. CAST, Ames, Iowa.

[17] Kabak, B., Dobson, A.D. and Var, I. (2006). Strategies to prevent mycotoxin contamination of food and animal feed: a review. *Critical Review in Food Science and Nutrition*, 46: 593-619.

[18] Taylor, W.J. and Draughon, F.A. (2001). Nannocystis exedens: a potential biocompetitive agent against *Aspergillus flavus* and *Aspergillus parasiticus*. *Journal of Food Protection*, 64: 1030-1034.

[19] Cao, H., Liu, D.L., Mo, X.M., Xie, C.F. and Yao, D.L. (2011). A fungal enzyme with the ability of aflatoxin B1 conversion: purification and ESI-MS/MS identification. *Microbiology Research*, 166, 475-483.

[20] Yi, P.J., Pai, C.K. and Liu, J.R. (2011). Isolation and characterization of a Bacillus licheniformis strain capable of degrading zearalenone. *World Journal of Microbiology and Biotechnology,* 27: 1035-1043.

[21] Zhao, L.H., Guan, S., Gao, X., Ma, Q.G., Lei, Y.P., Bai, X.M. and Ji, C. (2011). Preparation, purification and characteristics of an aflatoxin degradation enzyme from myxococcus fulvus ansm 068. *Journal of Applied Microbiology,* 110: 147-155.

[22] Gao, X., Ma, Q.G., Zhao, L.H., Lei, Y.P., Shan, Y. and Ji, C. (2011). Isolation of *Bacillus subtilis*: screening for aflatoxins B1, M1, and G1 detoxification. *European Food Research and Technology*, 232: 957-962.

[23] Lei, Y.P., Zhao, L.H., Ma, Q.G., Zhang, J.Y., Zhou, T., Gao, C.Q. and Ji, C. (2014). Degradation of zearalenone in swine feed and feed ingredients by Bacillus subtilis ANSB01G. *World Mycotoxin Journal,* 7: 143-151.

[24] Fan, Y., Zhao, L.H., Ma, Q.G., Li, X.Y., Shi, H.Q., Zhou, T., Zhang, J.Y. and Ji, C. (2013). Effects of *Bacillus subtilis* ANSB060 on growth performance, meat quality and aflatoxin residues in broilers fed moldy peanut meal naturally contaminated with aflatoxins. *Food Chemical and Toxicology,* 59: 748-753

[25] Fan, Y., Zhao, L.H., Ji, C., Li, X.Y., Jia, R., Xi, L., Zhang, J.Y. and Ma, Q.G. (2015). Protective effects of *Bacillus subtilis* ANSB060 on serum biochemistry, histopathological changes and antioxidant enzyme activities of broilers fed moldy peanut meal naturally contaminated with aflatoxins. *Toxins,* 7: 3330-3343

[26] Ma, Q.G., Gao, X., Zhou, T., Zhao, L.H., Fan, Y., Li, X.Y., Lei, Y.P., Ji, C. and Zhang, J.Y. (2012). Protective effect of *Bacillus subtilis* ANSB060 on egg quality, biochemical and histopathological changes in layers exposed to aflatoxin B1. *Poultry Science,* 91: 2852-2857

[27] Venkatesh, N. and Keller, N.P. (2019). Mycotoxins in conversation with bacteria and fungi. *Frontier in Microbiology,* 403(10): 1-10. Doi: 10.3389/Fmicb.2019.00403

[28] Da Costa, C.L., Geraldo, M.R.F., Arroteia, C.C. and Kemmelmeier, C. (2010). In vitro activity of neem oil on *Aspergillus flavus* growth, sporulation viability of spores, morphology and aflatoxin B1 and B2. *Advances in Biosciences and Biotechnology,* 1: 292-299.

[29] Valchev, I., Kanakov, D., Hristov, T., Lazarov, L., Binev, R., Grozeva, N. and Nikolov, Y. (2014). Effects of experimental aflatoxicosis on renal function in broiler chickens. *Bulgarian*

Journal of Veterinary Medicine, 17(4): 314-324

[30] Banerjee, S. (2010). Climate of Eastern India and naturally infected with aflatoxins. *World Applied Sciences Journal,* 9: 1383– 1386.

[31] Oguz, H. and Kurtoglu, V. (2000). Effect of CLI on fattening performance of broiler chicken during experimental aflatoxicosis. *British poultry science,* 41: 512-517.

[32] Sur, E. and Celik, I. (2003). Effects of aflatoxin B1 on the development of the bursa of Fabricius and blood lymphocyte acid phosphatase of the chicken. *Britain Poultry Science,* 44(4): 558-566.

[33] European Food Safety Agency (2007). Opinion of the scientific panel on contaminats in the food chain on a request from the commission related to the potential increase of consumer health risk by a possible increase of the existing maximun levels for aflatoxins in almonds, hazelnuts and pistachios and derived products. *European Food Safety Agency Journal,* 446: 1-127.

[34] European Food Safety Agency (2009). Review of mycotoxin-detoxifying agents used as feed additives: mode of action, efficacy and feed/food safety. http://www.efsa.europa.eu/en/supporting/pub/22e.htm

[35] Zinedine, A. and Mañes, J. (2009). Occurrence and legislation of mycotoxins in food and feed from Morocco. *Food Control*, 20(4): 334-344.

[36] Yunus, A.W., Razzazi-Fazeli, E. and Bohm, J. (2011). Aflatoxin B1 in affecting broiler's performance, immunity, and gastrointestinal tract: a review of history and contemporary issues. Toxins 3, 566-590

[37] Corcuera, L.A., Veltorazzi, A., Arbillage, L., Gonzàlez-Peñas, E. and López de Certain, A. (2012). An approach to the toxicity and toxicokinetics of aflatoxin B1 and Ochratoxin A after simultaneous oral administration to fasted F344 rats. *Food and Chemical Toxicology*, 50: 3440-3445.

[38] Agriopoulou, S., Koliadima, A., Karaiskakis, G. and Kapolos, J. (2016). Kinetic study of aflatoxins degradation in the presence of ozone. *Food Control*, 61: 221-226.

[39] Danicke, S.K., Ueberschar, H., Halle, I., Matthes, S., Valenta, H. and Flachowsky, G. (2002). Effect of addition of a detoxifying agent to laying hen diets containing uncontaminated or Fusarium toxin-contaminated maize on performance of hens and on carryover of zearalenone. *Poultry Science,* 81: 1671-1680.

[40] Pandey, I. and Chauhan, S.S. (2007). Studies on production performance and toxin residues in tissues and eggs of layer chickens fed on diets with various concentrations of aflatoxin AFB1. *British Poultry Science,* 48: 713-723.

[41] Wu, F. and Munkvold, G. P. (2008). Mycotoxins in ethanol co-products: modeling economic impacts on the livestock industry and management strategies. *Journal of Agricultural and Food Chemistry*, *56*(11): 3900-3911.

[42] Zhang, Y. and Caupert, J. (2012). Survey of mycotoxins in US distiller's dried grains with solubles from 2009 to 2011. *Journal of agricultural and food chemistry*, *60*(2), 539-543.

[43] Makun, H. A., Dutton, M. F., Njobeh, P. B., Gbodi, T. A. and Ogbadu, G. H. (2012). aflatoxin contamination in foods and feeds: a special focus in Africa. Trend in vital food and control engineering, Ayman Hafiz Amer Eissa (Ed.) 953-978.

[44] Kurtzman, C. P., Horn, B. W. and Hesseltine, C. W. (1987). *Aspergillus nomius*, a new aflatoxin-producing

species related to *Aspergillus flavus* and Aspergillus parasiticus. *Antonie van Leeuwenhoek,* 53: 147-158.

[45] Reiter, E., Zentek, J. and Razzazi, E. (2009). Review on sample preparation strategies and methods used for the analysis of aflatoxins in food and feed. *Molecular Nutrition and Food Research,* 53: 508-524.

[46] Sarigiannis, Y., Kapolos, J., Koliadima, A., Tsegenidis, T. and Karaiskakis, G. (2014). Ochratoxin A levels in Greek retail wines. *Food Control,* 42: 139-143.

[47] Coppock, W.R. and Christian, R.G. (2007). Aflatoxins, In: Veterinary Toxicology – Basic and Clinical Principles, R. C. Gupta; Academic Press, San Diego, Pp: 939-950.

[48] Bennett, J.W. and Klich, M., 2003. Mycotoxins. *Clinical Microbiology Reviews* 16: 497-516.

[49] Reddy, C. S., Reddy, K. R. N., Prameela, M., Mangala, U. N., and Muralidharan, K. (2007). Identification of antifungal component in clove that inhibits *Aspergillus* spp. colonizing rice grains. *Journal of Mycology and Plant Pathology,* 37(1): 87-94.

[50] Enyiukwu, D. N., Awurum, A. N. and Nwaneri, J. A. (2014). Mycotoxins in Stored Agricultural Products: Implications to Food Safety and Health and Prospects of Plant-derived Pesticides as Novel Approach to their Management: *Greener Journal of Microbiology and Antimicrobials*, 2 (3): 32-48.

[51] Farag, D. M. E. (2008). Aflatoxins: Awareness and control. *Dubai International Food Safety Conference*, 24-27 February, 2008, Pp: 1-55.

[52] Verma, J., Johri, T. S., Swain, B. K. and Ameena, S. (2004). Effect of graded levels of aflatoxin, ochratoxin and their combinations on the performance and immune response of broilers. *Britain Poultry Science*, 45(4): 512-518.

[53] Fouzia, B. and Samajpati,N. (2000). Mycotoxins production on rice, pulses and oilseeds. *Naturwissenschaften*, 87: 275-277

[54] Gallagher, E.P., Kunze, K.L., Stapleton, P.L. and Eaton, D.L. (1996). The kinetics of aflatoxin B-1 oxidation by human cDNA-expressed and human liver microsomal cytochromes P450 1A2 and 3A4. *Toxicology and Applied Pharmacology*, 141: 595-606.

[55] Diaz, G.J., Murcia, H.W. and Cepeda, S.M. (2010a). Bioactivation of aflatoxin B1 by turkey liver microsomes: responsible cytochrome P450 enzymes. *British Poultry Science,* 51: 828- 837

[56] Diaz, G.J., Murcia, H.W. and Cepeda, S.M. (2010b). Cytochrome P450 enzymes involved in the metabolism of aflatoxin B1 in chickens and quail. *Poultry Science*, 89: 2461-2469.

[57] Doi, A.M., Patterson, P.E. and Gallagher, E.P. (2002). Variability in aflatoxin B-1-macromolecular binding and relationship to biotransformation enzyme expression in human prenatal and adult liver. *Toxicology and Applied Pharmacology*, 181: 48-59.

[58] Eaton, D.L. and Gallagher, E.P. (1994). Mechanisms of aflatoxin carcinogenesis. Annual Reviews in Pharmacology and Toxicology 34: 135-172.

[59] Henry, S. H., Bosch, F. X., Troxell, T. C. and Bolger, P. M. (1999). Reducing liver cancer—global control of aflatoxin. *Science,* 286: 2453- 2454

[60] International Agency for Research on Cancer (1993). Monographs on the evaluation of the carcinogenic risk of chemicals to humans: some naturally occurring substances. Food items and constituents, heterocyclic aromatic

amines and mycotoxins. Lyon, France. IARC Monogr Eval Carcinog Risks Hum 56.

[61] Hussain, S. P., Schwank, J., Staib, F., Wang, X. W. and Harris, C. C. (2007). TP53 mutations and hepatocellular carcinoma: insights into the etiology and pathogenesis of liver cancer. *Oncogene*, 26(15): 2166-2176.

[62] Railey, J., Mandel, J.H.G., Sinha, S., Judahand, D.L. and Neal, G.E. (1997). Invitro activation of human ras Proto oncogene by aflatoxin B1. *Carcinogensis,* 18: 905-910.

[63] Giambrone, J.J., Ewert, D.L., Wyatt, R.D. and Eidson, C.S. (1978a). Effect of aflatoxin on the humoral and cell-mediated immune systems of chicken. *American Journal of Veterinary Res*earch, 39:305

[64] Giambrone, J.J., Partadiredja, M., Eidson, C.S., Kleven, S.H. and Wyatt, R.D. (1978b). Interaction of aflatoxin with infectious bursal disease virus infection in young chickens. *Avian Dis*ease, 22:431

[65] Fernandez A, Hernandez M, Verde M T and Sanz M. (2000). Effect of aflatoxin on performance, hematology, and clinical immunology in lambs. *Canadian Journal of Veterinary Research,* **64**(1 and 2): 53-58.

[66] Methenitou, G., Maravelias, C., Athanaselis, S., Dona, A. and Koutselinis, A. (2001). Immunomodulative effects of aflatoxins and selenium on human natural killer cells. *Veterinary Human Toxicology*, 43(4): 232-234.

[67] Bondy, G. S. and Pestka, J. J. (2000). Immunomodulation by fungal toxins. *Journal of Toxicology and Environmental Health B Crit. Rev.,* **3**(2): 109-143.

[68] Kataria, J. M., Dhama, K. and Mahendran, M. (2005). Mycotoxicosis in poultry: Immunosuppressive effects and remedial measures for its control. National Seminar-2005, SRDDL, IAH&VB, Bangalore. Souvenir. pp. 25-28.

[69] Rossano, F., Ortega De Luna, L., Buommino, E., Cusumano, V., Losi, E. and Catania, M. R. (1999). Secondary metabolites of Aspergillus exert immunobiological effects on human monocytes. *Research in Microbiology*, 150(1 and 2): 13-19.

[70] Marin, D. E., Taranu, I., Bunaciu, R. P., Pascale, F., Tudor, D. S., Avram, N., Sarca, M., Cureu, I., Criste, R. D., Suta, V. and Oswald, I.P. (2002).Changes in performance, blood parameters, humoral and cellular immune responses in weanling piglets exposed to low doses of aflatoxin. *Journal of Animal Science,* 80(5): 1250-1257.

[71] Kadian, S. K., Monga, D. P. and Goel, M. C. (1989). Effect of aflatoxin B1 on the delayed type hypersensitivity and phagocytic activity of reticuloendothelial system in chickens. *Mycopathologia,* 104: 33-36.

[72] Anjum A D. (1994). Outbreak of infectious bursal disease in vaccinated chicken due to aflatoxicosis. *Indian Veterinary Journal,* 71: 322- 324.

[73] Jand S K, Kaur P and Sharma N S. (2005). Mycoses and mycotoxicosis in poultry: A review. *Indian Journal of Animal Science*, 75(4): 465- 476.

[74] Glahn, R. P., Beers, K. W., Bottje, W. G., Wideman, R. J., Huff, W. E. and Thomas, W. (1991). Aflatoxicosis alters avian renal function, calcium, and vitamin D metabolism. *J. Toxicol. Environ. Health,* 34: 309-321.

[75] Hegazy, S. M. and Adachi, Y. (2000). Comparison of the effects of dietary selenium, zinc, and selenium and zinc supplementation on growth and immune response between chick groups that were inoculated with Salmonella and aflatoxin or Salmonella. *Poultry Science,* 79: 331-335.

[76] Edwards, S.G. (2004). Influence of agricultural practices on fusarium infection of cereals and subsequent contamination of grain by trichothecene mycotoxins. *Toxicology Letters*, 153: 29-35.

[77] Codex Alimentarius, 2002. Proposed draft code of practice for prevention (reduction) of mycotoxin contamination in cereals, including annexes on ochratoxin A, zearalenone, fumonisins and trichothecenes, CX/FAC02/21. Joint FAO/WHO Food Standards Programme Rotterdam, The Netherlands.

[78] Schrodter, R. (2004). Influence of harvest and storage conditions on trichothecenes levels in various cereals. *Toxicology Letters*, 153: 47-49.

[79] Jard, G., Liboz, T., Mathieu, F., Guyonvarc'h, A. and Lebrihi, A. (2011). Review of mycotoxin reduction in food and feed: from prevention in the field to detoxification by adsorption or transformation. *Food Additives and Contaminants Part A*, 28: 1590-1609.

[80] Kolosova, A. and Stroka, J. (2011). Substances for reduction of the contamination of feed by mycotoxins: a review. *World Mycotoxin Journal,* 4: 225-256.

[81] Gerbaldo, G.A., Barberis, C., Pascual, L., Dalcero, A. and Barberis, L. (2012). Antifungal activity of two Lactobacillus strains with potential probiotic properties. *Fems Microbiology Letters,* 332: 27-33.

[82] Dalie, D.K.D., Deschamps, A.M. and Richard-Forget, F. (2010). Lactic acid bacteria - Potential for control of mould growth and mycotoxins: A review. *Food Control,* 21: 370-380.

[83] Chowdhury, S.D., Ray, B.C., Khatun, A., Redoy, M.R.A. and Afsana, A.S. (2020). Application of probiotics in commercial layer diets: a review. Bangladesh Journal of Animal Science, *49 (1):1-12*

[84] World Health Organization (2018). Antimicrobial Resistance. Geneva: World Health Organization.

[85] Kabir, S.M.L. (2009). The Role of Probiotics in the Poultry Industry, *International Journal of Molecular Sciences* 10:3531-3546.

[86] Ray, B.C. (2018). Effects of single and multi-strain probiotics on laying performance and egg quality of commercial layers. MS Thesis, Department of Poultry Science, Bangladesh agricultural University, Mymensingh-2202, Bangladesh.

[87] Chichlowski, M., Croom, J., Mcbride, B.W., Havenstein, G.B. and Koci, M.D. (2007). Metabolic and physiological impact of probiotics or direct-fed microbials on poultry-A brief review of current knowledge. *International Journal of Poultry Science* 6: 694- 704

[88] Aalaei, M., Khatibjoo, A., Zaghari, M., Taherpou, K., Gharaei, M.A and Soltani, M. (2018). Effect of singleand multi-strain probiotics on broiler breeder performance, immunity and intestinal toll-like receptors expression. *Journal of Applied Animal Research* 47(1): 236-242.

[89] Ribeiro, V.J., Albino, L.F.T., Rostagno, H.S., Barreto, S.L.T., Hannas, M.I. and Harrington, D. (2014). Effects of the dietary supplementation of *Bacillus subtilis* levels on performance, egg quality and excreta moisture of layers. *Animal Feed Science and Technology* 195:142-146.

[90] Sobczak, A. and Kozłowski, K. (2015). The effect of a probiotic preparation containing *Bacillus subtilis* ATCC PTA-6737 on egg production and physiological parameters of laying hens. *Annals of Animal Science,* 15:711-723.

[91] Peralta-Sánchez, J.M., Martín-Platero, A.M., Ariza- Romero, J.J., Rabelo-Ruiz, M., Zurita-González, M.J., Baños, A., Rodríguez-Ruano, S.M., Maqueda, M., Valdivia, E. and

Martínez-Bueno, M. (2019). Egg production in poultry farming is improved by probiotic bacteria. *Frontiers in Microbiology,* 10: 1042.

[92] Neijat, M., Shirley, R.B., Barton, J., Thiery, P., Welsher, A. and Kiarie, E. (2019). Effect of dietary supplementation of *Bacillus subtilis* DSM29784 on hen performance, egg quality indices, and apparent retention of dietary components in laying hens from 19 to 48 weeks of age. *Poultry Science* 98(11): 5622-5635.

[93] Kalavathy, R.N., Abdullah, N., and Jalaludin, S. (2003). Effect of lactobacillus cultures on growth performance. Abdominal fat deposition, serum lipid and weight of organs of broiler chickens. *British Poultry Science* 44:139-144.

[94] Moataz, F.B., Ibrahim, A.H., Abdelaziz, A.D., Tarek, E., Osama, A.E. and Ahmed, A. (2018). Effects of dietary probiotic (*Bacillus subtilis*) supplementation on productive performance, immune response and egg quality characteristics in laying hens under high ambient temperature. *Italian Journal of Animal Science,* 17:804-814.

[95] Kanani, P.B., Hosseintabar, B.G., Youvalari, S.A., Seidavi, A., Ragni, M., Laudadio, V. and Tufarelli, V. (2018). Effects of using *artemisia annua* leaves, probiotic blend, and organic acids on performance, egg quality, blood biochemistry, and antioxidant status of laying hens. *The Journal of Poultry Science* 56:120-127.

[96] Yan, F.F., Murugesan, G.R. and Cheng, H.W. (2019). Effects of probiotic supplementation on performance traits, bone mineralization, cecal microbial composition, cytokines and cortico-sterone in laying hens. *Animal,* 13(1): 33-41.

[97] Ahlberg, S. H., Joutsjoki, V. and Korhonen, H. J. (2015). Potential of lactic acid bacteria in afaltoxin risk mitigation. *International Journal of Food Microbiology*, 207: 87-102.

[98] Park, J.W., Jeong, J.S., Lee, S.I. and Kim, I.H. (2016). Effect of dietary supplementation with a probiotic (*Enterococcus faecium*) on production performance, excreta microflora, ammonia emission, and nutrient utilization in ISA brown laying hens. *Poultry Science,* 95:2829-2835.

[99] Farzaneh, M., Shi, Z. Q., Ghassempour, A., Sedaghat, N., Ahmadzadeh, M. and Mirabolfathy, M. (2012). Aflatoxin B1 degradation by Bacillus subtilis UTBSP1 isolated from pistachio nuts of Iran. *Food Control*, 23(1): 100-106.

[100] Peltonen, K., El-Nezami, H., Haskard, C., Ahokas, J. and Salminen, S. (2001). Aflatoxin B1 binding by dairy strains of lactic acid bacteria and bifidobacteria. *Journal of Dairy Science,* 84(10): 2152-2156.

[101] El-Nezami, H. S. and Gratz, S. (2011). Control of mycotoxin contamination in foods using lactic acid bacteria. In, A volume in woodhead publising series in food science, technology and nutritionProtective cultures, antimicrobial metabolites and bacteriophage for food and beverage biopreservation (pp. 449-459).

[102] Cox, A. and Pavic, J.M. (2009). Advances in enteropathogen control in poultry production. *Journal of Applied Microbiology* 108:745-755.

[103] Chowdhury, S.D. (2018). Good Husbandry Practices in poultry production to ensure environment and food safety. In: *Technical Seminar on Food and Environment Safety in Commercial Poultry Production,* World's Poultry Science Association, Bangladesh Branch, pp. 4-7.

[104] Elsanhoty, R. M., Ramadan, M. F., El-Gohery, S. S., Abol-Ela, M. F. and

Azeke, M. A. (2013). Ability of selected microorganisms for removing aflatoxins in vitro and fate of aflatoxins in contaminated wheat during baladi bread baking. *Food Control*, 33(1): 287-292.

[105] Khan, R.U. and Naz, S. (2013). The application of probiotics in poultry production, *World's Poultry Science Journal* 69:621-631.

[106] Jadhav, K., Sharma, K.S., Katoch, S., Sharma, V.K. and Mane, B.G. (2015). Probiotics in Broiler Poultry Feeds- A Review. *Journal of Animal Nutrition and Physiology* 1:4-16.

[107] Yang, Y.P.A. and Choct, M. (2009). Dietary modulation of gut microflora in broiler chickens: a review of the role of six kinds of alternatives to in-feed antibiotics. *World's Poultry Science Journal,* 65:97-103.

[108] Timmerman, H., Koning, C., Mulder, L., Rombouts, F. and Beynen, A. (2004). Monostrain, multistrain and multispecies probiotics-a comparison of functionality and efficacy. *International Journal of Food Microbiology* 96: 219-233.

[109] Shephard, G.S., Thiel, P.G., Sydenham, E.W. and Savard, M.E. (1995). Fate of a single dose of 14C-labelled fumonisin B1 in vervet monkeys. *Natural Toxins,* 3: 145-150.

[110] Prelusky, D.B., Trenholm, H.L., Rotter, B.A., Miller, J.D., Savard, M.E., Yeung, J.M. and Scott, P.M. (1996). Biological fate of fumonisin B1 in food-producing animals. *Advanced Experiemental Medical Biology*, 392: 265-278.

[111] Gumbiner, B.M. (1993). Breaking through the tight junction barrier. *Journal of Cell. Biology*, 123: 1631-1633.

[112] Hashimoto, K. and Shimizu, M. (1993). Epithelial properties of human intestinal Caco-2 cells cultured in a serum-free medium. *Cytotechnology,* 13: 175-184.

[113] Bouhet, S. and Oswald, IP. (2005). The effects of mycotoxins, fungal food contaminants, on the intestinal epithelial cell-derived innate immune response. *Veterinary Immunology and Immunopathology* 108: 199-209

[114] Fleming, S.E., Youngman, L.D. and Ames, B.N. (1994). Intestinal cell proliferation is influenced by intakes of protein and energy, aflatoxin, and whole-body radiation. *Nutr. Cancer* 22: 11-30.

[115] Kimura, R., Hayashi, Y., Takeuchi, T., Shimizu, M., Iwata, M., Tanahashi, J. and Ito, M. (2004). Pasteurella multocida septicemia caused by close contact with a domestic cat: Case report and literature review. *Journal of Infection and Chemotherapy*, 10: 250-252.

[116] Moon, E.Y., Rhee, D.K. and Pyo, S. (1999). *In vitro* suppressive effect of aflatoxin B1 on murine peritoneal macrophage functions. *Toxicology*, *133*: 171-179.

[117] Jiang, Y., Jolly, P.E., Preko, P., Wang, J.S., Ellis, W.O., Phillips, T.D. and Williams, J.H. (2008). Aflatoxin-related immune dysfunction in health and in human immunodeficiency virus disease. *Clinical and Developmental Immunology*, *2008*, doi:10.1155/2008/790309

[118] Neldon-Ortiz, D.L. and Qureshi, M.A. (1992). Effects of AFB1 embryonic exposure on chicken mononuclear phagocytic cell functions. *Developmental and Comparative Immunology*, *16*: 187-196.

[119] Cusumano, V., Rossano, F., Merendino, R.A., Arena, A., Costa, G.B., Mancuso, G., Baroni, A. and Losi, E. (1996). Immunobiological activities of mould products: Functional impairment of human monocytes exposed to aflatoxin B1. *Res. Microbiol.*, *147*: 385-391.

[120] Silvotti, L., Petterino, C., Bonomi, A. and Cabassi, E. (1997).

Immunotoxicological effects on piglets of feeding sows diets containing aflatoxins. *Veterinary Record*, *141*: 469-472.

[121] Jakab, G.J., Hmieleski, R.R., Zarba, A., Hemenway, D.R. and Groopman, J.D. (1994). Respiratory aflatoxicosis: Suppression of pulmonary and systemic host defenses in rats and mice. *Toxicology and Applied Pharmacology, 125*: 198-205.

[122] Gratz S., Taubel, M., Juvonen, R.O., Viluksela, M., Turner, P.C., Mykkanen, H. and El-Nezami, H. (2006). *Lactobacillus rhamnosus* strain GG modulates intestinal absorption, fecal excretion and toxicity of aflatoxin B(1) in rat. *Applied and Environmental Microbiology,* 72: 7398-7400